Your Pregnancy Companion

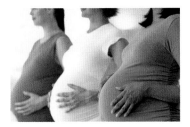

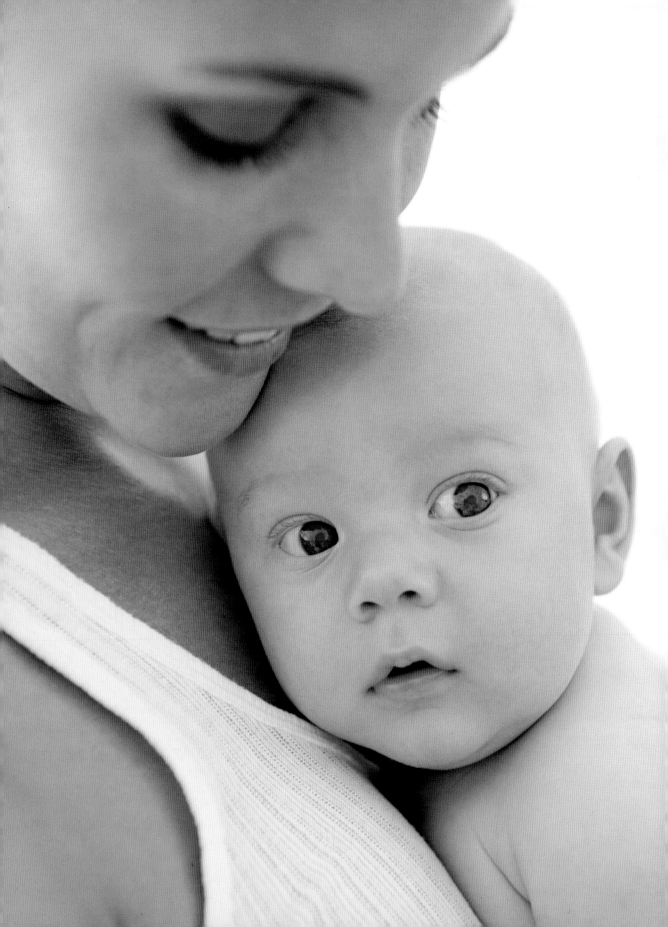

Your Pregnancy Companion

Zita West

Vermilion
LONDON

To my husband Robert West and my children Sofie and Jack West
for all their love and support – in all that I have achieved

10 9 8 7 6 5 4 3 2 1

Published in 2012 by Vermilion, an imprint
of Ebury Publishing
A Random House Group company

Edited by Claire Tennant-Scull

Produced by Bookworx:
Project editor Jo Godfrey Wood
Project designer Peggy Sadler

The Random House Group Limited Reg. No. 954009

Addresses for companies within the Random House Group
can be found at www.randomhouse.co.uk

The Random House Group Limited supports The Forest
Stewardship Council® (FSC®), the leading international forest
certification organisation. Our books carrying the FSC label
are printed on FSC® certified paper. FSC is the only forest
certification scheme endorsed by the leading environmental
organisations, including Greenpeace. Our paper procurement
policy can be found at www.randomhouse.co.uk/
environment

Printed and bound in China by Toppan Leefung

ISBN 9780091929350

To buy books by your favourite authors and register for offers
visit www.randomhouse.co.uk

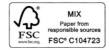

Praise for Zita West and her book

"Zita is a truly special woman. Her understanding and passion about all aspects of pregnancy and childbirth are second to none. I was so blessed to have her hold my hand throughout my pregnancy, both at her clinic and through her books. She became part of our extended family." Anne-Marie Duff

"Zita's support and advice helped me through the early days of my pregnancy, and this book will be a great companion to all pregnant women." Natasha Kaplinsky

"Zita West helped me at a point when I was really low and found it hard to believe I would get pregnant again. She gave me the belief and confidence I needed." Amanda Holden

"Pregnancy is a notoriously tricky time – most reference books deal only with worries and concerns in a traditional way. What every woman needs at a time like this is a confidante. Zita West is just that – and more. She treats the individual with the greatest scope of understanding and, most importantly, without prejudice and with the utmost insight. She is fazed by nothing and the naturalness in her approach is extremely calming. Zita has become a true friend and her generosity and concern know no bounds." Ulrika Jonsson

your pregnancy companion

CONTENTS

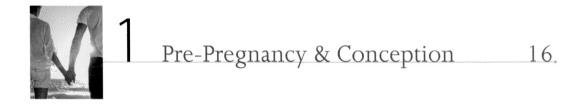

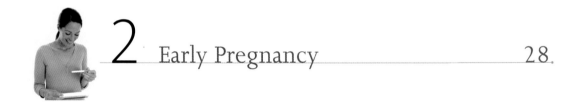

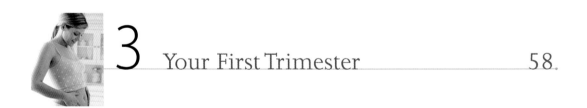

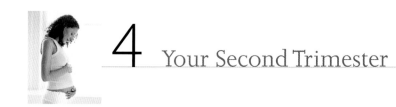
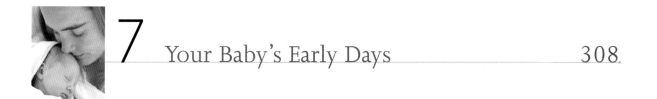

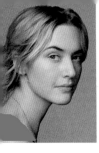

foreword by

KATE WINSLET

Zita West has written a wonderful book that offers help and support to mothers – from start to finish. Actually, even before the start she offers great advice on how to prepare yourself emotionally and physically for getting pregnant and then takes you through every step of the incredible journey of pregnancy, birth and the early days of looking after your new baby.

She is knowledgeable and smart about all the things you can do during pregnancy to give your baby the best possible start in life. At her suggestion, for instance, I took omega-3 throughout both my pregnancies. It's much more widely recommended now than it was then – Zita was ahead of her time with her insistence that it was invaluable for healthy brain development and I am sure that my children, Mia and Joe, are brilliant as a result!

I know that there is nothing in the world that prepares you for having a child. It doesn't matter how much advice you get, it's all just theory until you are holding your baby. And at that point you are exhausted, vulnerable and suddenly clueless. I went through the same concerns as all new mums and this book addresses these really well. One piece of advice that I found particularly helpful is to avoid the tyranny of all those well-meaning voices telling you what you should and shouldn't do. Zita's approach is calm, sensible, down-to-earth and often inspirational.

Among many things that I love about this book is the fact that it is a companion that offers help and support from beginning to end and gets you thinking about a lot of things. I especially like the mind-body-baby sections about making connections with your baby and thinking ahead to how you are going to be as a parent, and I like the integration between natural remedies and mainstream medicine.

I have followed Zita's work over the last 11 years. She looked after me for both of my pregnancies, births and beyond. She was present at Joe's birth and has been a part of both my children's lives while they were growing up. She has become a close family friend to me and to my children and I still look to her for advice and support as a mum.

Kate Winslet

Zita West – an introduction

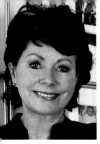

MY LIFE AS A MIDWIFE

In my thirty years as a midwife many events, people, places, patients, colleagues, doctors, midwives and mothers – not to mention the babies themselves – have enriched and shaped my career.

I grew up surrounded by my mother's friends, who were all nurses and midwives, and I am still learning from midwives and mothers today. We chat about our experiences and continue to share our knowledge. But looking back, I am aware of how we go through different phases of learning that affect how we practise, and it is the key aspects of that learning that I want to pass on in this book.

When I trained as a midwife, I loved the work more than anything I'd previously done in nursing. I was fascinated by every aspect of how a baby develops month by month and the whole journey through labour. At that time, in the 1980s, the experience of having a baby was usually a happy outcome for couples, though of course there was sadness for some. The focus at the time was very much on the medical side. The business of having a baby was highly medicalised and the health of the mother and baby was seen primarily in terms of new technologies that were available for monitoring both pregnancy and labour. For many of us involved with pregnant women, thoughts were limited to getting a baby through a pregnancy and delivered safely. There have been many more developments since I qualified that might make pregnancy even more hi-tech, but I have learnt that really being with a person on every level – mind, body and spirit – is what is most important. This means listening to the woman, meeting her emotional needs, reassuring and guiding her and giving her the confidence that

she can get pregnant in the first instance, carry a baby and, finally, give birth to him or her safely.

Today women have access to so much more information that, if anything, their fears have increased. Attitudes to being pregnant are changing, too, with more attention on the whole experience: what your baby experiences in the womb, how you can have a healthy baby and how you can influence his or her development physically, mentally and emotionally. Much work has been done recently on the influence conditions in the womb can have on the future health of your baby – nutritionally, physically and emotionally – such responsibility adding another layer to parents' anxieties! But I would like parents to see this as a positive change. You, as a future mother, have control over the environment your baby is growing in through your thoughts and emotions, in the way you react and deal with circumstances, in the food you eat for your baby's nutrition and through bonding with him or her. Mindset plays a huge role here and that is why I have included the mind-body-baby pages (see pages 110–11, 144–5, 236–9).

Phase One: The newly qualified midwife

The first phase of my learning was on a highly medical labour ward as a student midwife. Women were encouraged to endure their labour lying on their backs, so that they could be monitored throughout. After the birth, bottlefeeding was

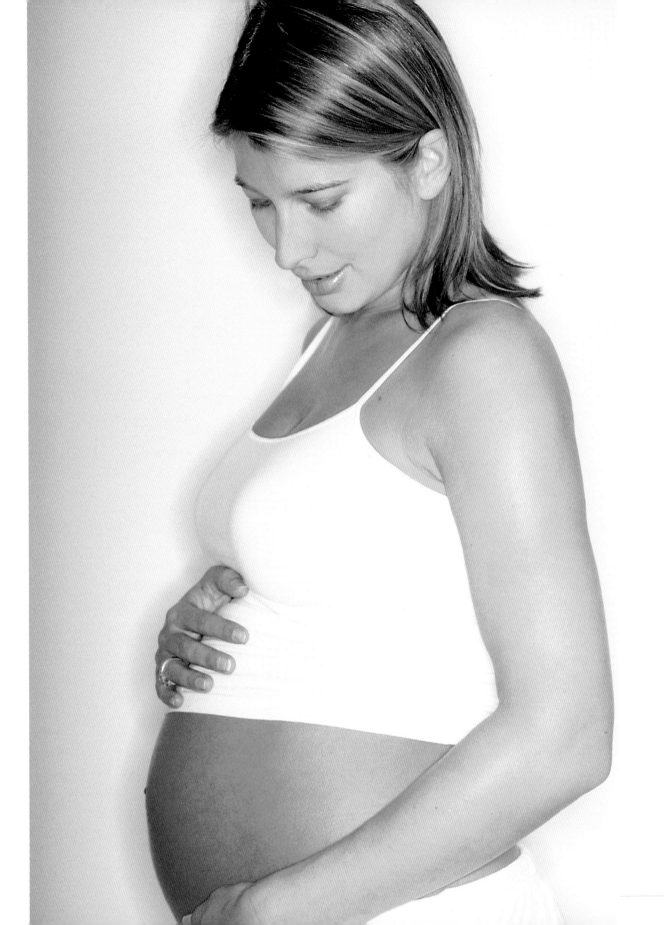

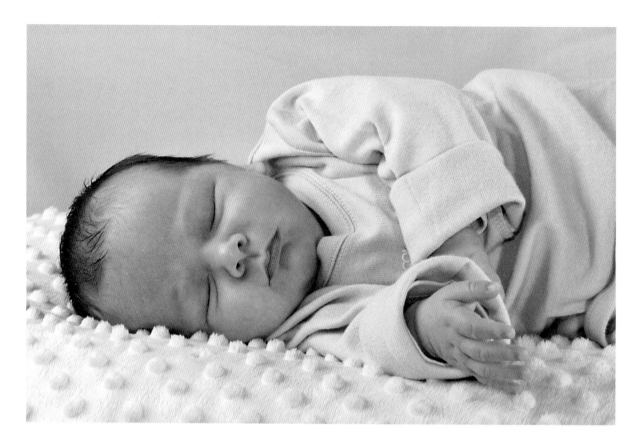

promoted – many mothers chose not to breastfeed at all. Babies were taken into the nursery, away from their mums, where as student midwives on night duty, we woke them every four hours for feeding.

Men were allowed to stay with their partners in labour, though as an aside, I don't think that it suits all men to be present at the birth. Some don't want to or are squeamish, and I have seen many couples with subsequent sexual problems as a result of the man's experience at the birth, when he felt obliged to be present, but would much rather not have been. Initially when men were first permitted in the labour ward they had to leave when examinations were being done. After that we went through a phase of them being encouraged to be highly involved. Other practices, such as artificially rupturing membranes, made birth a very difficult process for many women. All in all, what I learnt during this time was that I did not want to practise as a midwife in this way.

Phase Two: Real midwifery

I was glad to take up a post as a midwife in Oman – an opportunity that arose because of my husband's work. It was an amazing experience, which shaped my practice as a midwife and taught me skills for life. I really began to understand how to be with a woman in labour, away from a technical environment. Yes, there were monitors, but most of the time they were away being repaired! We had to monitor the babies using old-fashioned listening devices and came to understand the behaviour of women as they laboured and how their breathing patterns let us assess how labour was going. It was acceptable for the baby to sleep with the mother from the moment of birth and most breastfed very easily. I gave birth to my daughter, Sofie, there in a very simple local hospital. I had to work as a midwife right up to my waters breaking at 39 weeks and I gave birth to her with the help of life-long friends Serena and Jan Wilson.

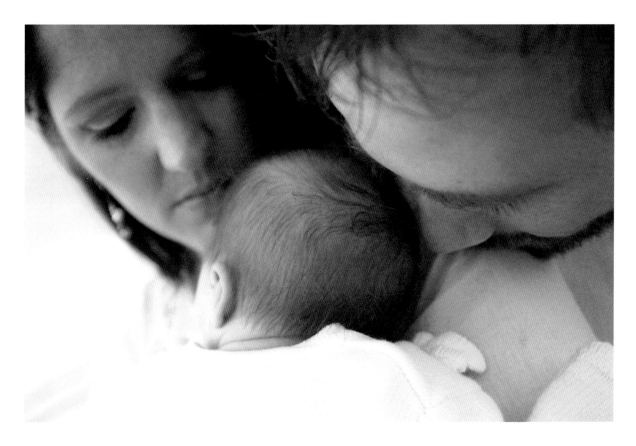

I laboured with a dozen other women in the same room, some of whom I had delivered the day before!

Phase Three: Maturing

Returning to the UK, I was very rusty technically. I was not used to setting up epidurals and I had only done one episiotomy in three years. I worked on a labour ward to get back into the swing of things, but decided that I really wanted to be a community midwife. I loved looking after mothers and babies in their homes and doing home births. I was also pregnant with my son, Jack. Sadly I suffered postnatal depression, so the condition is something I empathise strongly with. Working as a community midwife was hard at this stage as Jack was awake a lot at night, things were tough with my husband's work and we had a lot of worries. My doctor was fantastic, but all he could offer was antidepressants, which I didn't want to take, so I started to seek alternative

therapies. The area of complementary medicine was not as developed as it is today and I saw some good people, but also some who were not. I eventually stumbled on acupuncture and this had a huge impact on me. The therapist was excellent – I felt listened to, nurtured and more energetic than before and I decided to train in five-element acupuncture.

Phase Four: Integrating

The next stage of my life was three years' training to become an acupuncturist while working in a special care baby unit. This was a wonderful experience. I loved the ancient arts of five-element acupuncture and Traditional Chinese Medicine (TCM), particularly the notion of living within natural laws to stay healthy (pages 38–9). This was a completely different model of medicine, based on the art of listening to and understanding the patient as a complete human being, not just a body to be fixed. It introduced some very different ideas: such as the treatment of disharmony in the body, palpating to see how heat is distributed, looking at the tongue and taking pulses. Underlying all was the concept of 'qi' energy and the five elements, providing a unified theory of a person's health in mind, body and spirit.

While all this might have seemed strange in terms of mainstream medicine, it made such sense to me that I began to think about how I could combine acupuncture with midwifery. So many women experience common ailments in pregnancy that are considered 'par for the course', such as morning sickness, and I was aware that pregnant women are reluctant to take medication – and I was also interested in using acupuncture during labour. It was obvious that there was a gap in the range of treatments available that acupuncture could fill.

Once qualified in acupuncture, I had to persuade consultants to allow me to use it and I was delighted when I got the go-ahead to start up a service giving acupuncture alongside mainstream midwifery in the National Health Service (NHS). At that time the only other unit using acupuncture was in Plymouth, run by Sarah Budd and Sharon Yell, and I am very grateful to them for letting me observe them at work. I learnt a huge amount working in the NHS because I treated so many women and I was able to use acupuncture for all sorts of pregnancy-related conditions. Acupuncture took me in a different direction and I still use it today.

Phase Five: Professors & learned people
I developed a great interest in nutrition and micro-nutrients,both pre-conceptionally and during pregnancy, and this is now an important part of my practice. I became very interested in this area 20 years ago, through the work of Professor Barker on how the future health of a child can be influenced in utero. His concept is that the baby's growing organs have a critical window of development, when key nutrients need to be in place for optimum development of that organ. I also followed the work of Professor Michael Crawford in the importance of essential fatty acids. I developed a range of supplements and have been spreading the word about the benefits of omega-3 for 12 years. At my clinic we test for essential fatty acid status, micro-nutrients and antioxidant deficiencies and we have done much work on vitamin-D deficiency, testing over 1,000 patients.

Phase Six: 'Sage femme'
The influence of mind and body on your baby, and what you can do to have a healthy pregnancy and baby, is where I am now and understanding what your baby is aware of in utero and what you can do to influence will form the next chapter of my working life. I suppose my career has been spent looking at how to improve on what we already know about care and treatment in fertility and pregnancy. The final phase is to put it all together to help couples become pregnant, using the knowledge colleagues and I have gathered. Often that means looking where there is little evidence. Our skill is pulling the strands together, offering a holistic approach to include the mental and emotional aspects of pregnancy. The integration of current scientific thinking with therapies that offer women better well-being for themselves and their babies is the way forward.

The final phase has included setting up my own clinic. I established it a decade ago and until then worked as a sole practitioner offering acupuncture, nutritional advice, fertility awareness and counselling. The approach has always been: working with couples to formulate a plan of action for conception and pregnancy. Using acupuncture, nutrition, fertility awareness and counselling, we bring together a programme tailored to the individual's needs. My vision was a midwife-led clinic combining all I have learnt and offering the best advice available. I now have a fantastic team of therapists, and in 2011 we set up Zita West Assisted Fertility, offering IVF treatment within a holistic practice. The first Zita West IVF baby is due in June 2012.

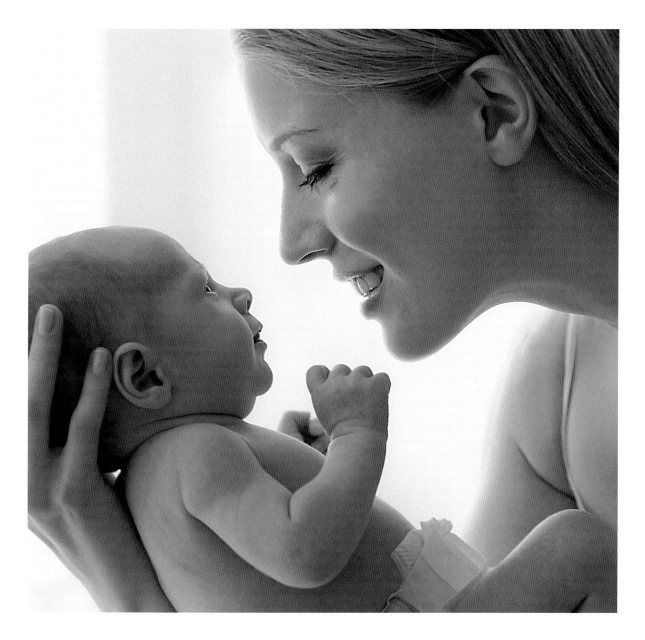

Like any venture into new territory, you can't do it on your own. I am eternally grateful to my great friend and colleague Anita O'Neill and also to Sarah Bearman and my team, who started with me ten years ago. I would like to thank Kate Winslet, an inspirational mother and friend, for writing the foreword (see pages 8–9).

Zita West

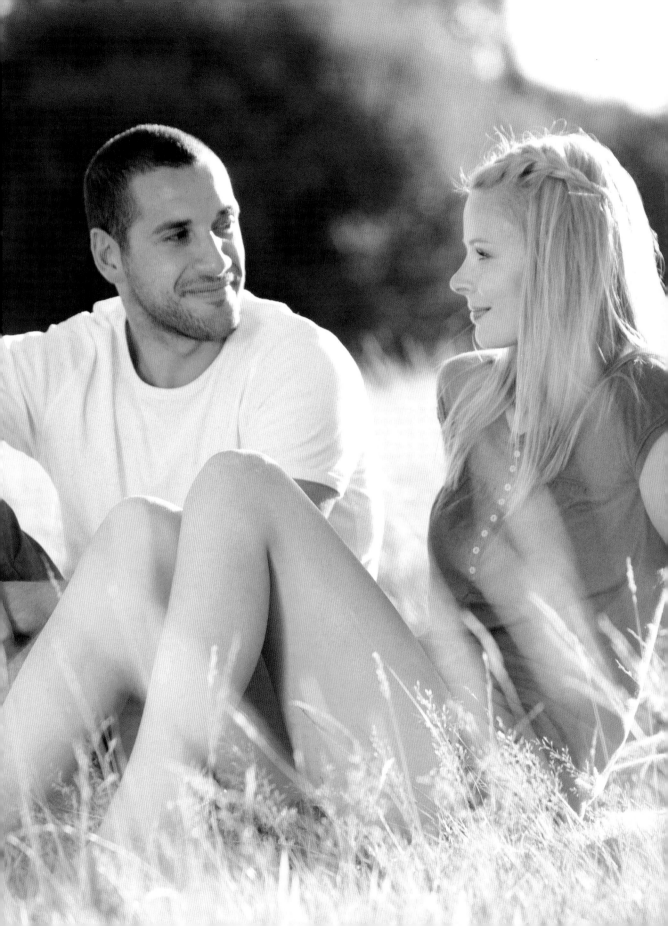

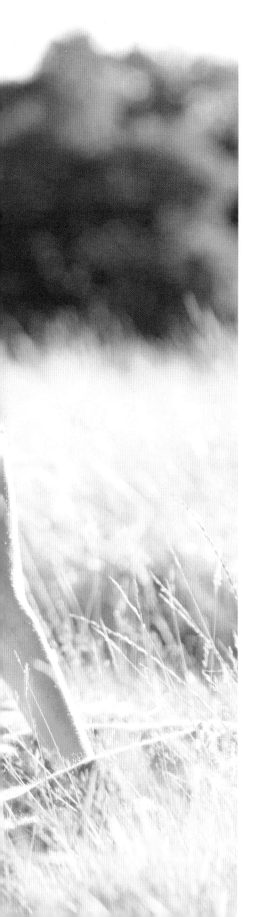

chapter 1

pre-pregnancy &
CONCEPTION

Laying down the foundations for a
healthy pregnancy and a healthy baby is
vital – and there are plenty of things you
can do to make sure things go well.

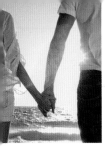

PRE-CONCEPTION

In days gone by, the baby's development as a healthy individual was assumed to start seriously only after the birth. We now know that factors during the preparation for pregnancy and the baby's development in the uterus are of enormous significance and can affect him before birth, after it and for the rest of his life.

A really good diet will help your body to stockpile the nutrients that are essential to the development of your foetus. If you and your partner stop smoking and/or drinking before trying to conceive it will give you the best chance of having a healthy egg, sperm and ultimately baby. So it's not just during your pregnancy that these things matter: the period before conception is important, too.

The theory of 'foetal origins'

The idea of 'foetal origins' focuses on how the interactions between the expectant mother's body and her developing baby has implications for the child in later life. David Barker, a physician and professor of epidemiology at the University of Southampton, has carried out much of this research. What has become known as the 'Barker Hypothesis' argues that quality of life in the womb is what determines how healthy a person will be during the rest of their life. Research has been conducted on how a range of factors in pregnancy can affect adult health. It considers how, for example, maternal stress, malnutrition, low birth weight and other environmental factors affect development in the womb and how this can cause long-term changes to the way the baby's body will function through childhood and then on into adulthood.

Much of this research is focused on how deprivation leads to poor health in later life and, thankfully, in the UK there are safety nets in place for those who are less well off. So although many people could improve their diet, what doctors would call 'malnutrition' is not a common feature here. However, the relevance of this research to all babies is clear and provides us with important information.

Your baby's future health

We can see that the nine months spent in the uterus can positively or negatively affect the future health of the child. Perhaps the most critical time is the period between fertilisation and the first 12 weeks of pregnancy, when the organs are developing (see pages 63–5). There is an opportunity during this period for each organ to reach its maximum potential for development, and so your baby needs exactly the right nutrients at the right time to enable the organ to mature and function to its full capacity.

Your baby relies on not just what you eat, drink and are exposed to in any one day, but on the resources you already have and those you build on. The theory of 'foetal origins' has now moved beyond the specialist medical journals and is being discussed as a more mainstream theory of child development in popular publications.

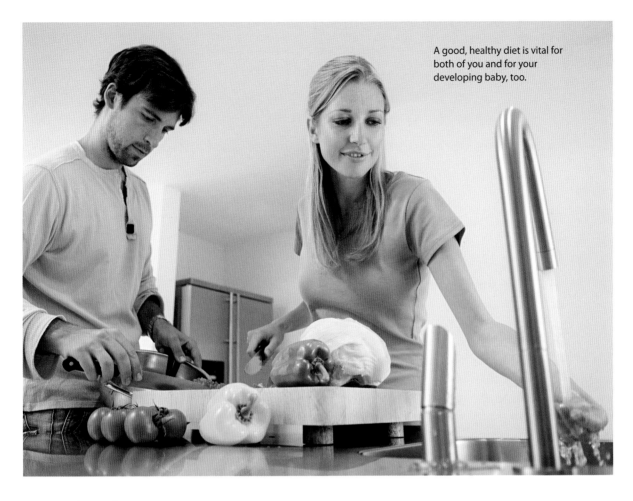

A good, healthy diet is vital for both of you and for your developing baby, too.

Passing down the generations

Good health is largely based on good nutrition and is passed on from one generation to the next. You and your baby have a nutritional inheritance stretching back through the generations – so you developed from an egg that formed in your mother's ovaries while she was growing inside her own mother. This means your nutritional inheritance stretches back, and the quality of nutrition in your own pregnancy reaches into the future. So it has an impact not only on your child, but on your grandchild, too. This means you can have a *positive* effect on your baby's health and development. If your pregnancy was unplanned, you may not have been thinking about improving your nutrition ahead of conception, but you can start now and make a real difference.

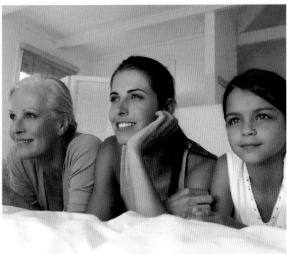

Good nutrition is passed on from one generation to the next, creating a legacy of good health in the family.

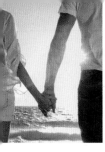

thinking about

GENES & INHERITANCE

At the point of conception, your baby inherits a set of genes that determine his physical and mental characteristics. Half of these come from your egg and half from your partner's sperm, so both of you contribute equally to your baby's inheritance.

The human genome is made up of 40,000, or more, genes that are arranged in pairs along chromosomes. Genes are the blueprint that carry small parts of deoxyribonucleic acid (DNA). It is the DNA that will decide how your baby will look – whether he will have brown eyes or blue or possess straight or curly hair. It will also dictate what your baby's blood type is and determine the specialised function of cells.

When your baby was conceived, your egg and your partner's sperm passed on a set of 23 pairs of chromosomes to your embryo, making a total of 46. Apart from identical twins, every baby receives a unique package of genes because each egg and sperm carries a different combination, so if you go on to have more babies, each one will be unique.

Genetic counselling

Some genes fail to form properly and if both genes in a pair do this it can result in problems such as Tay-Sachs disease or cystic fibrosis. These are thought to be inherited recessively. Dominant abnormal genes can also cause problems such as Huntingdon's disease, even if one of the pair is normal. Some disorders, such as haemophilia, are carried on the X chromosome and cause problems for boys rather than for girls. If you think you may be at risk of having a baby with a genetic abnormality, ask your doctor to refer you for genetic counselling.

Will it be a boy or a girl?

Your baby's sex is also determined at the point of conception – by just one pair of those genes that you passed on. These are the X and Y sex chromosomes. Boys have one X and Y chromosome, while girls have two X chromosomes. In former times women were blamed for 'failing' to produce a male, though we now know it is the man's sperm that determines sex. If the sperm contains the X chromosome the baby will be a girl and if it carries the Y it will be a boy.

EPIGENETICS (ENVIRONMENT & GENES)

Environmental factors, such as smoking, alcohol and lack or excess of certain nutrients (e.g. low folic acid) may affect the development of your baby's spinal cord. These factors can cause changes in the order of the genetic codes in genes, resulting in abnormalities. Genes go through several stages before producing the protein that gives the person their characteristic features. Environmental chemicals may cause permanent changes in the genetic code, which can be passed on to future generations. Epigenetics has shown that such factors increase or decrease chemicals vital for normal development. The subject adds a whole new layer to genes beyond the DNA. It proposes a control system of 'switches' that turn genes on and off and suggests that things people experience, such as nutrition and stress, can control these switches and cause heritable effects in humans.

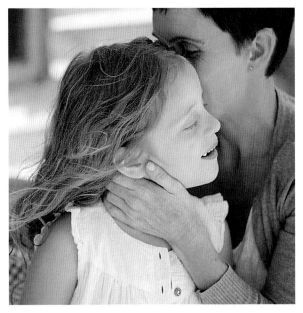

If both parents carry the recessive gene for red hair, then your child can turn out to be a redhead.

What colour eyes?

Eye colour is the most obvious sign of inherited traits involving dominant and recessive genes because the brown-eye gene is the dominant one, while the blue-eye gene is recessive. This means that the brown-eye gene is stronger.

You and your partner each carry a pair of genes that determine eye colour and these two pairs mean that there are four possible combinations of genes that could be passed on to your children.

To find out what colour eyes your baby is likely to have you need to think about your own genetic inheritance, if you know it. Even if both you and your partner have brown eyes, if one person in each set of your own parents has blue eyes, you may be carrying the recessive gene and if these combine, your baby will have blue eyes.

If both you and your partner have blue eyes then neither of you will carry the dominant gene and so your baby will definitely not have brown eyes. However, if one of your parents has brown eyes, your child may have grey or light-green eyes. You can use the chart (right) to help you get to grips with this.

DOMINANT & RECESSIVE GENES

The colour of the eyes is used as an example of how dominant and recessive genes work. The genes of two parents give four possible combinations of eye colour.

1 Both parents have brown eyes, with one parent possessing the recessive blue-eye gene.

Their children will always have brown eyes.

Parents

Children

2 One parent has brown eyes with a blue-eye recessive gene and one parent has blue eyes.

If the brown-eye gene dominates – the children will have brown eyes or if the blue-eye genes combine they will have blue eyes.

Parents

Children

3 Both parents have blue eyes.

The children will all have blue eyes as there is no dominant brown-eye gene to override the recessive blue.

Parents

Children

4 Both parents have brown eyes, but they each carry a recessive blue-eye gene.

There is a one-in-four chance that the children will inherit blue eyes.

Parents

Children

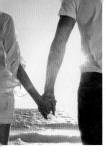

the miracle of

CONCEPTION

Life for your baby begins when your tiny egg joins with your partner's microscopic single sperm, but the conditions for such a momentous event have to be just right for conception to take place.

Conception (fertilisation of egg and sperm) happens in three stages: ovulation, fertilisation and the division of the fertilised egg before it implants in the wall of the uterus. This sequence is delicately balanced and the creation of a new life seems truly miraculous.

Women are born with around two million ova (eggs) already present in their ovaries, but from the moment of birth, a girl's eggs begin to die off, so that by the time she reaches puberty, the number has probably decreased to around 400,000. Of these, between 400 and 500 will mature and be released during her reproductive lifetime. The numbers have shrunk dramatically, but are still more than enough to create a family if all else goes well.

Men do not produce sperm until they reach puberty and there will be an astonishing 50–150 million sperm in each millilitre of the 2–6 ml of semen that a healthy young man will typically produce with each ejaculation. Each sperm measures around just 0.5 mm in length, yet to fertilise the woman's egg it will have to make a journey that in proportion to its size would be the equivalent of a man swimming a mile-long race.

Ovulation

Every month, on average, a woman's body is triggered to mature approximately 20 eggs in response to a hormone called follicle-stimulating hormone (FSH) that is released by the pituitary gland

(a pea-sized gland that is sited in your brain just behind your eyes). Usually, only one of these eggs will reach the necessary stage of maturity and when this happens, oestrogen is sent into the bloodstream to prevent the other eggs from developing any further and to prepare the uterus for the possibility of implantation (see pages 24–5).

The egg is released

Halfway through the monthly menstrual cycle the pituitary gland releases a short burst of luteinising hormone (LH), which will prompt the release of the now mature and dominant egg. Around 36 hours later, the egg will break out of its protective sac (follicle). The follicle will then form the corpus luteum, which will nourish the developing embryo until the placenta takes over the task. The egg is then

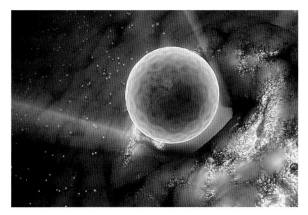

An ovum being released.

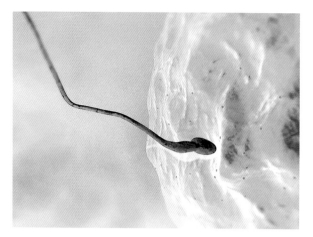

The sperm about to penetrate the egg.

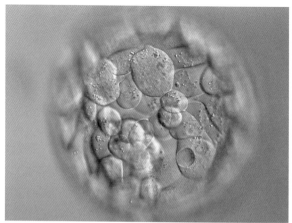

The blastocyst.

released by the ovary (ovulation) and is gently sent along the fallopian tube by the tiny hair-like strands (cilia) that line the passage. While the egg is in the fallopian tube fertilisation may take place, but for that to happen, the sperm has to complete an arduous and difficult journey.

The journey towards fertilisation

Of the 100–150 million sperm that may be ejaculated at one time, only 100,000, or less, will manage to survive the acid conditions of the vagina to get through the cervix and from there just 200 or so travel along the fallopian tubes. Only one sperm can fertilise the egg, so as the sperm arrives, the egg needs to be travelling down the fallopian tube to meet it. Sperm can survive in the fallopian tube for up to five to seven days. So if you have sex at least three times a week, you ensure that there is plenty of sperm in the fallopian tubes when you ovulate.

Reaching the nucleus

Before fusing with the egg, the sperm must first penetrate the egg's outer layer (called the corona radiata) and then another inner layer (zona pellucida) in order to reach the nucleus. Once the head of the successful sperm has reached the nucleus the egg releases chemicals to prevent any other sperm from entering. The 'winning' sperm will now

lose the tail that propelled it along its journey and the head will enlarge. As the egg and sperm fuse they form a 'zygote'. This will go on to divide into further cells called 'blastomeres'. The zygote carries on dividing, so that by the time it arrives at the uterus it is made up of about 50–60 cells (a 'blastocyst').

Implantation

The blastocyst is also made up of two types of cell – the trophoblast (outer cells), which will form the placenta and the inner cells that develop into the foetus. Around five to seven days after fertilisation the blastocyst will start to implant and attach itself to the womb lining. (If you have had IVF your embryo may have got to the blastocyst stage before it is transferred back inside you.) It will have divided again into about 100 cells and will release the hormone human chorionic gonadotrophin (hCG) (see page 36), which triggers the corpus luteum to keep producing progesterone, to ensure the pregnancy continues (see pages 36–7). Week 2 sees the outer layer of trophoblast cells merge into the uterine lining to develop into the placenta, while the inner cells will have formed into an embryo. Your egg and sperm have each contributed 23 chromosomes (see pages 20–1) containing genetic codes, so even at this early stage, the tiny embryo that will grow into your '
is already a unique mix of both parents.

HOW TWINS (& MULTIPLES) ARE CONCEIVED

In the last 20 years, or so, the number of twins and triplets born in the UK has increased, so that around 16 babies in every 1,000 born are multiple births. This is partly because of improved health in the general population, but it is also the result of the increased use of fertility treatments such as *in vitro* fertilisation (IVF), where more than one embryo is commonly transferred to the uterus.

Twins and triplets are conceived in two ways:
Non-identical twins (sometimes called 'fraternal' twins) are the result of two or more of your eggs being released and fertilised.

Identical twins are created when one egg is fertilised by one sperm and then divides into two zygotes that then become two separate embryos. If the egg divides into three, they will become triplets and so on. Because they have evolved from the single egg and sperm they will be made from identical genetic structures, so they will have the same blood type, eye and hair colour.

Both types of twins will develop within an amniotic sac filled with amniotic fluid. Non-identical twins will each have their own placenta because they were conceived from two individual eggs, while identical twins, conceived from a single egg will share a placenta, but will each have a separate umbilical cord.

Might you be carrying twins or more?
If you are over 35 you have an increased chance of conceiving non-identical twins because you are more likely to release more than one egg per cycle. Non-identical twins run in families, too, so you may want to find out about your family history on your mother's side.

Identical twins

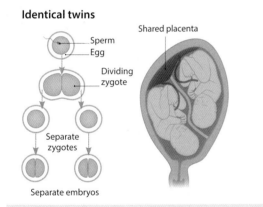

Sperm
Egg
Dividing zygote
Separate zygotes
Separate embryos
Shared placenta

Non-identical twins

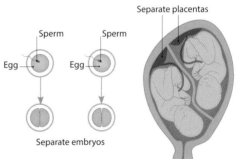

Sperm
Sperm
Egg
Egg
Separate embryos
Separate placentas

The process of implantation

The implantation of the fertilised egg in the uterus – which happens just five to seven days after conception – is a critical stage that sets up the foundation for your whole pregnancy.

The tiny bundle of energy, the blastocyst, attaches itself to the lining of the uterus – a process known as 'implantation'. At this point some women experience slight bleeding, which they may mistake for a light period. Some women feel mild pain, too, but for most the process of implantation is something that happens without them being aware of it, and so,

equally, they will be unaware if it fails. It is estimated that as many as 40 per cent of the eggs that are fertilised and which enter the uterus are lost and leave a woman's body as part of her menstrual period because they fail to implant. Successful implantation depends on a number of factors and timing is an important one, but so is the woman's health.

The blastocyst divides into two parts – one will form the embryo and become your baby, and the other will develop into the placenta (see pages 76–7). Implantation is a continuous process as the placenta is growing and developing. At implantation

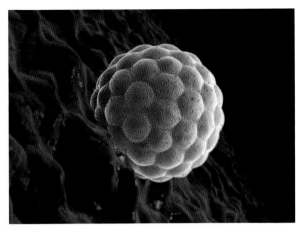

The implantation of the egg in the lining of the womb.

bringing the maternal and foetal circulation close together, but separated by a membrane. In the early weeks of pregnancy, the hormone hCG is secreted by the developing placenta and at the same time the developing embryo produces progesterone to encourage the endometrium to develop.

Early communication

The embryo is formed from both you and your partner, so it enters your body as a foreign protein and in a normal pregnancy your body accommodates it. But there are circumstances when it may be rejected (see pages 120–1). The embryo and the endometrium communicate by chemical messengers called 'cytokines' and there is a period during implantation when the uterus is most receptive to receiving the embryo and when the message from the embryo to the endometrium signals whether the pregnancy carries on. It is extraordinary to think that your baby is already 'communicating' with you.

the outer layer of cells that will become the placenta form finger-like structures called 'villi' that burrow into the womb lining. The embedding of the placenta determines the outcome of a pregnancy as it lays down foundations for the health of the developing baby. The mother's blood circulates between the villi,

HELPING THE WOMB ENVIRONMENT

For your blastocyst to implant, a number of factors are needed to develop a healthy womb lining. Here are some natural ways that may help:

Eat a diet rich in antioxidants from a variety of coloured foods. This will protect the womb from free-radical damage

Essential fatty acids, especially omega-3, help with immune and inflammatory responses and the healthy development of the embryo

You may also want to increase your consumption of foods that contain certain vitamins, or take a supplement, but be sure to check the dosage with your doctor or midwife before you consider taking anything

Selenium is a trace mineral that can help to guard against free-radical damage. Fish and seafood can be a rich source of selenium, but during pregnancy you may need to avoid certain species of fish and types of seafood (see page 87), so a balanced supplement may be helpful

Vitamin C is essential for the healthy formation and function of cells and connective tissue and can be found in citrus fruits, kiwi fruit and tomatoes, among others (see page 84)

Vitamin B1 (also known as 'thiamin') is good for the maintenance of tissue and improving blood flow, but it cannot be stored by your body, so you need to eat foods that contain it every day. You can find it in wholegrain breads and fortified cereals as well as some vegetable and fruits, cheese and eggs. You need to have a balance of all B vitamins

Vitamin E helps to protect cell membranes and its richest forms can be found in olive oil and soya, as well as nuts, seeds and wheatgerm

There are many vitamin and mineral supplements that are designed to be taken during pregnancy. Make sure that you take one that contains folic acid and omega-3 and vitamin D

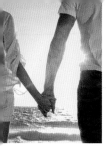

looking at the signs

AM I PREGNANT?

You might be one of those women who just instinctively knows when they are pregnant – or it may have taken you quite by surprise. Whichever category you fall into, you're likely to be experiencing at least one or two of the following common symptoms.

Missed periods

If your periods are normally irregular, it may be more difficult to know whether that missed period really has been missed or is just a little late. You might have been unwell, have lost weight or been under stress recently – any of which may explain delayed menstruation. You might even have had a very light bleed, but still assumed it was a period. It's also possible that you experienced some bleeding as the fertilised egg (blastocyst) implanted itself in your uterus. This is quite often mistaken for a 'light' period, so if you also have one or more of the other symptoms, do a pregnancy test to be absolutely sure.

Breast changes

Tenderness, an increase in size and weight of your breasts or even a tingling sensation are common early symptoms and are the result of the hormones released into your bloodstream after conception (see pages 36–7). You may also notice changes in their appearance, with bluish veins more noticeable and colour darkening in your nipples and areola.

Sensitivity to smells and tastes

You may be aware of an unfamiliar taste in your mouth that is slightly sweet or metallic and find that you are less keen on certain foods, drinks and even smells. This may be due to your pregnancy hormones and as coffee, alcohol, tobacco and fried foods are

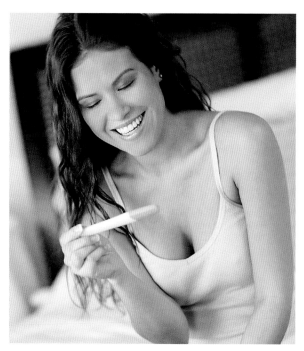

A do-it-yourself pregnancy-testing kit will give you accurate information on whether you are pregnant or not.

commonly the most offensive, it may be nature's way of protecting the growing foetus.

Frequent urination

Just a fortnight after conception, you may notice that you need to urinate more often. This is because your uterus is already expanding, pressing on your bladder and so limiting its capacity. At the same time, the blood supply to the kidneys steadily increases during the first trimester by about 30 per cent, so as the extra blood is filtered, it creates extra urine. Although the urge to urinate can be inconvenient, don't cut down the amount you drink. It is really important for you and your baby's health that you keep well hydrated. By the second trimester, your uterus will rise further up in your abdomen and this should relieve some of the pressure on your bladder.

Feeling tired

You may never have experienced such an overwhelming feeling of exhaustion as that of early pregnancy. You looking worn out can be alarming for friends and family if you are normally bursting with energy. Your tiredness may be because of the high levels of pregnancy hormones (especially the soporific effect of progesterone) or simply the result of the changes that are going on in your body. Your cardiac output will increase by 40 per cent before you reach week 20 and your blood volume will increase from about 5 litres (8¾ pt) before pregnancy to 7–8 litres (12¼–14 pt) by the time your baby is born. You will also have increased oxygen consumption and your tiny embryo will be growing at an astonishing pace, so is it any wonder you feel tired? By about week 14, you should begin to regain energy levels, but in the meantime, the best thing that you can do is to get as much rest as you possibly can.

Nausea & vomiting

Feeling sick, or even vomiting, is one of the most common symptoms of early pregnancy and it usually begins in the fifth or sixth week, though it can occur as early as the second. Most women experience a degree of nausea, which can happen at any time of the day. There may be several reasons for it. Straight after conception, the classic pregnancy hormone human chorionic gonadotrophin (hCG) surges through your system to maintain the pregnancy before the other hormones take over. The production

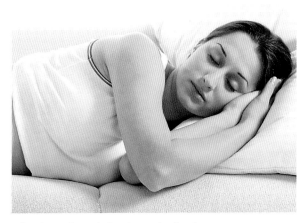

Take plenty of rest during the weeks of early pregnancy.

of hCG sharply decreases around weeks 13 to 14, so it may explain why nausea often ceases shortly afterwards. You may also feel sick when your blood-sugar levels are low, such as first thing in the morning, or you may be tired and need food at the end of a busy day. Another possible reason is that the hormone progesterone relaxes the muscles in the digestive tract, meaning that food is not digested as quickly as usual, causing you to feel, or be, sick. There are several things that you can do to relieve nausea (see pages 114–15) and it usually subsides after the first trimester. Occasionally, some women experience a severe form known as hyperemesis gravidarum, which requires help to prevent dehydration, but it is rare, occuring in only one in 200–500 pregnancies.

DON'T WORRY

Ordinary 'morning sickness' is certainly unpleasant, but it will not harm your baby. Rest assured that however little food or drink you seem to be keeping down, your baby will be taking all the nutrition that he needs. If you do not have any nausea at all, it doesn't suggest that your pregnancy is any less viable and it is not a cause for concern – you are just lucky!

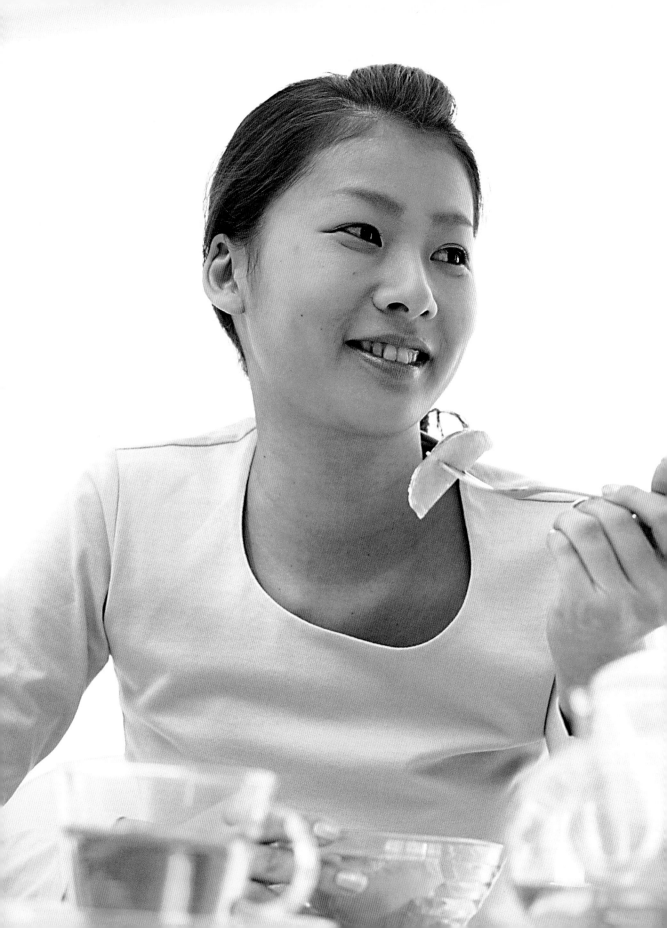

early
PREGNANCY

You're pregnant! Whether this moment has come out of the blue or you have been preparing for some time, this is an exciting time for you and your family and there is a lot that you can do by way of preparation.

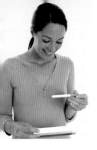

congratulations

YOU'RE PREGNANT!

This is the most miraculous news and whether you have been trying for a baby for some time or it has come as a complete surprise, stand by for your life to change for ever!

Sharing your news

Think about who you want to tell about your pregnancy and when. It may be wise to wait for a little while. Some pregnancies fail, but once you are 12 weeks' pregnant the risk of miscarriage falls dramatically. If you have other children, think about when is the best time to tell them. They are bound to be excited and while it is good to prepare them, if they are very young they might find it hard to understand about waiting for the baby to come.

Many women are nervous about telling their employers until they have had certain tests to make sure all is progressing well. However, this is an individual decision and is up to you.

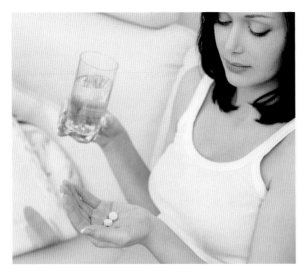

Take folic acid before conception and during pregnancy.

PRACTICAL THINGS TO DO NOW

Now's the time to get healthy. If you have been trying for a baby, you will have probably already looked at your lifestyle and made a few changes, but if not, now is a good time to start (see pages 102–3). If you smoke or take recreational drugs you need to stop now – speak to your doctor if you require help. The health professionals are there to help you, not to make judgements, and they will do all they can to ensure that your pregnancy continues as healthily as possible.

Alcohol is foeto-toxic, so in pregnancy, and before, it is important to stop drinking alcohol completely. There are some other drinks and foods that you may need to avoid, especially in the first trimester (see pages 86–7).

Take folic acid (vitamin B_9) – it's essential to your baby's development. Studies have shown that women who receive 400 mcg per day before conception and in the first 12 weeks of pregnancy can reduce the risk of neural tube defects in their babies by up to 70 per cent

Check with your doctor about your omega-3 intake. Many studies support the taking of supplements and it is hard to get all your requirements from your diet

Set up your first antenatal, or 'booking', appointment

Look for antenatal classes. There's no rush, but you might want to find out what's available and book a slot now

Begin a pregnancy diary to record the coming nine months. It may help you explore issues and to express your emotions

Your estimated delivery date (EDD)

Once you get that positive result from your pregnancy test, you'll probably be eager to know when your baby will be born. Make an appointment to see your doctor or midwife as soon as you can. They will be able to calculate your due date and you can begin to get to know them right at the start of your pregnancy. This will help to ensure that you receive the care you need.

Your last menstrual period (LMP)

First of all, you need to be able to tell your doctor or midwife the date of your last menstrual period (LMP) – keep a record in your diary.

Once the doctor or midwife knows this date, they can calculate your estimated delivery date (EDD). An average pregnancy lasts for 37 to 40 weeks, from the first day of your last period, so your doctor will use this to add on a standard 40 weeks, using the kind of chart shown below. However, conception usually occurs around two weeks after menstruation, so in effect, pregnancy usually lasts 38 weeks rather than 40. However, not every woman's menstrual cycle is strictly 28 days long – it might be longer or shorter, so doctors use an average. When you have a dating scan at around 10 to 14 weeks, your EDD may be adjusted. In the meantime use the chart below to determine your baby's approximate birth date.

ESTIMATED DATE OF DELIVERY (EDD) CHART

To use this chart, track the date of your last menstrual period (LMP) on the months and days shown in bold type below. The date that appears in lighter type underneath it is when your baby might arrive. To avoid confusion, it's best to stick to using weeks rather than months when you are discussing your pregnancy.

January	1	2	3	4	5	6	7	8	9	10	11	12	13	14	15	16	17	18	19	20	21	22	23	24	25	26	27	28	29	30	31
Oct/Nov	8	9	10	11	12	13	14	15	16	17	18	19	20	21	22	23	24	25	26	27	28	29	30	31	1	2	3	4	5	6	7
February	1	2	3	4	5	6	7	8	9	10	11	12	13	14	15	16	17	18	19	20	21	22	23	24	25	26	27	28			
Nov/Dec	8	9	10	11	12	13	14	15	16	17	18	19	20	21	22	23	24	25	26	27	28	29	30	1	2	3	4	5			
March	1	2	3	4	5	6	7	8	9	10	11	12	13	14	15	16	17	18	19	20	21	22	23	24	25	26	27	28	29	30	31
Dec/Jan	6	7	8	9	10	11	12	13	14	15	16	17	18	19	20	21	22	23	24	25	26	27	28	29	30	31	1	2	3	4	5
April	1	2	3	4	5	6	7	8	9	10	11	12	13	14	15	16	17	18	19	20	21	22	23	24	25	26	27	28	29	30	
Jan/Feb	6	7	8	9	10	11	12	13	14	15	16	17	18	19	20	21	22	23	24	25	26	27	28	29	30	31	1	2	3	4	
May	1	2	3	4	5	6	7	8	9	10	11	12	13	14	15	16	17	18	19	20	21	22	23	24	25	26	27	28	29	30	31
Feb/Mar	5	6	7	8	9	10	11	12	13	14	15	16	17	18	19	20	21	22	23	24	25	26	27	28	1	2	3	4	5	6	7
June	1	2	3	4	5	6	7	8	9	10	11	12	13	14	15	16	17	18	19	20	21	22	23	24	25	26	27	28	29	30	
Mar/Apr	8	9	10	11	12	13	14	15	16	17	18	19	20	21	22	23	24	25	26	27	28	29	30	31	1	2	3	4	5	6	
July	1	2	3	4	5	6	7	8	9	10	11	12	13	14	15	16	17	18	19	20	21	22	23	24	25	26	27	28	29	30	31
Apr/May	7	8	9	10	11	12	13	14	15	16	17	18	19	20	21	22	23	24	25	26	27	28	29	30	1	2	3	4	5	6	7
August	1	2	3	4	5	6	7	8	9	10	11	12	13	14	15	16	17	18	19	20	21	22	23	24	25	26	27	28	29	30	31
May/June	8	9	10	11	12	13	14	15	16	17	18	19	20	21	22	23	24	25	26	27	28	29	30	31	1	2	3	4	5	6	7
September	1	2	3	4	5	6	7	8	9	10	11	12	13	14	15	16	17	18	19	20	21	22	23	24	25	26	27	28	29	30	
Jun/July	8	9	10	11	12	13	14	15	16	17	18	19	20	21	22	23	24	25	26	27	28	29	30	1	2	3	4	5	6	7	
October	1	2	3	4	5	6	7	8	9	10	11	12	13	14	15	16	17	18	19	20	21	22	23	24	25	26	27	28	29	30	31
Jul/Aug	8	9	10	11	12	13	14	15	16	17	18	19	20	21	22	23	24	25	26	27	28	29	30	31	1	2	3	4	5	6	7
November	1	2	3	4	5	6	7	8	9	10	11	12	13	14	15	16	17	18	19	20	21	22	23	24	25	26	27	28	29	30	
Aug/Sept	8	9	10	11	12	13	14	15	16	17	18	19	20	21	22	23	24	25	26	27	28	29	30	31	1	2	3	4	5	6	
December	1	2	3	4	5	6	7	8	9	10	11	12	13	14	15	16	17	18	19	20	21	22	23	24	25	26	27	28	29	30	31
Sept/Oct	7	8	9	10	11	12	13	14	15	16	17	18	19	20	21	22	23	24	25	26	27	28	29	30	1	2	3	4	5	6	7

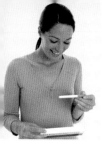

when you need

A LITTLE EXTRA HELP

It is a life-changing moment when you see the positive result on the pregnancy test and many women will be absolutely thrilled. However, some may have very different emotions.

You may have been trying to get pregnant for a while or it may have happened unexpectedly, but the news that you are expecting is the beginning of a new and exciting stage of your life. If you have only just started trying for a baby and you are pregnant within a couple of months, it can be a bit of a shock because it has happened so soon, when you might not have expected it to. However, for many other women it may have taken well over a year.

The threat of miscarriage

If you are unfortunate enough to have suffered a miscarriage, you may experience bitter-sweet emotions. The news of your pregnancy may be accompanied by the thought 'what if I miscarry again?' It is completely normal to have mixed emotions and for your feelings to fluctuate between elation and anxiety. You may feel that you are bursting to tell everyone. However, you and your partner will need time to adjust to the news, whatever your circumstances – so the best plan is to try to take things gently.

Egg donation & surrogacy

Significant numbers of women now enter pregnancy on their own and some may be a little apprehensive about how they will cope. Many will have had egg donation or they may be involved in a surrogacy arrangement. Circumstances differ, but the one thing

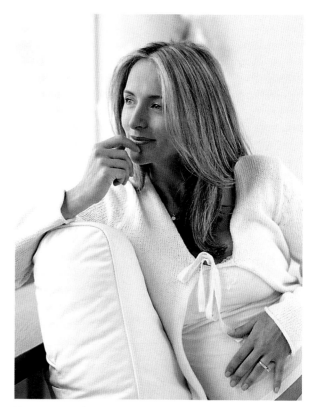

However you achieved your pregnancy, you will have much to contemplate as the months leading up to the birth go by.

that everyone wants is to have a happy, healthy baby. So, however you got pregnant, concentrate on the positive now. It may seem hard to believe, but the next nine months will fly by – try to enjoy your pregnancy and focus on the baby. You will soon be holding him in your arms.

High-risk pregnancy

If you need extra assistance to get through a difficult pregnancy, there is much help available these days. So, whether you are going to be an 'older' mum, perhaps have suffered miscarriages in the past or have received IVF or donor insemination – there's much to reassure you.

Being an older mother

If you want to become a mother over the age of 40, you are far from alone these days. Some older women become pregnant naturally, while others go through IVF or egg donation. You may want emotional and psychological support, as statistics may lead you to believe that you are more likely to have a difficult time. You'll be constantly reminded about high miscarriage rates and the start of your pregnancy could leave you feeling quite negative. Although older mums often do face increased risks of placenta failure, miscarriage or genetic abnormalities, it is important to remember that most women have no difficulties – and if you are an older expectant mum, your antenatal care will be tailored to your particular needs. You will be offered all the help you need and it is good to get an early scan.

Recurrent miscarriages

Some women find that they can get pregnant easily, but can't hold on to the pregnancy. This can be almost unbearable, as there's an uncomfortable feeling that they are just waiting to miscarry again. However, there have been huge advances in this field, especially in the area of immune response. Nevertheless, women may still feel that they cannot connect with pregnancy because of previous disappointments and natural fear of being hurt again. It is thought that around three out of every ten pregnancies will result in miscarriage – but if you are one of those women who is anxious about suffering from one, just look at that statistic again. You can see that seven out of ten pregnancies are actually successful – so why shouldn't yours be one of them?

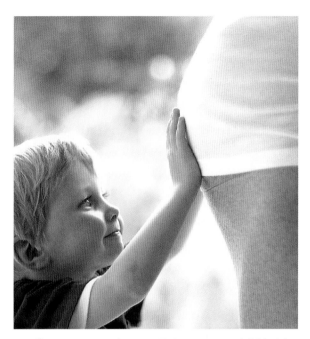

Not all pregnancies are the same. Having your second child might mean that different concerns come to the fore.

HIGH-RISK PREGNANCY Q&AS

"Help! I'm healthy, 38 and expecting twins. I've read that I'm in a 'high risk' category. What does that mean?"

Women over 35 are more likely to have twins and multiple births. There are certain risks, but these days you can be reassured that antenatal care is much better attuned to the needs of older mothers and multiple births.

"This is my second baby and I'm rhesus-negative; my partner is rhesus-positive. My doctor says I need anti-D injections, but my first baby was fine. Why the fuss?"

The rhesus factor in blood and negative/positive incompatibility doesn't usually present a problem in first pregnancies, but some of your first baby's Rh-positive blood could have got into yours, meaning your body will make antibodies that will attack your next baby if they too are Rh-positive. During pregnancy and after, you will be offered anti-D injections to destroy any Rh-positive cells and prevent your body from creating antibodies. If antibodies are found, you and your baby will need special care.

In vitro fertilisation (IVF) pregnancies

Many women go through IVF these days. Some are lucky the first time around, but others may have to try again and again. Once the embryos have been transferred to the uterus, you will have to go through a two-week waiting period and that time can feel like an emotional rollercoaster as your body seems to play tricks on you – one day you 'feel' pregnant, while the next you do not.

When you do get a positive pregnancy-test result, it could be quite a surprise. You may be so highly experienced in the medical procedures you have had so far that you now know a great deal about IVF and fertility, but next to nothing about pregnancy itself. You might feel highly anxious because you have suffered so many negative experiences and you cannot believe that things are going to go well for you. Try not to worry as you may find that you do perfectly well after you have received early pregnancy support. You need reassurance and it's important to feel that you are doing all the right things.

The early days and weeks of an IVF pregnancy can be fraught and it is very common to spot or bleed. (If you have had bleeding you must abstain from intercourse.) If you have gone through several unsuccessful IVF cycles due to implantation failure, you may be offered a cocktail of drugs that includes heparin (to prevent blood clots), steroids (to suppress the maternal immune system) and intralipid. You will need guidance and advice about when to reduce these drugs and will be monitored carefully. Don't be afraid to ask for information and advice if you need it.

IMMUNE ISSUES & IVF

Some women who are pregnant following miscarriages or who have been through unsuccessful IVF cycles may have been diagnosed with blood-clotting or immune disorders.

These women will be taking medication such as aspirin, heparin or low-dose steroids to help maintain the pregnancy, which needs careful monitoring by their doctor. Immune disorder is very a controversial area and the medical profession remains divided over certain tests.

However, these women may be extremely anxious early on in the pregnancy as they have already been through many disappointments along the way and need a lot of support to help manage their stress levels (see pages 108–9).

IN VITRO FERTILISATION (IVF) Q&AS

"My positive result came last week, but now I've had some spotting. Am I going to miscarry?"

Some bleeding is common with IVF pregnancies and may happen on implantation. Usually, more than one embryo is 'put back' and so bleeding occurs sometimes when one embryo comes away from the uterus. Stay calm and positive. Abstain from intercourse at least for the first trimester.

"My midwife says I'll have extra scans. Why?"

With IVF pregnancies there are usually more scans early on, to check where the embryo has implanted. This is important as ectopic pregnancies are more common with IVF. They will give you extra reassurance in the early days.

"After going through IVF three times, I thought I would feel fantastic if it worked, but now I'm pregnant I feel I'm just waiting for it all to go wrong. Why can't I be happy?"

Problems with fertility can leave lasting scars that take time to heal. You've had many disappointments and your negativity is simply your mind's way of protecting you against further hurt. Try to concentrate on looking after yourself – eat well, get plenty of fresh air (but perhaps avoid exercise and sex for now) and get lots of rest. Practise visualisation techniques (see pages 110–11). Once you have had your first scan and seen your baby's heart beat, you'll be able to believe the amazing news, and once you are reassured, you may feel more like sharing that news with those close to you.

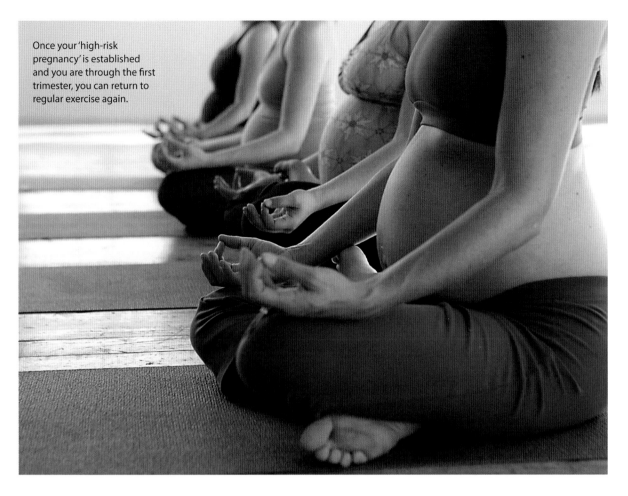

Once your 'high-risk pregnancy' is established and you are through the first trimester, you can return to regular exercise again.

USING DONOR EGGS

After exploring all other avenues, there will still be those who cannot give birth to their own genetic child. This includes many women who are in their forties, or younger women who have experienced premature ovarian failure or had to go through chemotherapy.

If this applies to you, egg donation offers a chance to have a much-longed-for baby. There is up to a 60 per cent success rate, compared with the less than five per cent chance that you would be likely to have using your own eggs. However, it is vital that you and your partner have proper counselling before you embark on egg donation and it is important to discuss all the issues and implications of the process.

EXISTING MEDICAL CONDITIONS

If you have an existing significant medical condition, such as heart disease or diabetes, you may be able to manage it well in normal circumstances, but now that you are pregnant you may worry about how it may affect your baby. It is important to realise that your pregnancy may also affect your condition, so you need to inform your doctor or midwife as soon as you can.

You may require further investigations or be referred to another specialist. Your medication, too, might need to be changed. Depending on your condition, you'll probably be asked to have more frequent antenatal appointments and checks if you are considered to be in the high-risk category.

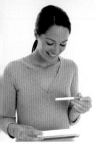

information about

PREGNANCY HORMONES

From conception, your body is undergoing dramatic but tiny, unseen changes. These are triggered and controlled by the production of key hormones. At first, your own body is responsible for these surges, but as your pregnancy progresses they are increasingly stimulated by your placenta and your growing baby.

The placenta is unique as an organ produced by two individuals. It has about 60 sets of enzymes of its own and produces hormones, nutrients, and the molecules and antibodies necessary to maintain a pregnancy and to help with the growth of the foetus.

THE KEY HORMONES

Human chorionic gonadotropin (hCG)

Produced in large quantities by the developing placenta after implantation, hCG is thought to be the hormone responsible for the nausea that may occur in early pregnancy (see page 27). Although this side-effect can be unpleasant, morning sickness rarely lasts beyond the first trimester and hCG is a vital element in a successful pregnancy because it triggers the release of other essential hormones such as oestrogen and progesterone.

HCG is the first hormone to make its presence known. It can be detected as soon as eight days after conception, but the amount produced begins to climb dramatically at week 5 and reaches a peak at around weeks 10 to 12. This hormone is detected by the type of pregnancy test that you might use yourself at home.

Oestrogen

The levels of this hormone increase throughout pregnancy and boost the flow of blood to the body's organs, giving you the pregnancy 'glow' of the second and third trimester. At the early stages of your pregnancy, oestrogen helps to thicken the lining of the uterus, a process that is vital for the successful implantation of the fertilised egg. It also promotes the growth and development of your breasts and uterus and softens the collagen fibres in your connective tissue so that your ligaments become more flexible as your baby grows.

Progesterone

This hormone has a wonderfully relaxing effect on so many parts of your body, including your brain, where it induces feelings of well-being. Pregnancy causes an increased

Increasing hormone concentration

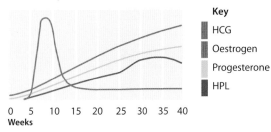

Key
- HCG
- Oestrogen
- Progesterone
- HPL

blood flow throughout the body and progesterone relaxes the blood vessels in the digestive and urinary tracts to help them to cope. Your muscles will be more relaxed, too, and progesterone helps tendons and ligaments to soften and become more elastic, to allow the uterus to expand. Later in pregnancy, progesterone prepares the birth canal for delivery, but importantly prevents the uterus from contracting until the baby is ready to be born. If you have conceived with the help of techniques such as IVF (see page 34) you will be given progesterone suppositories or injections to help sustain your pregnancy.

Human Placental Lactogen (HPL)
HPL accounts for 10 per cent of the production of protein by your placenta. It also sends glucose stored in your body to your baby and affects your insulin production to aid the transfer of nutrients to your baby. It helps your breasts to develop, too, and prepares them for milk production and breastfeeding.

Thyroxine (T4 and T3)
Necessary for the development of your baby's central nervous system, this hormone interacts with other hormones to stimulate your baby's growth and also helps him to process carbohydrates and proteins.

Calcitonin
This enables your body to store calcium and absorb vitamin D so that your own bone density is not adversely affected by the demands for calcium of your growing baby.

Cortisol and adrenocorticotropic hormone (ACTH)
The end of the first trimester of pregnancy sees an increase in the production of this hormone, which helps your baby's lungs to develop. It can also cause high levels of blood glucose and stretch marks.

Insulin
This is essential for your baby to store food (and therefore energy) in his body and it regulates glucose levels. If you are diabetic and your glucose levels are not carefully managed, it can result in your baby growing excessively and problems maintaining steady glucose levels.

Prolactin
Although prolactin levels increase throughout pregnancy, their effect is held in check until after your baby's birth, when they stimulate your breasts to produce milk.

Relaxin
This helps to soften the pelvic ligaments ready for the delivery of your baby. It also stimulates the cervix to 'ripen' – the process during labour when it softens and thins in preparation for dilatation and birth.

Oxytocin
Levels of oxytocin rise during the first stage of labour and cause the uterus to contract. As the birth canal widens, more oxytocin is produced to stimulate stronger, more effective, contractions. After childbirth, it is oxytocin that helps your uterus to contract and this process is stimulated by your baby feeding from your breast (see page 328).

Androgens (testosterone and similar hormones)
Some testosterone is necessary for the development of the male genitalia and helps to stimulate the production of oestrogen that is so essential throughout pregnancy.

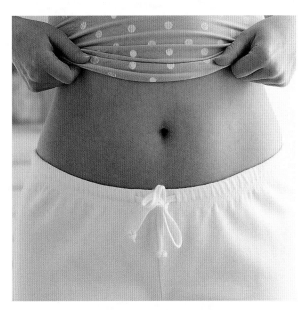

The unseen changes of pregnancy are initiated by a whole range of important hormones.

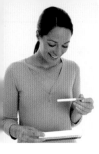

THE POWER OF QI

The care of mothers and babies has changed vastly in the last 30 years and one of the most important developments is a wide interest in the holistic approach of Traditional Chinese Medicine (TCM).

The ancient Chinese had the original holistic approach to health and well-being. They saw that physical, mental and emotional factors were linked and that they influenced one another, affecting the body at every level. They made acute observations and developed a whole medical system, being particularly interested in the relationships between people's physical, mental and emotional characteristics and how they were influenced by their environment.

Qi & the meridians

The whole concept of Chinese medicine is based on balance, harmony and conserving 'qi' (pronounced 'chi'), or dynamic energy, rather than depleting it. This is one of the most important concepts in TCM. Qi, along with 'jing' (essence energy) and 'shen' (the spirit) are known as the Three Treasures and form the basis of all energetic transactions in the body. Qi energy follows pathways through the body called 'meridians', of which there are twelve. The way qi runs through the body is influenced by many factors that can block or influence its flow, such as heat and cold, and mental, physical and emotional influences.

Qi & the elements

Qi and the idea of the fundamental elements has always been a difficult concept for Western medicine, but it is not entirely foreign to Western thinking. We use words like 'phlegmatic' to describe personal

YOUR QI LEVELS

What can deplete your levels of qi?

Working long hours without taking enough rest

Having a very short gap between children's births

Going without a spare minute in the day to relax

Eating on the run and trying to accomplish other tasks while you are eating

Not getting enough proper sleep

Eating too many raw foods

How can you build up your levels of qi?

Getting plenty of good-quality, restful sleep

Setting aside time to eat relaxed meals and digest your food properly

Practising techniques such as meditation, tai chi, chi gong, yoga, visualisation and relaxation

Eating a balance of both 'warming' and 'cooling' foods

characteristics or phrases such as 'green about the gills', and they derive from early European medicine, when the 'humours' provided a link between physical ailments and their causes.

The concept of the 'five elements' in TCM are associated with particular physical, mental and emotional characteristics. They are: water, fire, wood, earth and metal. Each meridian is related to one of

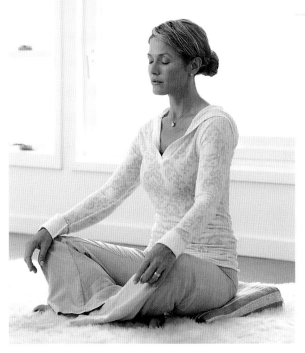

Practising meditation is a good way of increasing your levels of qi.

Acupuncture points

Acupuncture points lie along the meridians, which reflect the physical, emotional and spiritual characteristics that they connect with. Acupuncture is perfect for many of the common ailments of pregnancy, but it is important to find a properly qualified acupuncturist. It can be used to treat morning sickness, backache, carpal tunnel syndrome and migraines (see pages 116–17) and it can also be used to help emotional problems such as anxiety and depression and is especially beneficial alongside other complementary treatments (see pages 40–1). Through diagnostic techniques, the acupuncturist distinguishes where that pattern of disharmony lies and which organ is out of harmony in terms of its energy. They will then stimulate acupuncture points along the meridian to the organ linked to influence the flow of qi.

The connection between the heart and uterus

The heart in Western medicine is seen as the vital organ for keeping us alive. In TCM it is known as The Emperor because it stores our spirit and emotions. In pregnancy it is important for the qi to flow to the uterus (called the Palace of Infants). The Chinese believe that emotions such as worry, fear and anxiety can stop this flow, and visualisation can really help you to connect with your baby and restore the smooth flow of energy (see pages 110–11).

The kidneys and the heart are also mutually dependent and TCM holds that the kidneys store jing. This energy affects all aspects of reproduction, growth and development, and is considered to be the most refined constituent of our bodies. Jing can be described as constitutional health: it is both inherited from your parents and affected by your own lifestyle. It follows then, too, that building up your jing benefits your baby, since you pass it on to him in pregnancy. Shen is the most difficult to define, but it is essentially the mind or spirit of a person. In TCM, shen is believed to reside in the heart, so if the heart is unbalanced the shen will become disrupted.

the five elements and each of the elements is related to an organ or body system. For example, the fire element is linked to the heart and the element of water to the kidney.

The importance of environmental factors

Environmental factors are also critical – the Chinese believe that you should try to live in harmony with the laws of nature. So, for example, the 'yin' time of year is the winter, when we should rest, sleep and conserve energy, while the 'yang' time is the summer, when we are more active.

We should try to balance contraction and expansion, stillness and movement, and not resist the natural order of things. The purpose of traditional Chinese exercise such as tai qi gong (a form of tai chi) is to promote the smooth flow of energy through the meridians.

In TCM the body's organs have a physical function, but are also related to an emotion, which can affect that organ and influence the smooth flow of qi energy. Each of us has a unique pattern of disharmony related to an organ, which influences the way that qi flows.

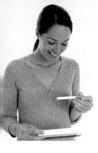

FINDING A REMEDY

Complementary therapies offer a wealth of remedies to promote relaxation and relieve common complaints. Although they are generally safe, check with your doctor or midwife first and always consult a qualified practitioner.

Consulting a complementary therapist can help make you feel less stressed, more listened to, more relaxed and better prepared for the birth of your baby. There is an enormous range of treatments and therapies available and everybody's needs are different. For many women, pregnancy is a time in their lives when they do not want to take conventional medicine for common ailments, but would rather try a holistic and natural approach. The most common therapies are outlined here. Treatments for specific complaints are detailed on pages 114–17, 160–3 and 204–7.

Safety of treatments in pregnancy

Be sure to tell the practitioner who is treating you that you are pregnant. You should exercise caution in pregnancy when using herbs or oils that may otherwise be used when you are not pregnant, as certain treatments are contraindicated. In fact, this is true for all therapies: for example, certain acupuncture points are unsafe to use during early pregnancy. Practitioners registered with an affiliated body will know this, so it is wise to establish that the practitioner is affiliated at the outset.

Take note

If you have pregnancy complications, a history of miscarriage (or threat), you must avoid some treatments. Check with your doctor or midwife first.

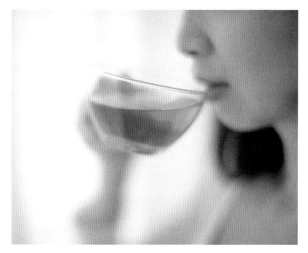

Opt for for delicious and refreshing herbal teas as an alternative to caffeine and alcohol during pregnancy.

Acupuncture

As long as the treatment is carried out by a fully qualified and accredited practitioner, this ancient Chinese practice should be safe during pregnancy. It can be helpful if you suffer from nausea and sickness, or lower back pain, but take care because certain acupuncture points may stimulate contractions.

Aromatherapy

'Essential', or concentrated, plant oils are applied through massage or aromatic infusion. They can be very effective in dealing with stress and pain relief, and promoting feelings of well-being and relaxation.

Some are unsafe to use in pregnancy, however, and generally it is best to avoid using all aromatherapy oils before 12 weeks. However, from week 13 the following oils are considered safe. Remember that they should always be diluted in a carrier oil (such as grapeseed oil) and used externally only.

Citrus	Lime	Ylang ylang
Grapefruit	Bergamot	
Lemon	Neroli	

Herbal remedies

Fruit teas can be a refreshing alternative to caffeine-containing coffee or breakfast tea, and a few slices of fresh ginger in boiling water can also relieve nausea, but take care with teas and remedies containing herbs as they can be very powerful, or even toxic (see the list below). Always consult your doctor or midwife before you take any herbal remedy or visit a herbalist. Clary sage has been linked to foetal distress in late pregnancy, so it is best avoided. If you choose to self-administer herbal remedies, you need to be aware that there are certain herbs you should not take during pregnancy. These include:

Arbor vitae	Mugwort
Barberry	Pennyroyal
Black and blue cohosh	Poke root
Cinchona	Rue
Golden seal	Sage
Greater celandine	Squaw vine
Juniper	Tansy
Marjoram	Wormwood
Motherwort	

Homeopathy

Homeopathic remedies can be helpful in treating the common complaints of pregnancy such as nausea, headaches and heartburn, and some women use them during labour (see pages 256–257). Homeopathic treatments are based on treating the individual with highly diluted substances that trigger

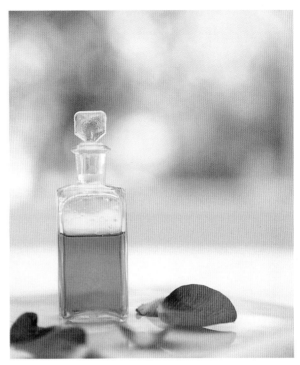

Aromatherapy oils are good to use, but it is vital to check whether they're suitable for pregnancy beforehand.

the body to heal itself. They are unlikely to cause side-effects because the amounts of active ingredient are tiny. Consult a qualified practitioner, though, because it can be difficult to identify the remedy that is exactly right for you. Keep your midwife or doctor informed of anything that you intend to take.

Hypnotherapy

This is usually a course (beginning around week 24) teaching self-hypnosis, relaxation and breathing techniques to help with labour and birth.

Reflexology

This works on the principle that points on the hands and feet correspond to other parts of the body, linked by energy pathways. Some styles of reflexology are based on the acupuncture meridians. Reflexology can be effective in improving circulation and treating back pain, but it is best avoided in the first trimester if you have a history of miscarriage.

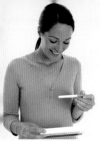

how diet affects your

BABY'S DEVELOPMENT

Recent research has shown that there is a window of opportunity for each of your baby's organs to develop to their full potential. To do so, exactly the right form of nutrition is needed, so what you eat and when can positively influence your baby's growth and development.

Twenty years ago Professor David Barker of Southampton University showed that babies who were born with a low birth weight had an increased risk of developing heart disease. Since then, further research has shown that the nutrition the unborn baby receives from the mother is crucial to his development and that there are critical windows of opportunity for each of the baby's organs to develop. If those opportunities can be grasped and made use of, then the baby's organs can develop to their maximum potential.

A nutrition-packed diet

Your body converts what you eat into nutrients for your baby, but it can only transfer as much as you take in, so you need to make sure that what you eat and drink is nutrient-packed. Ideally, you will have built up some reserves before you even became pregnant, but if your diet then was sometimes lacking, it is even more important now that you eat a varied and balanced range of foods.

The importance of protein

How much protein you consume at the start of pregnancy is strongly linked to the baby's size at birth. This is because proteins consist of amino acids, which your body needs to make hormones, and for the generation and repair of tissue. Proteins are the building blocks for the baby's organs.

Insulin

The hormones that you manufacture control your baby's growth and one of the most crucial hormones is insulin. As the embryo becomes a foetus, it begins to produce its own hormones, too, and if the mother is undernourished, it will produce less insulin in response, therefore slowing its own rate of growth.

Folic acid

All pregnant women are advised to take folic acid (preferably from pre-conception) as it is vital for the healthy development of the neural tube (see page 64). It is thought that folic acid helps the neural tube surrounding the spine to fold and close over.

Essential fatty acids (EFAs)

During the first trimester the embryo grows fast and just 18 days after conception your baby's brain has begun to develop (see page 64). For it to grow properly, the brain needs essential fatty acids (EFAs) from you. A crucial component of the brain, eyes and nerve cells is docosahexaenoic acid (DHA), which is an omega-3 EFA. It is also thought important for the healthy development of the signalling structures in the human brain, so your baby must receive an adequate supply. An omega-3 supplement will ensure that you build up a supply, ready for when your baby reaches 28 weeks and goes through the rapid development phase.

ESSENTIAL FATTY ACID (EFA) FOODS

EFAs are essential for the development of your baby's brain. You can make sure that he is receiving this important requirement by eating the following foods:

Avocados

Brazil nuts, pine nuts and walnuts

Fish such as cod, mackerel, salmon, tuna and herring (limit them to one portion per week because of the high levels of mercury in some fish – see page 87)

Eggs

Flaxseeds and flaxseed oil

Grapeseed oil

Hempseeds and hempseed oil

Olives and olive oil

Pumpkin, sesame and sunflower seeds

Dark-green, leafy vegetables such as spinach, mustard leaf and kale

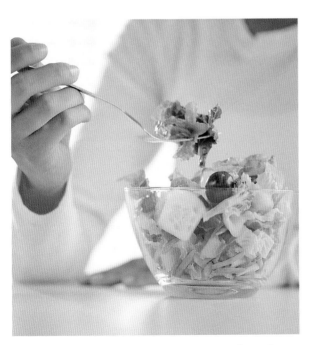

A good, healthy diet during pregnancy, containing plenty of nutrient-rich foods, will help your baby to grow and develop in the best ways possible.

FOETAL NUTRITION

The basic elements for foetal nutrition are glucose, amino acids, fats, water, minerals and vitamins. The placenta burns up large amounts of glucose to provide energy for the developing foetus.

Proteins are the building blocks for cells, tissue and organs, and are essential for bringing about repair

Zinc is important for many enzymes and is required for RNA and DNA, in the process of cell division and for the synthesis of proteins

Lipids and fats are essential for cell membranes and for brain development

Antioxidants protect against free-radical damage

Iron is needed to build a good blood supply from the placenta

Choline

Choline is essential for the production of cell membranes and cell division and it may be linked to the learning and memory centres in the brain. A well-balanced diet will usually supply you with enough choline because it is found in a wide variety of foods including bananas, barley, butter, cauliflower, corn, egg yolks, flaxseeds, lentils, milk, oats, oranges, potatoes, sesame seeds, soybeans and soybean products, tomatoes and wholewheat bread.

Iodine

Iodine helps to make the thyroid hormones that assist the brain in development and help keep cells and the metabolic rate healthy. A good basic diet should deliver all you need. Fish, shellfish and edible seaweeds contain the most iodine, but most seafoods should be avoided during pregnancy (see page 84). However, iodine is found in cow's milk, yogurt, cheese, eggs and strawberries.

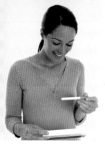

WEEK-BY-WEEK OVERVIEW

Over the next nine months your body will undergo miraculous changes in order to create a new person. Hold tight – this will be the most amazing journey of your life. These pages show a brief overview of what bodily changes to expect over the weeks.

First trimester

Although your body may not alter very obviously in the first trimester, it is, in fact, undergoing incredible changes that are vital to the healthy progression of your pregnancy. Use this chart as a quick reference.

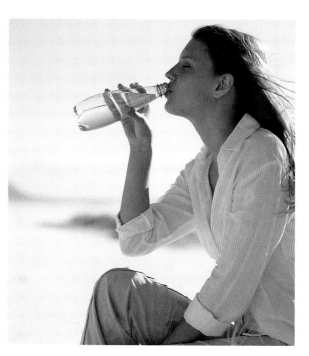

1 Your pregnancy is dated from this week.

2 Your ovaries have ripened an egg and released it – you may feel a very slight pain at this time or notice vaginal secretions being wetter and clearer.

YOUR ANTENATAL CARE TIMELINE

Week	6–8	10	10–12	10–14	11–16	16	11–16
	'First contact' with your doctor or midwife	Blood tests (see page 71)	'Booking' appointment with your doctor or midwife (see pages 70–1)	Routine scan to confirm EDD and check for twins or more (see page 75)	A nuchal translucency scan (NTS) may be offered if your pregnancy is considered to carry some risk factors	Routine antenatal check	You may be offered a 'triple 'or 'quadruple' blood test to check for Down's syndrome, Edward's syndrome or spina bifida (see pages 74–5)

3 Conception has now taken place. Your egg has joined with a single sperm to create the unique group of cells that will eventually become your baby.

4 The fertilised egg has travelled along the fallopian tube to your uterus and as it attaches itself to the endometrium you may notice slight bleeding. Your uterus is about the size of a plum.

5 It's now about the right time to make an appointment to see your doctor or midwife.

6 Your breasts may be feeling heavier and perhaps a little sore as your newly released pregnancy hormones stimulate the milk-producing glands.

7 You may be feeling extremely tired and experience some nausea and sensitivity to certain smells, foods and drinks.

8 You may feel hotter than usual and are urinating more frequently. Your uterus is now about the size of an orange.

9 Your tummy is becoming rounder and your waistband may be feeling a little tight.

10 You may be feeling thirstier than usual as your body needs extra fluids. Extra blood is being pumped around your body and your hands and feet quite possibly feel much warmer than usual. It could be that your skin seems different and even displays a few spots caused by hormone increase.

11 Changes in blood pressure may cause dizziness, especially when you get out of bed or stand up quickly.

12 Your breasts may feel very tender and are rapidly increasing in cup size. Your uterus will now be around the size of a grapefruit.

13 This week marks the end of the first trimester. Your tiredness should start to wear off and you'll regain some of your old energy. Any nausea or sickness should start easing now.

18–20	25	28	31	34	36	38	40	41
Routine scan to check the baby's development and the position of the placenta	Routine antenatal check	Routine antenatal check	Routine antenatal check	Routine antenatal check	Routine antenatal check	Routine antenatal check	Routine antenatal check	Further antenatal checks if you are overdue

Second trimester

During this stage of pregnancy you should begin to feel and look in the bloom of good health. You will look pregnant as your baby is rapidly growing and your body is changing to accommodate him.

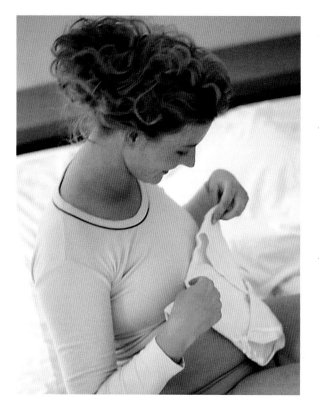

14 You may notice your nose feeling stuffy and your ears blocked, due to increased blood flow. It's possible that you also have bleeding gums, so go for a dental check-up. If you are slightly constipated, drink more water and eat more fruit, vegetables and wholegrain breads and cereals.

15 Your placenta is now fully formed. Your clothes probably feel tight as your bump continues to expand.

16 You might now experience food cravings and your hair and skin texture may seem different to normal.

17 You may feel a slight fluttering of your baby's first movements around this time.

18 Now that your energy levels are improving, you may also notice changes in your libido as more blood is pumped around the pelvic area, making you feel more easily aroused.

19 Your hair and nails are probably looking stronger and shinier. Any freckles and moles will appear darker. You may have skin patches, called 'chloasma', caused by increased levels of oestrogen. These will fade after the birth. Always protect your skin from the sun.

20 If you haven't already felt your baby move, you should do so in the next few weeks. See your doctor or midwife if you are concerned.

21 You will probably gain around 5.4 kg (12 lb) during this trimester, so you may find that you are perspiring more easily because you are carrying some extra weight.

22 By now your uterus will have expanded outwards and upwards in your abdomen and you may have a prominent 'linea nigra', which will fade after the birth.

23 As your uterus takes up more space it leaves less room for your digestive system, so you may experience indigestion and heartburn. Try eating a little and often rather than just a few large meals.

24 Your hormonal activity will have become more settled now, so you should have far fewer mood swings, if you have been suffering these. In fact, by this time you may find that you feel much more relaxed and calm altogether.

25 You may notice that you are sometimes short of breath. Improving your posture and using relaxation techniques may help (see pages 140–1).

26 Your bump really will feel much heavier now and you may have some backache. Perhaps you notice that you have some developed some stretch marks on your abdomen, hips or breasts, although not everyone gets them.

27 The size of your bump depends on your height and weight and whether this is your first baby. It will also be affected by the amount of amniotic fluid. You may find that you have some stress incontinence because your pelvic floor muscles are being stretched. If you haven't already started them, now is the time to begin regularly practising your pelvic floor exercises (see page 141).

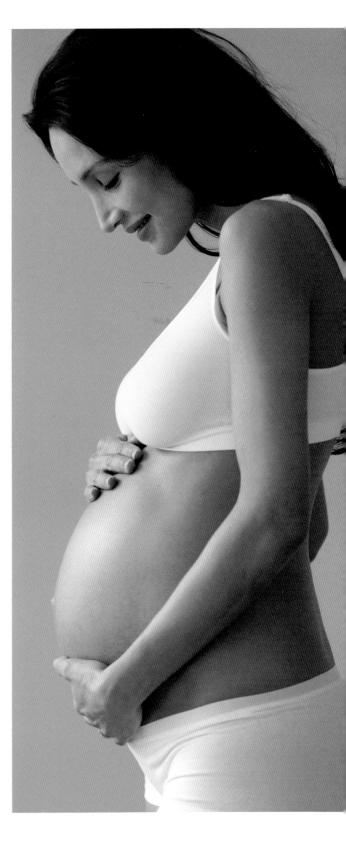

Third trimester

It won't be long now… in these last three months of your pregnancy your bump will expand at an extraordinary rate and you will notice all kinds of changes as your body prepares for your baby's birth.

28 Your tummy button is possibly either flattened or sticking out now and your uterus will be pushing up against the lower part of your ribcage, which can feel uncomfortable. You may be able to feel, or even see, your baby kicking now.

29 Your legs may feel heavy and swollen ankles are all too common at this stage. You may need to try to raise your lower legs whenever you sit down.

30 Backache is common at this stage of pregnancy because of your growing bump. Lengthening your spine and back to get your pelvis into a good position may help.

31 Moving around really does seem more of an effort this week and you might feel very short of breath at times. Try to rest as much as you possibly can.

32 You are probably putting on weight at quite a rate by now. You will now be able to feel the top of your uterus about 12 cm (5 in) above your navel.

33 You perhaps feel increased pressure in your pelvic area as your baby moves into the 'head-down' position. Shortness of breath and indigestion should improve when he does move down, but you may have to urinate more frequently.

34 Your hands and feet quite possibly feel swollen. This is commonly due to fluid retention and may ease when you have rested, but notify your doctor or midwife if it is severe and accompanied by a headache. It could be a symptom of pre-eclampsia and so prompt treatment needs to be given.

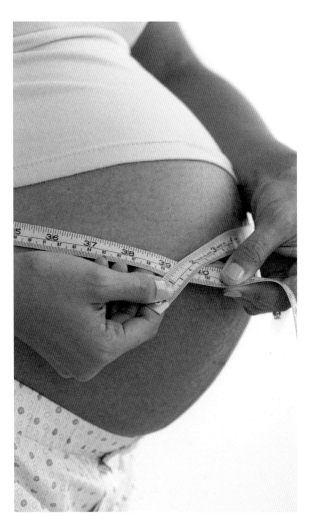

35 Your nipples will have noticeably enlarged and become much darker. Your breasts will feel much heavier. You may be finding it hard to sleep. Try sleeping on your side and place a pillow between your legs.

36 You will be putting on weight more rapidly than ever as your body prepares for labour. Your baby's weight is increasing, too. He is now fully developed, but 'filling out' and laying down vital fat stores in his body.

37 You might experience Braxton Hicks' (practice) contractions. They will be noticeable, but should not be at all painful. If the pain is very strong, contact your doctor or midwife.

38 Your weight gain will probably level off now. Your appearance might be flushed as your circulation is working harder than ever.

39 You will probably feel quite uncomfortable by now. Your uterus is taking up almost all the space in your abdomen and pressing against your ribcage.

40 This is the week that you may expect to give birth, but don't be too surprised if nothing happens just yet. You might not give birth for another two weeks yet, but in the meantime, your doctor or midwife will keep a close eye on you.

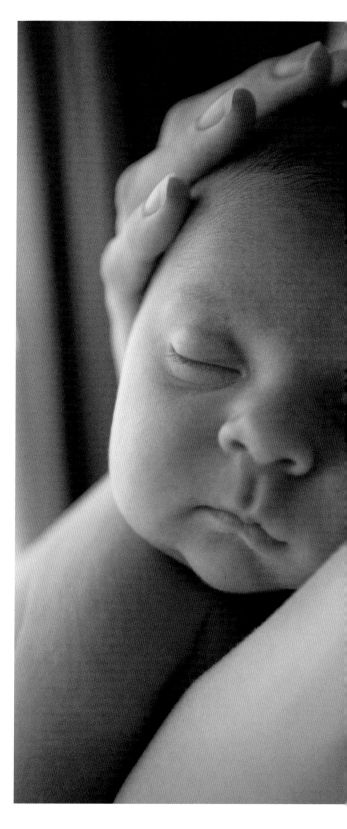

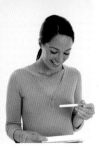

WEEK-BY-WEEK OVERVIEW

In just nine months your baby has transformed from a simple cluster of cells to a complete, new, human being. From the moment of conception, your baby will develop at an amazing rate and he will change almost daily. Knowing what is going on can make it easier for you to take really good care of yourself and your baby.

Your pregnancy will be dated from the first day of your last menstrual period (LMP), so if your last period was eight weeks ago, you will be said to be in your eighth week of pregnancy, even though your baby may only be six weeks old. Pregnancy is considered to last for approximately 40 weeks, so babies born before 37 weeks will be treated as premature, while babies delivered after 40 will be regarded as postmature.

First trimester

4 The blastocyst embedded in your uterine wall divides, the inner half developing into the baby, the outer half into the placenta and umbilical cord.

5 The 'ball' of cells has started to elongate and the brain, spinal cord, liver and kidneys are beginning to develop. The eyes and ears can be seen. The heart walls are starting to form and the bones and muscles are beginning to form.

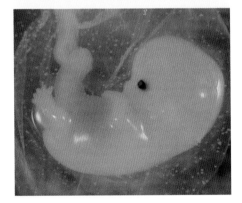

YOUR BABY'S SIZE & WEIGHT

Week	Length crown to rump	Week	Length crown to rump	Weight
4	0.36–1 mm (¹⁄₇₀ and ¹⁄₂₅ in)	9	22–30 mm (1 in)	
5	1.25 mm (¹⁄₂₀ in)	10	31–42 mm (1¼–1²⁄₃ in)	
6	2–4 mm (¹⁄₁₂ to ¹⁄₆ in)	11	44–60 mm (1¾–1¼ in)	8 g (¹⁄₃ oz)
7	4–5 mm (¹⁄₆ to ¹⁄₅ in)	12	61 mm (2½ in)	8–14 g (¹⁄₃–½ oz)
8	14–20 mm (½ in)	13	65–78 mm (2²⁄₃–3 in)	13–20 g (½–²⁄₃ oz)

6 The head is beginning to take shape. Chest and abdominal cavities are forming and tiny buds for arms and legs are appearing.

7 The 'tail' has almost gone and the head is taking shape. The eyes are dark spots and nostrils have begun to form. The heart has divided. The arm and leg buds are beginning to lengthen and the hands and feet are forming.

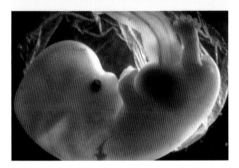

8 Most of your baby's organs have formed at a basic level. The heartbeat is beginning to normalise. The skeleton is beginning to ossify. Tiny facial features can be seen and your baby may begin to move around.

9 The embryo now looks more like a baby. The arms, legs, hands and feet are growing rapidly and the tiny toes and fingers are clearly visible.

10 This week your baby officially changes from 'embryo' to 'foetus'. The head is much larger than the body and facial features are more recognisable. Arms and legs have elongated and ankles and wrists have formed.

11 Your baby's vital organs have formed and are functioning. Now his body will rapidly elongate.

12 Your baby can smile, frown and even suck his thumb. He looks fully formed and his fingers and toes are no longer webbed. The brain and organs continue to develop and the genitals become more visible.

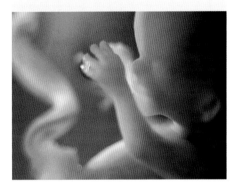

13 Your baby may look fully formed, but the major internal organs are still developing. He can support some head movements and the eyes are gradually coming to the front of the face. The ears may begin to sense sound.

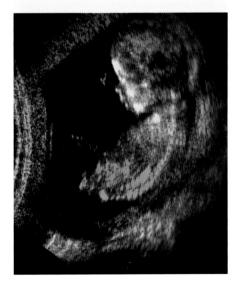

Second trimester

14 This week sees your baby 'practising' breathing (see opposite). His growth rate increases. His nervous system has begun to function and he has nails.

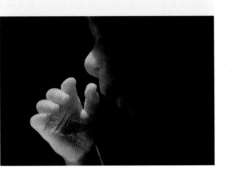

15 Hearing mechanisms are developing. In just a few more weeks he will be able to hear your heartbeat and voice. Lanugo (see page 178) is beginning to form a covering over your baby's paper-thin skin and he is growing eyebrows.

16 Ultrasound scans can now detect your baby's sex. His bones continue to harden and his joints work. His nervous system is functioning.

17 Your baby is beginning to lay down fat, giving him the energy to roll over and wave or kick. He can hear sounds and sudden noises may make him jump.

18 The baby is entering his most active phase and he is trying out movements. His eyes are now in the correct position; there are touch pads on his fingers and his fingerprints are forming.

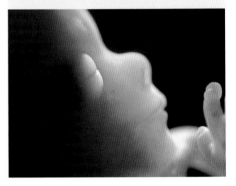

19 Glands in the skin secrete vernix, which covers your baby's skin and the nerves are being coated with myelin. The placenta is still taking away waste products, but the kidneys are beginning to function.

YOUR BABY'S SIZE & WEIGHT

Week	Length crown to rump	Weight	Week	Length crown to rump	Weight
14	80–93 mm (3¼–4 in)	25 g (1 oz)	**21**	16 cm (7¼ in)	300 g (10½ oz)
15	104–114 mm (3¼ to 4 in)	50 g (1¾ oz)	**22**	19 cm (7½ in)	350 g (12¼ oz)
16	108–116 mm (4⅓–4⅔ in)	80 g (2¾ oz)	**23**	20 cm (8 in)	455 g (1 lb)
17	11–12 cm (4½–5 in)	100 g (3½ oz)	**24**	21 cm (8½ in)	540 g (1¼ lb)
18	12.5–14 cm (5–5¾ in)	150 g (5¼ oz)	**25**	22 cm (8¾ in)	700 g (1½ lb)
19	13–15 cm (5¼–6 in)	200 g (7 oz)	**26**	23 cm (9¼ in)	910 g (2 lb)
20	14–16 cm (5½–6½ in)	255 g (9 oz)	**27**	24 cm (9½ in)	1 kg (2 lb)

20 An important stage for sense development. Also the nerve cells linking sight, hearing, touch and smell are developing. Complex connections are being made that will be needed for memory and thinking.

21 Your baby can respond to touch. Taste buds have developed. He may stroke his face and suck his thumb. Your baby has enough room to make large movements.

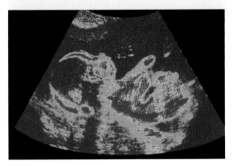

22 The skin is becoming less transparent. The brain is still developing at a phenomenal pace and the germinal matrix is producing brain cells.

23 Talk to your baby as much as you can – when he is born, he will be able to recognise his parents' voices.

24 Your baby is practising breathing by taking in amniotic fluid and his lungs are beginning to produce surfactant, a substance that prevents the air sacs within them sticking together.

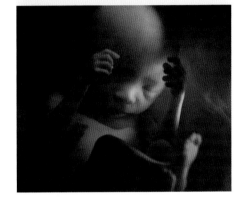

25 White blood cells are now being produced that are vital for fighting infection. Brown fat under his skin will help him regulate temperature after birth. Adult teeth are developing in buds.

26 Your baby reacts to sounds now and studies have shown that unborn babies' pulses will quicken in response to certain sounds.

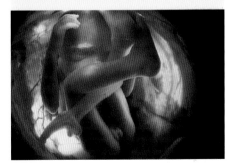

27 Your baby is getting much rounder and plumper. The eyelids have grown eyelashes and the retinas are forming. Your baby will be able to sense changes in light.

Third trimester

28
Your baby can easily raise his feet above his head, so you may feel a kick at the top of your abdomen.

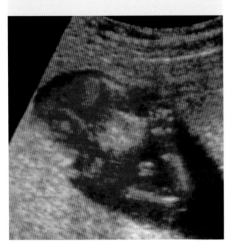

31
As your abdomen is stretched, more light is let into the uterus and your baby will be more aware of it. His pupils will dilate occasionally.

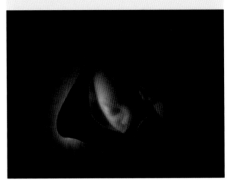

32
Your baby is sleeping for as much as 90 per cent of the day. He can now turn his head and all his five senses are functioning.

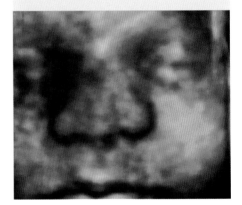

29
Your baby's head is in proportion to the rest of his body.

30
You may feel strong kicks under your ribcage and pressure on your pelvic floor as your baby moves into the head-down position for birth.

YOUR BABY'S SIZE & WEIGHT

Week	Length crown to rump	Weight	Week	Length crown to rump	Weight
28	25 cm (10 in)	1.1 kg (2½ lb)	35	32 cm (12¾ in)	2.55 kg (5½ lb)
29	26 cm (10½ in)	1.25 kg (2¾ lb)	36	33 cm (13 in)	2.75 kg (6 lb)
30	27 cm (10¾ in)	1.36 kg (3 b)	37	34 cm (13½ in)	2.95 kg (6½ lb)
31	28 cm (11¼ in)	1.59 kg (3½ lb)	38	35 cm (14 in)	3.1 kg (6 ¾ lb)
32	29 cm (11½ in)	1.8 kg (4 lb)	39	36 cm (14½ in)	3.25 kg (7 lb)
33	30 cm (11½ in)	2 kg (4½ lb)	40	37–38 cm (14¾–15¼ in)	3.25 kg (7 lb)
34	31 cm (12½ in)	2.26 kg (5 lb)			

33 Whatever you do prompts activity or slumber. Your baby is lulled by rhythmic movement as you walk about.

34 Your baby's movements will be slower because there is much less room. His immune system is developing and by the time he is born it should be able to fight mild infections.

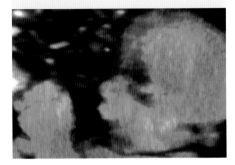

35 The lungs are mature and so a premature baby delivered now is unlikely to suffer breathing difficulties.

36 Your baby's movements will seem more deliberate now and they are strong, though increasingly constricted.

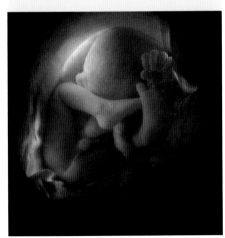

37 Your baby is now considered full term. Your midwife will be able to tell the position of your baby (see pages 212–15).

38 Labour may start at any time. Your baby's immune system is developing and will continue to do so after delivery, when it is boosted by the antibodies and nutrients in the colostrum.

39 Your baby may have swallowed some lanugo via the amniotic fluid. It will form part of the 'meconium', the first 'solid' waste that he will pass after he is born.

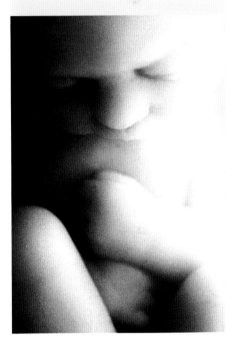

40 Your baby will leave the fluid-filled uterus and take his first breath of air any time now. Breathing will prompt changes within his heart and arteries that will send the blood supply to his lungs.

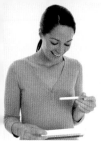

adjusting to your new life

STARTING OUT TOGETHER

It may take a little time for you both to get used to the idea of being parents, so try to remain patient if one or both of you are finding things difficult. Stay positive – you are a team and you are about to become a family.

You will have all kinds of decisions to make over your lifetime as parents, and if you are just in the first trimester of pregnancy, you may be feeling a little overwhelmed. Take things one step at a time and keep all the channels of communication open between you. Your worries, concerns and needs may differ, so you need to at least respect each other's feelings – even if you have trouble understanding them.

Ups & downs

After the initial feelings of elation at the news of your pregnancy, you may find that the first trimester is quite a trying time for you and your partner. Everyone enters pregnancy with a unique set of baggage, so talking through problems may help enormously. On the physical side, you might be feeling nauseous, or even actually vomiting, and it is likely that you will be experiencing overwhelming fatigue. Your body is busy laying down the foundations for your baby's development and so extreme tiredness is not at all surprising.

However, in these early days you won't appear especially pregnant and so it may be hard for others to feel sympathetic. Getting a seat on the bus may be even harder! Add to the physical symptoms, fluctuating emotions intensified by hormonal changes and you may wonder what has hit you, while your partner may not know whether to expect

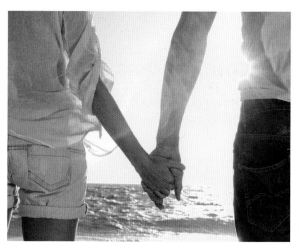

A new experience for both of you – it's important to stay close.

laughter or tears. Try to remember that it may be difficult for your partner to know how you are feeling. He may find it quite hard to anticipate what you need and so either 'fuss' around you or else seem oblivious to your altered state.

It might be useful to look at how your relationship is at the moment and consider what changes you might make in these first 12 weeks that could make a difference. Look at your work–life balance and consider carefully how you could achieve more free time to spend together. Perhaps you could build in a few treats for yourselves. Whatever you do, it's important to be as patient as possible and to communicate how you are feeling.

Changing needs

Your needs will change throughout your pregnancy, so in the second trimester you may feel a bit like superwoman: perfectly well and strong – perhaps ready and willing to deal with anything. But as the size of your bump increases, you may find simple physical tasks, such as emptying the kitchen bin, far too strenuous. If your partner fails to take the initiative with such tasks, don't suffer (or sulk) in silence, but be prepared to ask for help. As the years go by, your lives as parents will involve plenty of negotiating and compromise on both sides, so pregnancy is an excellent time to start practising these skills.

For dads-to-be

Although you are not undergoing all the physical and hormonal changes that your partner is, you may be feeling a little confused. Among all the excitement, perhaps a little anxiety has crept in. You may be thinking about practical issues such as juggling finances, but try not to think of these as 'your' problems, for you to solve on your own. You are embarking on family life together and issues need to be solved together. Attention may seem focused on your partner and it may be hard to see how you can be involved before your baby arrives. But don't worry, there will be plenty for you share. Even at this early stage, your contribution is invaluable.

WAYS FOR EXPECTANT DADS TO GET INVOLVED

Food

Nausea and tiredness may make it difficult for your partner to even think about food, so if she usually does most of the shopping and cooking, you could take over more responsibility. Make sure you know what she really doesn't want to eat and avoid eating it yourself. If the smell of cheese makes her feel ill, try to find another calcium-rich alternative. You can use the nutrition section to help you compose a balanced shopping list (see pages 78–85). Be prepared to have some other options to hand when you prepare a meal, too. What might have seemed a good idea to your partner a day or so ago, might now be nausea-inducing, so try not to take things personally if your menu is rejected.

Sleep

It may be hard to understand the numbing depths of your partner's tiredness in these first few months, but try to be sympathetic. Eating meals earlier in the evening and slowing down your social life together for a little while will help to give her the best chance to get enough rest. A gentle massage or a soothing bath may also help her to drift off peacefully – sex may not be on the agenda just now (see pages 106–7), so either option will give you some intimate time together.

Emotions

You will probably be feeling an extraordinary mix of feelings at the prospect of being a father: elation, pride and excitement, but perhaps also anxiety, fear and isolation, too. This is absolutely normal and you will need time to adjust. Try not to keep your feelings bottled up. You may feel concerned that you don't want to spoil things for your partner, but it's very likely that she will share some of your misgivings, too. Her emotions will also be heightened by the cocktail of hormones that will be released into her body as the pregnancy establishes itself, so do not be at all surprised if she seems a little unpredictable. The best way for you both to cope is to try to keep communicating with one another. Make time for a few treats – a trip to the cinema or a stroll in the park. Going out somewhere together, away from the daily chores, can help you both to put worries into perspective.

Lifestyle habits

If either of you smokes, takes recreational drugs or drinks alcohol, you need to make drastic changes. Your partner should stop smoking or using drugs and it is important not to drink alcohol at any time during pregnancy. If you smoke you should do your best to stop because your baby could be seriously affected just by your partner breathing in your smoke (see page 103). Ask your doctor for help with quitting and at least ensure that you go outside if you do have a puff. Long term, you need to give up smoking for the sake of your own health and that of your family. Babies and children suffer a range of health problems if they are exposed to smoke, including an increased risk of cot death (see page 340), so the health and well-being of your baby is surely the best incentive to quit you could ever have. If you take recreational drugs, you also need to stop and your doctor can help with this, too. Drinking alcohol moderately is OK, but bear in mind that your partner will be relying on you as pregnancy progresses, so when she is closer to her delivery date, you may need to be able to drive her to the hospital at very short notice. If she has stopped drinking, then you could support her by stopping, too.

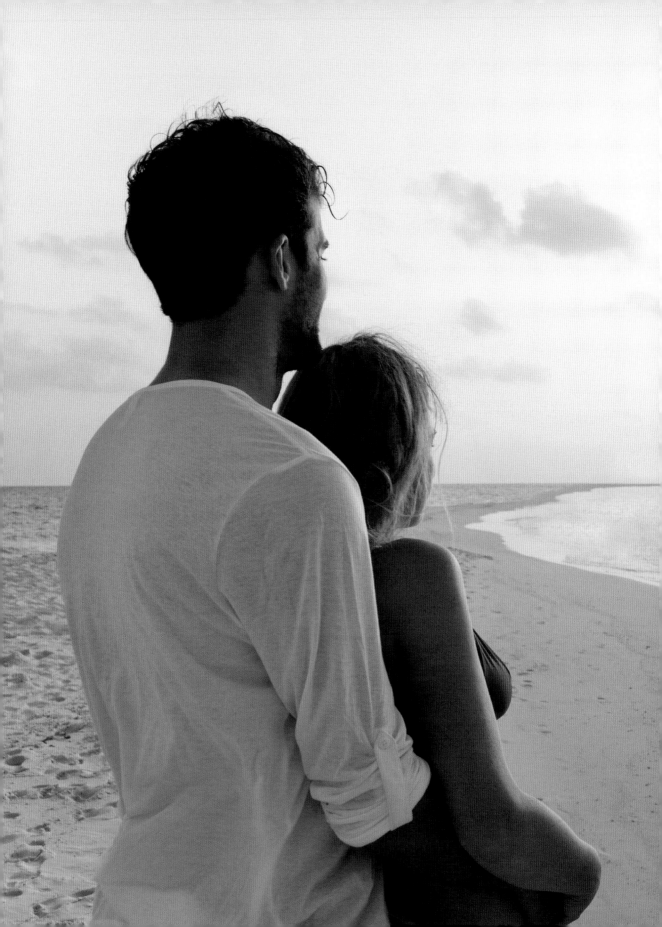

chapter 3

your first
TRIMESTER

You and your partner will be getting
used to the news of your pregnancy –
these next few pages let you know
what to expect.

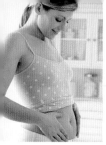

YOUR CHANGING BODY

Although you may not look very pregnant in this first trimester, with so many changes happening to your body, you will certainly feel that something momentous is going on.

Week 1
The first day of your last menstrual period (LMP) and the day that your pregnancy will be officially dated from on all your documentation is sometime this week, though conception may not actually have taken place for another two weeks yet. Pregnancy usually lasts for about 40 weeks, though in fact this is just an average time. Some pregnancies are slightly longer; others are shorter.

Week 2
Your ovaries will have ripened an egg and released it. You may experience a very slight pain at this time or have noticed that your vaginal secretions are becoming wetter and clearer. If you have been trying to get pregnant for some time, you may have already been taking a folic acid supplement regularly, but if not, don't worry – just start now.

Week 3
The egg has now connected with a solitary sperm, which has formed a particular cluster of cells that will develop into your baby.

Week 4
The fertilised egg (blastocyst) has now found its way to your uterus, which is already beginning to enlarge and soften. As the blastocyst attaches itself to the lining of the uterus (endometrium) you may experience some slight bleeding.

Week 5
You have probably noticed that your period is late by now and you have probably used a home pregnancy test. Once you have a positive result, you need to make an appointment to see your doctor or midwife.

Week 6
Your breasts may be feeling slightly heavier, fuller and a little tender as your newly released pregnancy hormones stimulate the milk-producing glands (see pages 328–9). You might notice that the veins under the skin of your breasts are more visible, as the blood supply to your breasts increases. Your nipples have possibly become more prominent and the areola (the circles of pinkish brown skin around your nipples) will probably have increased in size and have darkened in colour.

Week 7
You are probably feeling extremely tired and may already be experiencing the nauseous feelings and perhaps even vomiting of early pregnancy (see page 27) because the classic pregnancy hormone hCG (see pages 36–7) is surging through your body. You may also have found that you are now far more sensitive to smells, have gone off certain foods completely or that you have an unfamiliar, metallic taste present in your mouth.

Before you became pregnant your heart pumped about two per cent of the total blood in your body to

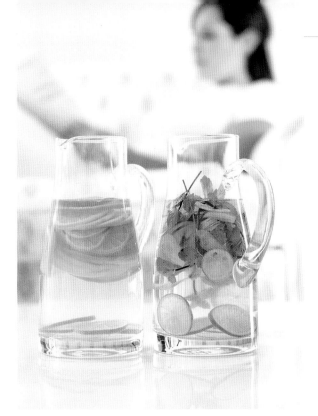

Try to drink as much as you can. If you find drinking plain water tedious, add oranges, lemons, limes and mint.

your uterus, but by the end of the first trimester your heart rate will be sending up to 25 per cent of your circulating blood to your rapidly developing placenta and baby. The muscles in the walls of your heart and your blood vessels will be relaxed by the hormone progesterone (see pages 36–7), so that they can cope with the increased volume of blood without dramatically increasing your blood pressure.

Week 8

Whether or not you have already had a first 'contact' meeting with your doctor or midwife, your 'booking' visit should be scheduled to take place between now and week 12. Your metabolic rate will rise by up to 25 per cent, which means that you may find that you feel much hotter than you usually do. You are also probably urinating more frequently because your kidneys are filtering your blood more efficiently. Your uterus has now reached double its original size, so that it is now approximately the size of an orange.

Week 9

If you feel unusually emotional, you can probably blame at least part of it on those pregnancy hormones. You might not have a noticeable bump just yet, but your waistband may be getting a little tight. Time to change into something looser?

Week 10

Your body needs extra fluids, so you are likely to feel thirstier than usual. With the increase in the volume of blood being pumped around your body, your hands and feet will probably feel much warmer than usual and your skin tone and texture may be changing. You might even break out in spots as your body adjusts to the increase in hormones.

Week 11

You may feel dizzy or even faint as you get out of bed in the morning or rise from a chair quickly. This is due to fluctuations in blood pressure and is very common in pregnancy.

Week 12

You or your midwife may now be able to feel your swelling uterus, which by this time will be about the size of a grapefruit. Your breasts may have increased by several cup sizes and around your nipples you may now see small raised bumps called Montgomery's tubercles. Your breasts may feel tender and you might feel more comfortable if you wear a soft non-wired bra at night.

Week 13

Many pregnant women will have gained around 1 kg (2½ lb) or more by now, but if you've had a lot of nausea you may have lost a little. However, the nausea should begin to ease, so you should soon feel better. Week 13 marks the end of your first trimester and as you pass this point the risk of miscarriage is reduced by around 65 per cent. You should also feel less tired, have regained energy and have begun to acquire the fabled 'bloom' of pregnancy.

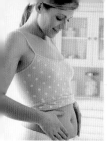

your baby in the first trimester

STAGE BY STAGE

This first trimester is one of the most crucial periods in your pregnancy. It is the time when your baby will grow and develop at a dramatic rate, but this is also when she is at her most vulnerable – so take good care of yourself and your growing baby.

Early on, you may not even know that you are pregnant, but dramatic changes are going on in your body and this first trimester is one of the most crucial periods in your baby's development. What was a simple cluster of cells will develop into an embryo and by week 8 into a foetus. By the end of week 13 your baby will be fully formed, so development rate in this first trimester is astonishing.

The blastocyst

Your newly fertilised egg has divided repeatedly to become a blastocyst that has hatched and implanted in the lining (endometrium) of your uterus. It will have divided into two, so that the half that attaches itself to the endometrium will become the placenta and the other, inner half of the blastocyst will become your future baby. At the same time, the hundreds of cells that will make up the baby have become specialised so that they will be assigned to develop into particular parts of her body.

Within this part of the blastocyst, there are three different layers of cells known as 'germ layers', and each of these is 'programmed' to create different parts of your baby's body. The ectoderm (outer layer) forms the hair, skin, nails, nipples, tooth enamel, eyes, inner ear, nervous system and the brain. The mesoderm (middle layer) develops into the skeleton, cartilage and muscles along with the arteries, veins and heart and the reproductive organs. The endoderm (inner layer) will become the digestive and respiratory system and includes the formation of the stomach, bowel, liver, urinary tract, bladder and the lungs. The process is irreversible, so that once a cell has been allocated a function, it cannot change.

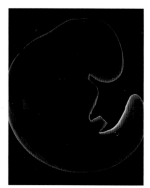

3 weeks

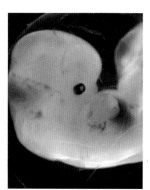

6 weeks

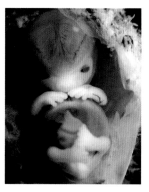

7 weeks

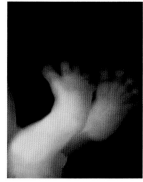

10 weeks

MEASURING YOUR BABY

In the first trimester, babies grow at a common and predictable rate. Measuring their body length can be done as early as seven weeks and is the most reliable method of working out their age. At this stage, babies are measured from the top of the heads to their bottom, known as 'crown to rump'. This is because their legs are often bent, so it's easier to measure every baby in the same way. As they grow, their legs (particularly their thigh bones) will be measured, too, but as a separate figure, so that your midwife or doctor can check that their limbs are developing normally.

Week 5

The embryo only measures around 125 mm ($^1/_{20}$ in) in length from crown to rump, but it already has all the elements in place for the growth of the baby's vital organs.

There is now a distinct head and tail and the row of cells that will become the spinal cord can be seen along the back of the embryo, which still looks remarkably like a tadpole or a prawn. The brain has now begun to form and traces of what will become the eyes and the ears are just beginning to be visible. Cartilage is growing and will eventually turn into the bone that will form your baby's skull and skeleton. The heart is also beginning to form and by the end of this week it will start to circulate blood.

Week 6

The liver and kidneys continue to develop and the neural tube that connects the brain and spinal cord closes over. A digestive system also starts to form as a tube that stretches from the mouth to the rump. In time this will become the stomach, liver, pancreas and bowels, but it will be many months before it functions properly. Tiny buds appear on the body and these will grow to be arms and legs. What will eventually become your baby's ovaries or testes begin to form, too.

Week 7

The embryo is beginning to look less like a comma and more human: the tail has almost disappeared and in the next four weeks the embryo will quadruple in size. The back of the head is still growing more quickly than the front, though, which is why it looks as if it is curled over. The embryo may also begin to move its body and tiny arm and leg buds, but although this can be detected by an ultrasound scan, the embryo is still so tiny (4–5 mm/$^1/_6$ – $^1/_5$ in) that you will be unable to feel any movements yet.

Week 8

Paddle-shaped hands are now visible and the cartilaginous limbs are gradually lengthening. The embryo's facial features are continuing to develop and the eyes already contain some colour pigment. The ear canals deepen and the middle ear, which will be responsible for hearing and balance, develops. Most of your baby's organs have formed at a basic level at least. Her heartbeat is beginning to normalise and her circulatory system is becoming more efficient (tiny blood vessels can be seen under the translucent skin). Her skeleton is slowly beginning to ossify (to harden from cartilage to bone). Tiny facial features can be seen and in the next eight days your baby's eyes and inner ears will go through a crucial stage of development. Floating in amniotic fluid, your baby may begin to move around, but she is still only the size of a peanut and weighs less than a gram (0.3 oz) so you cannot yet feel her.

BE CAREFUL

As all her major organs form, your baby is particularly vulnerable at this point in her development, so you need to take great care to try to avoid potential problems by steering clear of alcohol, drugs, viruses and environmental hazards (see pages 96–7 and 102–3). Take care, but try not to be too anxious; it is rare for congenital foetal abnormalities to develop after the first trimester.

Week 9

The webbed paddles that formed the hands and feet are now separating into fingers and toes. By the end of week 10 the fingers will also have developed touch pads at their tips. The embryo has also developed some basic sensory perceptions and may respond to touch. Although her head is still bent forwards the embryo looks more like a baby now. In the next few days her diaphragm will develop and her intestines will move into the abdominal cavity from the umbilical cord, where they began to form.

Week 10

The embryo is now recognisably human and has officially become a foetus. Her brain has expanded so rapidly that the head is still bigger than the body and her facial features are becoming more recognisable. Her arms and legs have elongated and ankles and wrists have formed.

The heart has divided into four chambers and is beating at twice the rate of yours (around 180 beats per minute). Two atria receive blood from the foetus's rapidly forming circulatory system, while the ventricles pump oxygenated blood back into the system. Valves are forming in the heart, too, which will ensure that the blood is always pumped in one direction. The digestive system is rapidly developing from the simple tube that it consisted of at week 6. In fact it grows so rapidly that as loops in the intestines form, they even protrude through the abdomen. The stomach, spleen and liver are now all in place and will continue to grow. Your baby is now 10,000 times bigger than the egg was when it was first fertilised and her facial features are becoming more recognisable.

Week 11

All the vital organs – the brain, heart, lungs, liver, kidneys and intestines are formed and already beginning to function. The outer ears (pinna) have grown on the lower part of the sides of the head, but will not be fully working yet. Your future baby can

BRAIN DEVELOPMENT

Between week six and ten the neural tube separates into the brain and spinal cord. At the same time, the nerve cells multiply and travel to the brain, where they start to form connections. This is the beginning of the neural network that will transmit messages from the brain to the rest of the body.

As the brain grows, it has to fold in order to fit into the comparatively small skull, so that in cross-section its rippled surface looks rather like a walnut. The cells (neurons) within it will multiply at a rate of 250,000 per minute and the unborn baby's brain will generate twice as many cells as it will need, so many of these will naturally die away by the time the baby is eight months old.

How many neurons survive really depends on the number of them that make functioning connections and this is made possible by axons (long extensions from the cells) that link together rather like an electrical wiring system. Billions of neurons are loosely connected, but if they are unused, they will fail to make further connections and so will die away.

By the 24th week in the uterus, your baby's brainwave patterns are comparable to those of a newborn. In the third trimester, myelin, the protective sheath that coats the nerve fibres in the rest of the body also covers the nerve fibres that enter and leave the brain. The myelin makes the transmission of impulses much smoother, and therefore faster, so your baby is capable of making finer, more precise, movements and is able to acquire new skills.

already open her mouth, swallow and yawn. From now on until the birth, she simply needs to grow. In fact your baby has passed the most critical stage of her development and the risk of a congenital abnormality (a defect that occurs before or at birth, but is not necessarily genetically inherited) or of her being adversely affected by an infection lessens. Now her body will rapidly elongate so that by the end of the week, it will have doubled in length.

COMPARING SIZE

At six weeks the foetus is about 2–4 mm (1/12–1/6 in) long, or a bit smaller than your fingernail. At 12 weeks it is about 61 mm (2½ in) long, or about the size of your little finger.

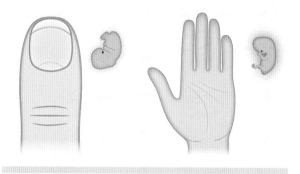

Week 12

The foetus's limbs are slowly ossifying (changing from cartilage to bone). Hair and nails are growing and the genitals are beginning to be recognisable as the pituitary gland starts to manufacture hormones. The digestive system can now process and absorb glucose. The jaw has 32 tiny tooth buds and the foetus can now open her mouth, yawn and hiccup. Just 10 weeks after conception, your baby can smile, frown and even suck her thumb. She looks fully formed and her fingers and toes are no longer webbed but have separated so that she can move them, too. The brain and organs continue to develop. The umbilical cord is circulating blood between the baby and placenta that is both providing her with nourishment and taking away any waste products.

Week 13

This week is considered to be the end of the first trimester and although your baby may look fully formed, the major internal organs are still developing and so she would not yet be able to survive outside the uterus. Her neck has formed so that it can support some movements of the head and her eyes (which are still developing behind closed lids) are moving into position on the front of her face, while her ears may begin to sense some sound. The ears

won't be fully developed until 24 weeks or so, but it is thought that babies can 'hear' sounds through the vibrations they sense in the uterus. The heart rate has begun to slow as it matures and pumps blood with greater efficiency. The liver has begun to release bile and the pancreas is starting to produce insulin.

During the early weeks of pregnancy blood cells were produced in the yolk sac, but by week 12 or 13, they will be manufactured by the foetus's liver until the bone marrow and spleen contribute to this task later in the second trimester. The stomach is now properly connected to the mouth and intestines and the foetus now swallows amniotic fluid, perhaps in preparation for excreting it as urine when her kidneys begin to operate.

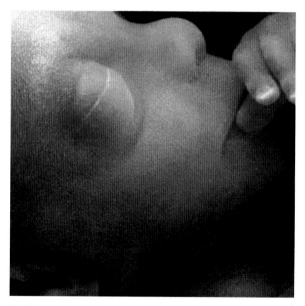

The face at 12 weeks.

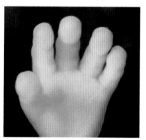

The hand at 12 weeks.

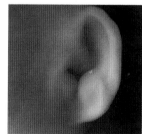

The ear at 12 weeks.

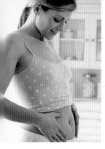

All about your

ANTENATAL CARE

It is vital that you take good care of yourself and your baby and one of the most important things that you can do is to sign up for your antenatal care – as soon as you can.

Why you need antenatal care

The aim of your antenatal care programme is to support a healthy pregnancy that will result in the successful birth of your baby. It's perfectly true that the 21st century is the safest time in human history to have a baby and if you are generally healthy you have a 95 per cent chance of a successful outcome, but don't assume that this means that your medical care can be taken for granted. Studies show that early antenatal care and regular check-ups are strongly linked with the delivery of healthy babies.

Information is power and your antenatal care is designed to provide you with the knowledge and support you need to see you through the next nine months and to parenthood beyond. So take advantage of all the information and help that is on offer.

Assessments & monitoring during your pregnancy

Your general health If you have any underlying health problems, these will be taken into account and your care will be adjusted accordingly.

Your well-being Both your physical and emotional health will be monitored thoughout your pregnancy and you will be encouraged to discuss any issues that might be troubling you.

Your baby's well-being Antenatal tests are scheduled and designed to check the normal development and growth of your baby at all the crucial stages of your pregnancy. If there is anything unusual, further tests

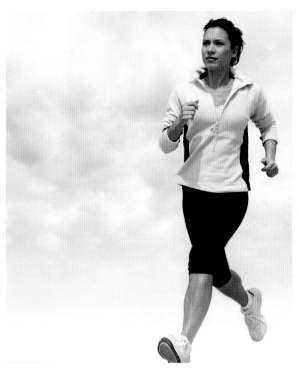

Whatever your general levels of health and fitness, you will need to arrange good antenatal care.

will be offered to confirm the problem and possible options discussed with you.

Any complications Common complaints such as nausea and haemorrhoids are inconvenient, but relatively minor, and your doctor or midwife can give you advice on dealing with them, or you may find alternative remedies helpful (see pages 40–1). In later pregnancy there is the chance of developing

KEEPING APPOINTMENTS

You are legally entitled to take time off work to attend your antenatal appointments. Although you may wish to keep the news of your pregnancy to yourself for a little while longer, you may need to inform your employer once you have had your booking appointment.

'invisible' conditions such as pre-gestational diabetes, but again the examinations and tests in antenatal care are designed to detect and treat them so that they have minimum impact on your baby's development. If you have had egg donation, you will need to tell your doctor as scan results will be different.

Support you can expect to receive during antenatal care

Preparing for parenthood At the early stages of your pregnancy, it may be hard to think beyond the next nine months and it may seem as though the birth is your ultimate goal, but of course that's only the start of your new role as a parent. There's a great deal to learn, but a parenting class is a good place to start and this can be a great way to make new friends for you and your baby. Your antenatal care provider may be able to recommend a good local class to join.

Preparing for birth Your baby's birth might seem a long way off just now, but the day will arrive surprisingly quickly. Your antenatal team will help you to make informed choices about the sort of birth you want (and whether it's at home or in hospital), and will also be there to support you throughout what will undoubtedly be a life-changing experience.

Options for antenatal care

When making decisions about the kind of antenatal care and birth you would prefer, it is helpful to understand more about what is on offer. In the UK, the NHS has both hospital midwives and community midwives. Both types are fully qualified, though the way they perform their jobs is slightly different.

You may not actually look pregnant during the first trimester, but you will be only too aware that there is a lot going on.

Hospital midwives work within a hospital, where they may run antenatal clinics, help women during labour and birth and look after women staying in the antenatal and postnatal wards. They often work closely with teams of doctors and are usually experienced in dealing with interventions such as induction and continuous monitoring.

Community midwives usually give maternity care outside the hospital, although they are also normally attached to a hospital or a doctor's surgery. Antenatal care may take place in local clinics or sometimes in women's homes. They can attend women who are in labour or giving birth at home and they sometimes accompany women to hospital during labour. Community midwives also visit women and their new babies at home post-birth.

Types of antenatal care

Shared care is the most common and popular form of antenatal care programme for both hospital and home births in the UK. If you opt for this your doctor will share your care with the local hospital, so that your regular check-ups take place at your doctor's surgery or health centre and you attend the hospital outpatients' clinic for scans or investigations when necessary.

At 8–12 weeks you will have your 'booking' appointment with your community midwife and some routine tests at the hospital. If no problems arise as a result, you will continue your antenatal care with your doctor and your community midwife.

Community midwife care is most commonly offered to expectant mothers whose pregnancies are

BE PREPARED: ASK QUESTIONS

You might like to compile a list of questions or concerns before your first appointment, so that you don't forget the issues you want to discuss. Your doctor or midwife is there to help and if you don't understand something, ask. Your partner might want to come along and ask questions, too.

ASK YOUR MIDWIFE

What are my antenatal care options?

Are my pregnancy symptoms normal?

Which natural or complementary remedies can I use during my pregnancy?

Which conventional medications and analgesics are safe for me to take during pregnancy?

Does my pregnancy carry any high-risk factors?

If I do have a pre-existing condition, how will it affect my pregnancy?

Where can I give birth?

What should I do if I experience some spotting?

likely to be free of complications. The birth can take place at home or in hospital and the same midwife (or team) will carry out the postnatal checks, too. If any complications do arise, the plan can be changed and the midwife will refer you on to a consultant, so that you can have the remainder of your check-ups at a hospital.

Hospital-based consultant care will probably be advised if you have an existing medical condition or health problems, have had a previous pregnancy or delivery with difficulties or there are other factors that might make your pregnancy 'high risk'. This means that you will have all your antenatal care and delivery at a local hospital. Your doctor or community midwife will arrange for you to be cared for by a consultant obstetrician and to have your regular check-ups carried out at the hospital.

Private care is also available and you can be attended by a consultant obstetrician at a private hospital or by a private midwifery team, who will carry out all antenatal checks in your home. An independent midwife will also be with you during the labour and delivery – whether this takes place at home or in hospital – and then carry out the early days of postnatal care, too.

Home or hospital birth?

If you opt for a home birth (see page 199) through the NHS you will probably be looked after by a small team of community midwives. Although you will be assigned a named midwife from the team who will give you your antenatal care throughout your pregnancy, you will also meet the other team members. Your antenatal appointments will usually take place at your local clinic or perhaps at home. When labour begins, you can contact your midwife and she will care for you until your baby is born. Your midwife or one of the other team will also visit you and your baby regularly at home for up to 10 days after the birth. However, if there are problems these visits may be extended up to 28 days.

If you book a hospital birth (see pages 198–9), then your care may be carried out by hospital or community midwives. If you would like to have your baby at a particular hospital, you should ask who would be responsible for your care. You may also be able to choose to give birth at an NHS birthing centre, (see page 199) where you will have the care of community midwives, who will provide a certain continuity of care. Birthing centres do not have doctors or specialists on site, however, so some forms of pain relief, such as epidurals, are not available. Bear in mind, too, that if problems do arise you may need to be transferred to the nearest hospital.

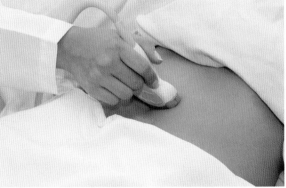

Routine scans will be offered as part of your continuing antenatal care package.

APPOINTMENTS – WHAT TO EXPECT

During your pregnancy you can expect to have between 7 and 10 routine appointments, as well as tests and scans.

6–8 weeks
Routine appointment with your doctor or midwife – your 'first contact' – when you think you are pregnant

10 weeks
Routine appointment with your doctor or midwife – your 'booking' appointment (see pages 70–1)

10–12 weeks
Blood tests (see page 71)

10–14 weeks
Routine scan – to confirm your baby's due date and to detect twins or multiple pregnancies

11–16 weeks
Screening tests – a 'triple' or 'quadruple' blood test to check for the presence of Down's syndrome, spina bifida or Edward's syndrome

A nuchal translucency test (NT) (see page 74) may also be offered if your pregnancy carries some risk factors (see pages 72–3) along with further blood tests

16 weeks
Routine scan – to check the 'lie', or position, of the placenta and your baby's development

18–20 weeks
Routine check-up with doctor or midwife

25, 28, 31, 34, 36, 38, 40 weeks
Routine check-ups with doctor or midwife

41 weeks
Further checks if your baby is overdue

Diagnostic tests
If the results of your screening tests suggest a high risk of chromosomal abnormalities (e.g. Down's syndrome) you will probably be offered further tests (see pages 154–5).

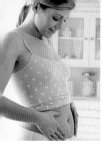

all about your

BOOKING APPOINTMENT

Once you have had your 'first contact' meeting with your midwife, you will have your 'booking' appointment, at which you will discuss your medical history and your antenatal care and birth options. You may also have some routine tests to establish that all is well.

These initial appointments allow your midwife to get a clear vision of your general health and medical history. She will use this information, along with your preferences, to tailor your antenatal care. She will also outline tests and procedures.

What you can do to prepare

- Ask your parents about your own childhood illnesses and immunisations.
- Note the first day of your last menstrual period so that your midwife can calculate your expected delivery date (EDD) (see page 31).
- Check your partner's blood type. If he is Rhesus-positive and you are Rhesus-negative your body could build up antibodies against your baby. You can have an anti-D injection to prevent this.
- You will also be asked about your lifestyle, so be honest about how much and how often you drink or smoke. Both could affect your baby's health and your midwife or doctor can help you stop.
- Note medication or supplements and their dosages.

Be prepared to discuss

- Your health and medical history – including your and your partner's families. Are there genetic conditions? Existing health problems?
- Your mental health in the past month – if you have felt down or depressed.
- Your ethnic background – some conditions such as

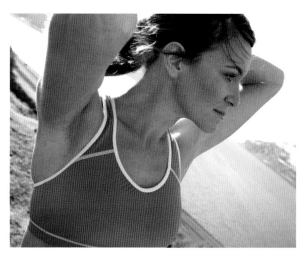

Your health is important now – eat a good, nutritious diet, get lots of good-quality sleep and take plenty of exercise.

thalassaemia or sickle-cell disease are more common among particular ethnic groups.
- Your obstetric health – any previous births, miscarriages or terminations? This helps your midwife determine care and delivery options.
- Your sexual partners – this is to check whether you are carrying a sexually transmitted disease that could be passed on to your baby.
- Your lifestyle – do you exercise? How much do you drink/smoke? Do you/have you taken drugs?
- Your job – do you work with chemicals or X-rays? Are there any other risks or potential hazards?
- Your preferences for your baby's birth.

Routine tests

You will probably have a few routine tests that will include giving a blood sample, being weighed, having your blood pressure taken and possibly producing a urine sample.

Weight Your midwife will take a baseline height and weight measurement so that she can work out your body mass index (BMI) (see page 91). This is to help identify certain risk factors and at subsequent appointments your weight will be fully monitored to ensure that you are gaining weight at a healthy rate.

Blood pressure This reading will be recorded as your baseline figure and at every appointment blood pressure will be taken again by way of a comparison. It is perfectly normal for your blood pressure to rise and fall throughout pregnancy, but your midwife will be looking for significant or dramatic changes.

Blood tests You will be asked to provide a blood sample so that it can be tested for a number of factors (some tests are optional and you can talk to your doctor or midwife about whether they might or might not be relevant to you):

• A full blood count test to check for signs of anaemia, which may be caused by low levels of iron, folic acid or vitamin B_{12}. If you are anaemic you'll be offered advice on eating iron-rich foods (see page 85) and you may need to take an iron supplement.

• A test to find out what blood group you are (A, B, O or AB) and to determine whether you are Rhesus-positive or Rhesus-negative (see page 33).

• Immunity to rubella, since infection in pregnancy can cause serious complications for the baby (see page 77). If you are not immune, you cannot be safely vaccinated until you have given birth.

• Your blood sample will also be tested for hepatitis B, a viral liver disease that can be passed to the baby during pregnancy and birth.

• You will also be offered a test for human immunodeficiency virus (HIV). If you do have HIV you can reduce the possibility of passing it on to your baby by taking antiviral agents, planning the method of delivery and not breastfeeding once the baby has been born.

• A test will also check whether you have ever suffered from syphilis. If the disease is still active it can cross the placenta and cause serious problems for your baby, so it's very important to address this issue now.

• Sickle cell disease, or thalassaemia, will be tested for, too. These are genetic disorders that affect the ability of red blood cells to carry oxygen around the body and are most common in people of African, Mediterranean and Hispanic origin. If you are found to be carrying it, your partner will also need to be tested and if he is carrying it, too, there is a chance that your baby could develop the disease.

Routine urine tests Your urine will be checked at each appointment for traces of protein that could indicate an infection, or more rarely, kidney disease. If an infection is found it can be treated with antibiotics suitable for use during pregnancy. Your urine will be tested again later on in pregnancy because the presence of protein in the later stages can be sign of pre-eclampsia (see pages 208–9).

DON'T WORRY

If this all sounds rather daunting, try not to worry. Most women sail through these tests without any problem at all and get their results at their next appointment. If there does seem to be a cause for concern, your doctor or midwife will contact you earlier to discuss the results and any necessary treatment.

If all is well, your next antenatal appointment in four weeks' time will be much shorter and involve fewer checks. Make sure that you keep your appointments, though, even if you feel fine. It is important to be seen regularly as it is the best way to check your progress and that of your baby.

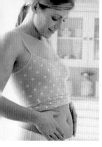

SPECIAL CARE

Your booking appointment may have identified factors that mean you need closer monitoring during your pregnancy. If this is the case, try not to worry and accept the help and advice of your doctor and midwife – it will be the best thing for you and your baby.

If you have an existing medical condition, such as heart disease or diabetes, are aged over 35, or have had a complicated previous pregnancy, you may be offered more screening tests than would otherwise be the case. If you are expecting twins, or more, you'll also be more carefully monitored, to ensure that you and the babies remain healthy.

Older mothers

In the UK one in five babies are now born to women who are aged over 35. If this applies to you, your chances of a trouble-free pregnancy and birth have never been better, thanks to improved health care and medical technology. However, there are some risks associated with older mothers, such as problems with the placenta (see page 209), chromosomal abnormalities (see pages 154–5), gestational diabetes (see opposite) or hypertension (see opposite).

Other complications
Epilepsy

It is especially important that you are closely monitored when you are trying to get pregnant and throughout the course of the pregnancy itself. Some anti-epilepsy drugs can cause abnormalities and so another drug needs to be substituted instead. Pregnancy can also alter the way that your body metabolises the drugs, so you may need to have the dosage adjusted, too. You may need extra folic acid.

Diabetes

Two types of diabetes can affect pregnant women – the pre-existing form (diabetes mellitus) and the pregnancy-induced form (gestational diabetes). If possible, women with diabetes mellitus should try to gain control of their blood-sugar levels before they become pregnant because hyperglycaemia (sugar levels too high) or hypoglycaemia (sugar levels too low) in the early stages of pregnancy can increase the risk of miscarriage and foetal abnormalities. Your medical team can help you to control the condition with careful monitoring, dietary measures and regular adjustments of your insulin dosage.

Gestational diabetes develops in between 1 and 3 per cent of pregnant women. Most of these women can manage the condition with dietary changes, but some will need to take medication. Careful monitoring is important, since although gestational diabetes is not associated with foetal abnormalities, it can cause complications in later pregnancy. Have a vitamin D check as it is very common to be deficient if you are diabetic.

Asthma

Around 3 per cent of pregnant women may have asthma, although careful diagnosis is necessary because most pregnant women develop breathlessness during pregnancy which may be unrelated to bronchial problems. If you have asthma

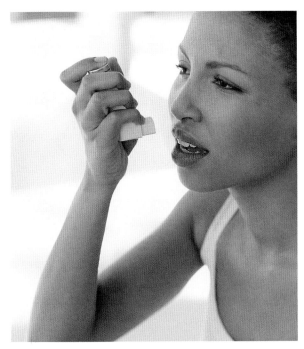

Be sure to inform your doctor and midwife if you suffer from asthma – your medication will need reassessing.

it is important to try to avoid whatever may trigger an attack, such as pollen, smoke, chemicals or dust. Asthma can often actually improve during pregnancy because the mother's body increases its production of cortisone. There is no risk to the foetus from inhaled steroids, but if you take oral steroids there is an increased possibility of developing pre-eclampsia or intra-uterine growth restriction (IUGR) in your baby (see pages 192–3), so you will need to have your medication reassessed.

Inflammatory bowel disease

Crohn's disease (inflammation of the small intestine) and ulcerative colitis (inflammation of the large intestine) cause chronic diarrhoea and abdominal pain. Pregnancy sometimes brings improvement as your body produces an increased amount of natural steroid hormones, but if possible it is best to try to get the condition under control before becoming pregnant. You will need to have your regular medication reassessed and monitored once pregnant.

Heart disease

Maternal heart disease during pregnancy is now rare, but it is important that mothers with this have specialist care. If you had congenital heart disease as a child you will also need to be closely monitored and have your blood pressure controlled and your labour managed – to keep it short.

Essential hypertension

If you already had high blood pressure when you were trying to get pregnant, you should ideally obtain medical help to get it under control. There is a risk of developing pre-eclampsia (see pages 208–9) or kidney damage, and once you are expecting, you may need to have your medication adjusted since some anti-hypertensive drugs are unsuitable to take during pregnancy.

Renal disease

Kidney problems can occasionally develop during pregnancy as a result of the extra filtering that your kidneys have to do for your baby. If you have an existing renal disease you should be aware that pregnancy may exacerbate your problems. You will need to discuss your condition with your doctor or midwife as soon as you get your positive pregnancy result, so that they can coordinate your care with the relevant specialists.

HIV

Screening for the human immunodeficiency virus (HIV) is now routinely offered to all pregnant women. If you are found positive, of course it is not good news, but be reassured that new drugs have greatly improved the life expectancy of patients and they can also significantly reduce the risk of the virus being passed on to your baby. Delivery by Caesarean section and antiretroviral treatment can reduce the risk of transmission to babies from 20 to just 2 per cent. If you already know that you are HIV positive, it is vital that you inform your antenatal carers so that they can offer you the best treatment and advice.

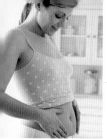

what you need to know about

YOUR SCANS

Your first ultrasound scan usually takes place between 10 and 14 weeks. It will allow your antenatal team to monitor the baby's development and offer you a first glimpse of your baby.

How scanning works

Ultrasound scans do not emit radiation. Instead, they work by sending out high-frequency sound waves that are sent through a pregnant woman's body using a hand-held device called a transducer. The sound waves bounce off the solid tissue of your growing baby and are then converted into images on a computer screen.

What to expect

Ultrasound dating scans usually take place at your local hospital and because this will be your first sighting of your baby, your partner will probably want to be there with you, too. Around an hour before your scan appointment you will be asked to

drink at least one pint of still water. After this, you should avoid emptying your bladder and although you may find this a bit uncomfortable, it is important because the urine acts as a 'window' over your uterus, allowing clearer images of your tiny baby to be visible.

You will be asked to lie down and uncover the lower part of your tummy, so wear it will help if you wear something comfortable and loose-fitting. The sonographer (the hospital ultrasound technician) will then smear a little lubricating gel over your abdomen to make it easier to move the transducer around smoothly. As it slowly moves over your abdomen you will see the image of your uterus and baby on a computer screen beside you.

NUCHAL FOLD TRANSLUCENCY SCAN

If you are an older mother, or carry some other risk factor, you may also be offered a nuchal fold translucency scan (NTS) between 11 and 14 weeks. This is a non-invasive screening test that measures the amount of fluid that is under the skin of the foetus's neck. The measurement gives an indication of the possible level of risk that the foetus has of having Down's syndrome. It is important to realise, though, that this is only an indication and does not give a definitive answer. If the measurements are found to be high or borderline you may be offered further screening and diagnostic tests (see pages 154–5), but it is up to you as to whether you have them or not.

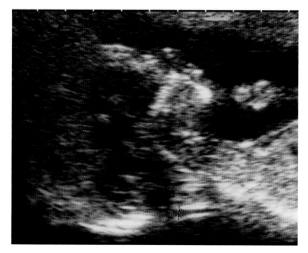

An example of a nuchal fold translucency scan.

What the scan can reveal

The dating scan can be especially useful if you have recently stopped using the contraceptive pill, your periods are irregular or you are simply unsure when you might have become pregnant. As well as pinpointing the duration of your pregnancy to within five to seven days, the scan will be an opportunity to take baseline measurements in order to monitor your baby's growth, but it can also reveal whether you are expecting twins, triplets or more.

More than one?

Twin pregnancies may be detected now, when two or more amniotic sacs may be visible. By 12 weeks the sonographer will examine the thickness of the membranes that separate the two amniotic sacs in the uterus and from that be able to tell whether you are carrying identical (monochorionic) or non-identical (dichorionic) twins. If two thin layers of the sac's inner part (amnion) separate the cavities, the twins will be identical. If a thicker membrane can be seen and it is made up of two layers of amnion (inner layer) and two layers of chorion (outer layer) then non-identical twins will be expected (see page 24).

Vital statistics

There are two key measurements that will be taken at the dating scan. This will be the crown-to-rump length (CRL), which is the length of your baby from the top of his head to his bottom, and the biparietal diameter (BPD). The parietal bones are the bones on the sides of the skull and the sonographer will measure the distance between them. This information, along with the CRL, will be used as the baseline figures, which will then be used for comparison with every subsequent measurement, to monitor your baby's growth. At this stage of your pregnancy, your baby will most often be lying in a curled up 'foetal' position, so it is not easy to measure limbs. By the middle of the second trimester, though, the thigh bone (femur) will also be measured at least twice, to check that your baby is growing at a healthy pace. If

you have had any bleeding or pain you may be offered a scan earlier than 10 weeks, so that your doctor or midwife can check for threatened miscarriage or ectopic pregnancy (see pages 120–1).

WHAT YOU MAY SEE

Your first glimpse of your baby can be an emotional experience and it may be the moment when your pregnancy actually begins to feel 'real'.

If at all possible, try to attend your scan with your partner, or at least with someone who is close to you. It is an experience to be shared and although you will probably be offered a printout of your scan, a still photograph is not quite the same thing as seeing your baby moving around in real time.

If your scan takes place at around 12 weeks, you should be able to see the outline of your baby's head and body. You may also see her tiny nose in profile and be able to see a little row of white dots along her back, which are the gradually hardening bones that will make up her spine. She may even wave her arms, hands and legs and the sonographer will also be looking for your baby's minute heartbeat. It is very unlikely, but if there is a problem (see pages 154–5) you will be informed straight away and this is another good reason to take someone along with you.

DON'T WORRY

Try not to be too concerned if your baby doesn't seem quite as well developed as you had expected. It may be that the estimated delivery date (EDD) that was based on your last menstrual period (LMP) was not quite right. The sonographer may revise your due date as a result of the scan's findings and if there is any cause for concern, such as poor foetal growth (see pages 192–3), your antenatal care will be revised accordingly.

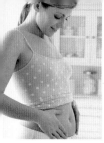

THE PLACENTA

The placenta acts as the vital link between you and your baby. It is actually created by both of you and it is an essential element in a healthy, successful pregnancy.

As soon as the blastocyst attaches itself to the wall of the uterus there is an exchange of chemical signals. It is as if your future baby is communicating with you already. Your body responds by beginning to set up a support system for the embryo. This support system will be the placenta, but it will take a little time to develop, so at this very early stage the embryo is being nourished by the yolk sac (see pages 22–5).

The placenta is an amazing organ. It will begin to support your baby from around week 8 and will be fully formed by around week 12. Until your baby is born, it will act as her lungs (by supplying oxygen)

THE LINK BETWEEN YOU

The placenta is linked to your baby by the umbilical cord, which contains a thick vein that carries oxygenated blood from the placenta to the baby. There are also two arteries that return deoxygenated blood and waste products, such as carbon dioxide, away from the baby and back to the mother for her body to dispose of.

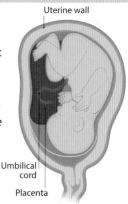

Uterine wall

Umbilical cord

Placenta

THE AMNIOTIC FLUID

Humans evolved from an aquatic environment, so it is interesting to note that babies spend the first nine months of life in 'water'. Amniotic fluid is rather more complex than water and it is vital to your baby's development. If the amniotic sac is ruptured and the fluid is lost early in pregnancy it is rare for the baby to survive. Towards the end of pregnancy, though, the spontaneous rupturing of the sac, known as 'waters breaking' (see page 232), can be one of the signs of the onset of labour.

Amniotic fluid performs several functions in the development of your baby. In early pregnancy, the amount of fluid in the amniotic sac that surrounds the embryo is quite small, but the volume of liquid increases every day.

Amniotic fluid not only shields the baby from impact by acting as a watery cushion and allows her to move around, but it also protects her from infection from the second trimester onwards. In addition it aids the development of her musculoskeletal, respiratory and digestive systems.

In the first trimester, the baby absorbs fluid through her paper-thin skin, but once the kidneys begin to develop, she will swallow it, so that some goes into the lungs and the rest passes through the gut and kidneys, to be excreted. Amniotic fluid also contains flakes of cells from the baby's body and it is these that can be used to check for abnormal chromosomes if you have an amniocentesis test (see page 155).

SUPERFOODS TO FEED THE PLACENTA

A healthy placenta will grow best from a thick, well-nourished uterine lining, but you can also help it by eating foods containing antioxidants, which include:

Asparagus	Cauliflower	Kidney beans
Avocado	Garlic	Plums
Blueberries	Grapes (red)	Prunes
Blackberries	Green peppers	Spinach
Broccoli	Red peppers	Strawberries
Brussels sprouts	Kale	Tomatoes

to her digestive system (by supplying nutrients that can be readily absorbed) and her kidneys (by filtering out and disposing of your baby's waste products). It will also supply the hormones that will stimulate your baby's growth and development. When you think of what it does, you can see why it is important to try to nourish it as best you can.

Tree-like structure

Think of the placenta as a growing tree, with its base forming root-like structures that embed deeply into the womb lining. Like a tree root reaching into the soil, if it is not fed, watered and nurtured it develops a poor root system, unable to draw the nutrients it needs to develop. This early development lays down the path for the healthy outcome of your pregnancy and helps you to avoid complications later on, such as foetal growth restriction and pre-eclampsia (see pages 192–3 and 208), both of which can result from a poorly developed placenta.

If all goes well, during the second trimester your placenta grows faster than your baby and the larger it becomes, the better nourished your baby. As well as providing nourishment, the placenta acts as a barrier, protecting the foetus from harmful substances, but there are some things, known as 'teratogens' that can still cross the placenta (see box right).

TERATOGENS

There are some harmful substances that are capable of crossing the placental barrier:

Drugs Certain medications, sedatives and tranquillisers, analgesics, antidepressant drugs, morphine, opium, marijuana, cocaine, nicotine and alcohol. Check with your doctor if you are taking any kind of medication

Chemicals Heavy metals (such as lead, mercury and arsenic) and environmental pollutants such as PCBs (see page 102)

Radiation Including X-rays, although modern X-rays are carefully targeted, so if they are really necessary doctors can minimise the risk to the unborn baby

Rubella Also known as 'German measles', this virus is especially harmful to the unborn baby and can cause miscarriage, still birth or damage to the baby that may include deafness, brain damage, cataracts or heart defects. Since 1970 there has been a nationwide childhood vaccination programme in the UK, so you should already be protected against it, but if you know that you may not be immune, keep away from anyone who has the virus (especially in the first 16 weeks of your pregnancy)

Toxoplasmosis A parasitic infection found in cat faeces and soil (see page 97). Infection in pregnancy is rare and most people will have acquired some immunity from a previous infection that will have had such mild flu-like symptoms that they will probably have been unaware of the cause. It can cause serious problems in pregnancy, however, such as brain damage to the foetus or miscarriage, so you should avoid contact with cat litter and always wash fruit and vegetables thoroughly (see page 86) and wash your hands carefully after handling soil

Sexually transmitted diseases For most of these, the highest risk of transmission from mother to baby is during delivery and so it is important that your carers are aware of your condition and can take steps to minimise the risk (see page 73). Syphilis can actually cross the placenta and infect the baby in the uterus. If untreated, the effects can be life-threatening to the baby, but a single dose of penicillin can treat the mother and prevent foetal infection

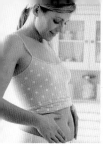

first trimester

NUTRITION

You have the best incentive ever to eat healthily now. By including a wide variety of fresh, wholesome, preferably organic, foods you will be giving your baby the very best start in life. The first trimester focuses on antioxidants; the second trimester focuses on vitamin D, calcium and magnesium and the third on essential fatty acids.

The aim prior to pregnancy and during the first trimester is on growing a healthy placenta and making sure you are getting key nutrients for your baby's developing organs. The better the

THE NUTRITION TRIANGLE

Think of your dietary requirements as a triangle: carbs form the largest part of your diet at the bottom, while oils, fats and sugars form the smallest part at the top.

Oils, fats and sugars Less than 30 per cent of daily intake

Proteins Two to three portions per day. One portion = 85 g (3 oz) meat, 115 g (4 oz) fish, or 140 g (5 oz) cooked lentils

Dairy products Three portions a day. One portion = 200 ml (½ pint) of milk, 40 g (1½ oz) cheese or 140 g (5 oz) yogurt

Fruit and vegetables At least five portions a day. One portion = one piece of fruit such as an apple, 3 tbs of cooked vegetables, or one glass of fresh fruit juice

Complex carbohydrates Four to six portions a day. One portion = two slices of wholemeal bread, 140 g (5 oz) potatoes, 4 tbs cooked rice or 6 tbs cooked pasta

placenta, the better the exchange of nutrients and oxygen. In the early weeks it can take a while to get used to your body's growing demands for nutrition, and you might assume that you need a significantly higher calorie intake. In fact, the additional amount you need is almost zero in the first trimester, around 200 extra calories per day in the second, rising to 400 extra calories a day in the third. Your body's use of calories becomes more efficient in pregnancy, in fact, so calorie-counting is not helpful. Your appetite is the best guide to how much food you need. Eat little and often: five or six small nutritious meals a day rather than one or two large ones.

Getting a balanced diet

A healthy, balanced diet is easy to achieve. If you make up your meals from a range of whole, fresh foods that include plenty of vegetables and fruits, wholegrains and some good proteins and fats they will contain a good mix of nutrients. Use the nutrition triangle (left) to select from the five food groups. Carbohydrates, in the bottom row, should make up the largest part of your diet (around six servings per day), closely followed by fruit and vegetables (five or more), then dairy products (two to four), proteins (two to three) and finally, oils, fats and sugars as the smallest proportion. You don't have

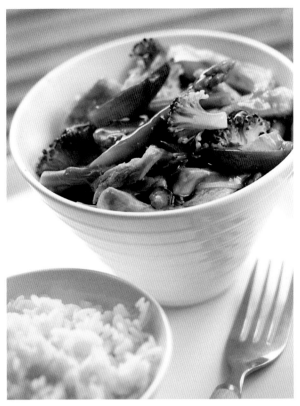

Stir-frying vegetables is a great way to cook them quickly, in order to conserve as many of the food's nutrients as possible.

HOW TO NET MORE NUTRIENTS

Fresh vegetables and some fruits lose their nutritional value quickly, so shop for these more frequently and eat them as soon as you can

Eat fruit when it is at the peak of its ripeness, slightly soft, because it will be at its most delicious and the vitamin and mineral content will be at its peak

Fruit and vegetables lose nutrients where they are cut, so try to eat fruit in larger pieces or whole, and cook vegetables such as broccoli florets with just the ends trimmed

Try steaming vegetables rather than boiling them, because nutrients leach out into the cooking liquid. If you do opt to boil vegetables, try to use a little less water than you are used to, cook them as quickly as possible and use the cooking liquid in gravies, sauces and soups

Many vegetables store a high proportion of their nutrients just under the skin, so try to scrub root vegetables such as carrots and parsnips and steam potatoes with their skins on, or bake them

If you cannot get fresh fruit and veg, opt for frozen ones over the tinned variety as they retain more of their nutrients

to measure out exact proportions, just try to create a balance over the day. If you do this, your diet will be well balanced through the week. By selecting fresh wholefoods and avoiding processed ones that fill you with 'empty' calories, you will find that your body functions more smoothly and you are far less likely to feel nauseous or shakily hungry between meals.

Carbohydrates

A craving for carbohydrates is common in pregnancy; they are converted into the glucose that powers your pregnancy and helps your baby to grow. There are two kinds of carbohydrate: 'complex' and 'simple'. Complex carbs tend to come directly from natural sources, so if you eat unrefined foods such as wholemeal bread or brown rice, it will take longer for your digestive system to process it and, therefore, the energy is released into your bloodstream slowly

– exactly what you and your baby need. Simple carbs have generally been produced through refining processes and so a good deal of the 'breaking down' has taken place before they reach your table. This means that food such as white bread is converted to glucose far more quickly and so produces a 'spike' of energy, but it is a short-lived type of fuel. Don't feel that you have to stop eating your favourite baguettes – just add more wholegrains to your overall diet and make sure that if you eat bread twice a day, one of those occasions includes the wholegrain type.

Vegetables & fruit

Aim for a rainbow of colours and you will be getting a variety of nutrients. Not only do fruit and vegetables provide you with essential vitamins and minerals, but they contain water and fibre, which your body needs to digest everything efficiently.

VEGETARIAN & VEGAN DIETS

Although a varied vegetarian diet can be very healthy, when you are pregnant you need to make sure that you are getting enough protein, iron, calcium and vitamins B_{12} and D. Some of the amino acids that make up proteins are more easily found in animal-derived proteins, so if you do not eat eggs or dairy you need to eat a more complex combination of plant-based proteins. Try eating more soya-based foods and legumes as well as extra portions of nuts and seeds. For vitamin B_{12}, try incorporating yeast extract and fortified cereals into your daily intake. To get enough iron, eat extra dried fruits and combine with a drink of fruit juice so that the vitamin C helps your body maximise the absorption of iron. Consult your doctor or midwife to see whether you might need supplements.

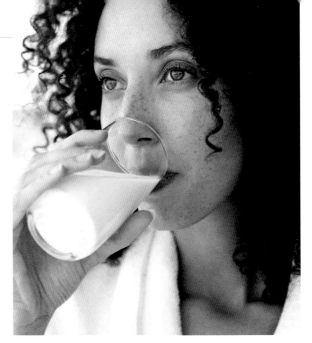

Milk is an excellent food choice during pregnancy – opt for semi-skimmed or skimmed types over full fat.

Dairy products

Milk, cheese and yogurt are packed with calcium, which is vital for the development of your baby's bones and teeth (see pages 136–7). Reduced fat or semi-skimmed versions retain all the nutrients you need, but some low-fat yogurts, for example, are simply bulked up with starches and artificial ingredients. Make sure the dairy products you eat or drink are pasteurised and take care because some cheeses are unsuitable during pregnancy because of the risk of food poisoning (see pages 86–7).

Proteins

Proteins are the building blocks for a healthy pregnancy. They help your baby's tissue and organs to grow, they repair and renew cells and transport hormones. They also make antibodies to fight infection. If you take in too little protein, this can easily affect your baby's development. Vegans and vegetarians need to balance their foods carefully to achieve the right mix of proteins (see above).

Meat is an excellent source of protein, but there are other, equally good, sources, such as fish, lentils and dairy products and you can improve the quality of your protein by varying its sources.

Oils & fats

Fats are essential for every cell and cell membrane in the body, and especially for brain development (see third trimester, page 185). There are three kinds of fats: saturated, monounsaturated and polyunsaturated. Don't fall into the trap of thinking that all fats are 'bad' – you and your baby particularly need the 'good' fats in polyunsaturated fats and oils. This group includes essential fatty acids (EFAs – see

RECOMMENDED DAILY PORTIONS

Ensure that your daily food intake is made up of the following portions:

Five or more portions of vegetables, salad and fruit (a variety of green, yellow, orange, purple and red)

Four to six portions of complex carbohydrates such as wholemeal bread

Two to three portions of protein such as fish, red meat, chicken or pulses

Two to four portions of dairy products (semi-skimmed milk)

One to two servings of iron-rich foods such as fortified cereals and eggs

MEAL IDEAS FOR THE FIRST TRIMESTER

Choose from the following (organic options if possible):

Breakfast

Porridge made with semi-skimmed milk, sweetened with a little honey

Fortified cereal with semi-skimmed milk, topped with fruit

Home-made muesli with oats, wheatgerm, nuts, dried fruit

Wholemeal toast with butter, cheese and yeast extract spread

Live, organic natural yogurt with fruit purée, or sliced or crushed fresh fruits

Scrambled egg on wholemeal toast

Lunch

Wholemeal bread or pitta sandwich filled with salad and roast chicken or tuna

Baked potato with cottage cheese and a mixed salad

Tomato and chickpea soup with wholemeal bread

Mushroom omelette with a salad of lettuce, raw spinach, tomato, cucumber and raw peppers, sprinkled with sunflower seeds and pine nuts

Grilled, steamed or roasted salmon steak with steamed potatoes (with the skins on) and salad

Supper

Roasted parsnips, butternut squash and sweet potatoes served with grilled or baked fish

Aubergines, peppers, courgettes and tomatoes, roasted in a little olive oil and served with brown rice or pasta

Lentil, chickpea, kidney bean and spinach curry served with brown rice, natural yogurt and steamed green beans

Stir-fried vegetables with ginger, pork, chicken, beef or lamb

Grilled chicken, courgette slices and peppers with rice, pasta or steamed potatoes

White fish steamed with ginger and served with egg fried rice and steamed broccoli, green beans or spinach

Desserts

Baked apples stuffed with cinnamon and dried fruits

Baked peaches sprinkled with crumbled amaretto biscuits

Panna cotta made with skimmed milk, served with fruit coulis

Yogurt with crushed fresh fruit, sprinkled with sliced almonds

Thin crêpes served with orange sauce

Fruit crumble made with unrefined sugar, a mix of wholemeal and white flour, and oats

---

page 43). Eating fats is also important for the absorption of fat-soluble vitamins A, D, E and K and all the immune-boosting carotenes in vegetables. Modern food processing often uses artificially modified fats, known as hydrogenated and trans fats, which can increase the risk of coronary heart disease. These types of fats are often present in processed breads, pastries, biscuits, crisps and margarines. Opt for fats or oils that are high in mono- or polyunsaturated fatty acids. These tend to come from plant and fish sources and as a general rule are liquid at room temperature. Saturated fats are usually derived from animal sources and are solid at room temperature. Small amounts of these, along with natural sugars, are not harmful.

DIETARY DO'S & DON'TS

Do eat organic foods – if you are able to choose

Do eat protein and carbohydrates together

Do eat snacks – don't leave long gaps between meals

Don't skip breakfast

Don't be tempted to have fizzy drinks

Don't eat refined carbohydrates

Don't eat sugar unintentionally. Read the food labels: there is a lot more sugar in many products than you might expect

Don't take sweeteners in hot drinks

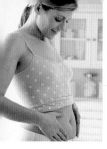

ESSENTIAL NUTRIENTS

The old saying 'eating for two' is commonly heard, though we are now aware that eating enough for two is not a good idea. However, it is worth bearing in mind that the quality of your nutrition is important – not just for your own health, but for your baby's, too.

Your body can manufacture a few vitamins, but it relies on the food you eat to provide the nutrients that you and your baby need.

Vital vitamins

There are 13 known vitamins and each one plays an important part in the health of you and your baby. Your body can store the fat-soluble vitamins such as A, D and E, but it cannot store the water-soluble variety, which are the B vitamins and vitamin C, so you need to consume them on a regular basis.

Vitamin A

Vitamin A is naturally found in two forms: retinol (which derive from animal products) and betacarotene (which the body converts from plant sources). Vitamin A is essential for the development of your baby's cells, circulatory system, heart and nervous system.

In the last trimester, especially, your baby needs an adequate supply, but take care not to consume too much of the animal form (retinol), which has been associated with birth defects. This is why pregnant women are strongly advised to avoid eating liver and liver pâté.

A normal diet should provide you with plenty of vitamin A, but if you are taking antenatal multi-vitamin supplement check that the vitamin A is derived from betacarotene rather than retinol.

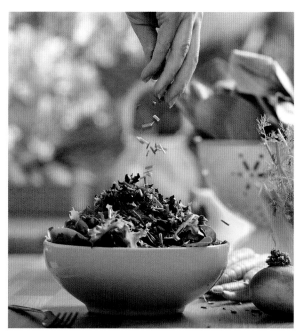

Green, leafy vegetables are a great source of vitamins and minerals including: vitamins A, B₂ and C, folic acid, calcium and magnesium.

B vitamins

B vitamins help your body to convert food into energy and are important in early pregnancy because they play a part in the formation of new cells. Other benefits are: the development of your baby's nervous system and brain function; the maintenance of healthy skin, hair and nails, and the production of red blood cells and antibodies to help fight infection.

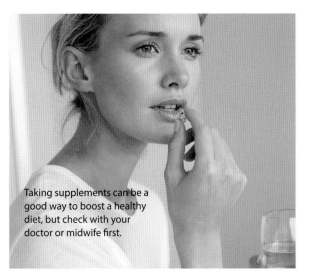

Taking supplements can be a good way to boost a healthy diet, but check with your doctor or midwife first.

SHOULD YOU TAKE SUPPLEMENTS?

Many women who have been eating healthily prior to becoming pregnant are often surprised that they don't eat well in the early part of pregnancy due to sickness, tiredness or cravings. If this is the case a multivitamin and mineral supplement designed for pregnancy might be the answer. Ask your doctor or midwife whether you need one. Remember that a good supply of vitamins and minerals is only part of a healthy diet, and that your body also needs essential fatty acids, protein, carbohydrates and fibre to function properly (see pages 78–81).

Vitamin C

Vitamin C is especially important in pregnancy because it helps to manufacture new tissue. Vitamin C also plays a vital role in helping your body to absorb iron, so you can maximise your iron intake by drinking fresh fruit juice with an iron-rich meal.

Vitamin D

Vitamin D is essential for the absorption of calcium, for you and your baby's bones and teeth. Your skin can synthesise vitamin D from sunlight (see page 137), but levels vary, so check your supplement.

Vitamin E

Vitamin E is an important antioxidant that helps to protect against cell damage and may help to prevent pre-eclampsia (see pages 208–9).

Folic acid

Folic acid belongs to the family of B vitamins and protects against neural tube defects such as spina bifida. It is vital to take a supplement in the first trimester and although it is found in wholemeal bread and fortified cereals, it is easier to absorb the synthetic version. It is recommended that women take a supplement before conception and throughout pregnancy.

Essential minerals

Your body has to obtain the minerals it needs from the foods you eat and some, such as calcium, iron and zinc, are vital during pregnancy (see page 85).

Calcium

Calcium is not only essential for strong bones and teeth, but also for blood clotting, muscle contraction and the smooth transmission of nerve signals. It is also thought to prevent high blood pressure and is therefore implicated in the prevention of pre-eclampsia. Your unborn baby will receive adequate supplies of calcium – deficiencies in your diet will be compensated for by being drawn from stores in your body, but this means that calcium levels in your bones and teeth can diminish, so you need to boost your intake (particularly if you are under 25, because your bones are not yet mature). Drink three 225 ml (8 fl oz) glasses of cow's milk per day to achieve 100 per cent of your RDA.

Iron

Iron is in greater demand during pregnancy because your blood volume may actually double. It is essential for the formation of new cells and haemoglobin, which is the substance in red blood cells that carries oxygen around your body and to your growing baby.

ALL ABOUT VITAMINS & MINERALS

This chart sets out a choice of foods, to give you all the vitamins and minerals you need in the first trimester of pregnancy. To ensure that you are receiving a full range of nutrients, choose a variety of different-coloured fruit and vegetables and make sure that your daily diet is always as varied as possible. Choose organic foods if possible.

Vitamin	Best sources	Benefits
Vitamin A (retinol/betacarotene)	Yellow, orange and red fruit and vegetables (apricots, mangoes, melons, peaches, carrots and peppers), dark-green vegetables, egg yolk, dairy produce, oily fish such as mackerel	Important for the bones, eyes, skin and hair. Helps to fight infections and is full of antioxidants. * Take care – it can be toxic in excess
B1 (thiamin)	Wholemeal bread, fortified breakfast cereals, eggs, milk, dried peas and beans, swede, turnips, carrots, pork, bacon and yeast extract	Works with other B vitamins to help break down and release the energy from food. Keeps muscles and nerves healthy
B2 (riboflavin)	Wholemeal bread and cereals, milk, cheese, egg yolk and green leafy vegetables	Keeps skin, eyes and nerves healthy. Produces red blood cells
B3 (niacin)	Wholemeal bread, fortified breakfast cereals, dried peas and beans, nuts, fish and lean meats	Helps to extract energy from food, keeps the digestive and nervous systems healthy
B6 (pyridoxine)	Fish, chicken, pork, eggs, wholemeal bread and fortified breakfast cereals	Helps the body to use and store energy from the carbohydrates and protein in food. Aids the production of haemoglobin (to carry oxygen around the body)
B12 (cobalamin)	Oily fish, lean meat, milk, eggs and cheese	The production of red blood cells, releasing energy from food, processing folic acid and maintaining a healthy nervous system
Folic acid/folate	Wholemeal bread, fortified breakfast cereals, peas, chickpeas, green vegetables such as broccoli, green beans, kale, spinach, bananas, orange juice and berries	Helps to prevent neural tube defects in the foetus, promotes red blood cell formation and helps the body to break down protein
C (ascorbic acid)	Citrus fruit and juices, kiwi fruit, blackcurrants, cranberries, strawberries, papaya, tomatoes, potatoes (especially cooked in their skins), sweet peppers, green vegetables, cauliflower	Promotes the growth and repair of tissue (including skin, bones and teeth), essential for the absorption of iron. Also full of antioxidants
D (calciferol)	Eggs, butter, polyunsaturated margarine, cheese, oily fish such as salmon, mackerel, sardines and herring. Sunshine	Aids absorption of calcium and increases the deposition of essential minerals in bone. If you have limited exposure to sunshine, or have a BMI of over 30 (see page 91) you should take a supplement
E	Nuts such as hazelnuts, pine nuts and almonds, sunflower seeds, avocado, eggs, vegetable oils, green vegetables such as broccoli, kale and spinach	Important for the maintenance of healthy nerves, skin, muscles, red blood and heart. A useful antioxidant, it also protects against free radicals

ALL ABOUT VITAMINS & MINERALS (continued)

Mineral	Best sources	Benefits
Iron	Red meat, tinned fish such as sardines and tuna, eggs, apricots, raisins and prunes, sesame seeds, fortified cereals (liver and kidney are rich in iron, but should be avoided in pregnancy)	Vital for the production of haemoglobin in red blood cells in you and your baby. Builds and maintains muscles
Calcium	Dairy products, small bony fish such as sardines, eggs, dried fruits such as apricots and figs, nuts, fortified breakfast cereals, tofu and other soya products, leafy green vegetables such as kale and broccoli	Vital for strong bones, teeth and muscles in you and your baby. Also helps with the transmission of nerve impulses
Zinc	Seafood (but take care in pregnancy, see page 87), beef, nuts, bananas, wholegrain foods, sweetcorn	Needed for growth and energy, helps wounds to heal, supports the immune system
Magnesium	Green, leafy vegetables such as spinach and kale, nuts, wholemeal bread, fish, meat and dairy products	Contributes to converting food into energy, works with calcium to help with muscle contraction and blood clotting, and helps regulate blood pressure. It assists keeping calcium in tooth enamel, supports the immune system.
Selenium	Brazil nuts, wholemeal bread, fish, meat, eggs	Plays an important role in the function of the immune system and helps prevent damage to cells and tissue.

Iron is found in both animal and plant sources. Red meat, fish and poultry contain haem iron, which is easier for the body to absorb than non-haem iron (from vegetables, fruit, grains, pasta, nuts, eggs and fortified cereals). Vegetarians and vegans should balance their diet carefully to extract enough iron from their food (see page 80).

Zinc

Zinc is vital for tissue growth and the repair. It is also vital for the immune system and the processing of fat, protein and carbohydrates. Get your zinc from food, but if you are taking an iron supplement it may interfere with the body's absorption of it, so perhaps eat more zinc-rich foods (see above).

Magnesium & selenium

Magnesium and selenium are also important in pregnancy. Magnesium (which we are often low in) works with calcium to help with muscle contraction and blood clotting, as well as regulating blood pressure and the functioning of the lungs. It also helps the body to make use of glucose for energy and absorb protein and fat. It helps to fix calcium in tooth enamel to prevent decay and supports the normal functioning of the immune system. Selenium is a trace element that is also important for the immune system and helps to prevent damage to cells and tissue. Take care, however, with both these trace elements.

CHOOSE A VARIED DIET

Be sure to eat as wide a range of foods as you can and don't always select your 'favourites'. When you are shopping, buy items and produce you haven't tried before to add to your repertoire. That way you will be certain of eating a good basic healthy diet, which will provide you and your growing baby with all the essential nutrients.

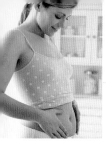

FOOD & DRINK CONCERNS

Good food hygiene is always important, but when you are pregnant you are more vulnerable to infections, so you need to choose and prepare all your food and drinks with extra care.

If you follow some simple rules it is unlikely that you'll suffer any episodes of food poisoning, but the risk from some bacteria, such as listeria, is potentially so dangerous that now may be a good time to reassess your food prep and hygiene habits.

- Food safety begins with selection and buying. Buy from reputable retailers and reject all food that has damaged packaging (including dented tins).
- Check sell- and use-by dates and select foods with the longest shelf life. Choose non-perishable goods first and refrigerated items last, so that they are out of the refrigerator for as short a time as possible.
- Unpack and put away refrigerated and frozen foods immediately after you return from shopping.
- Keep raw and cooked foods separately. Raw meat, poultry and fish should be covered and stored on the bottom shelf of the refrigerator to prevent raw juices from dripping on to other foods.
- If you save leftovers, cover them as soon as they are cool and place them on the upper shelf of the refrigerator or wrap them in a freezer bag or freezer-proof container before freezing.
- When defrosting food, put it in the refrigerator. Never re-freeze anything that has already defrosted.
- Before preparing food, wash your hands thoroughly and then wash utensils, boards and work surfaces with hot, soapy water before you begin cooking.
- Always use separate chopping boards to prepare meat, poultry and fish.

GOING ORGANIC

Food, especially during pregnancy, should be as free of pesticides and additives as possible, so try to buy some organic foods. Pesticides can contain 'gender-bending' or hormone-disrupting chemicals – their composition being similar to human oestrogen. These chemicals accumulate in fatty tissue, so the fattier the food is (e.g. butter, cheese, fatty meats), the more important to buy organic. In addition, certain foods contain more pesticide residues than others and buying organic enables you to avoid ingesting them. The 'top ten' list of foods to be concerned about are: flour, potatoes, bread, apples, pears, grapes, strawberries, green beans, tomatoes and cucumbers.

Another reason to opt for organic is that research suggests that organic foods may contain more nutrients, probably due to farming methods. However, you will need to weigh up the issues of cost, whether the food is locally grown and its seasonality. Your best bet is to try buying organic when purchasing animal products, wholegrain products and vegetables grown in the ground.

- Wash all fruit and vegetables thoroughly under cold, running water and take care to remove traces of soil. Top and tail, and peel root vegetables such as carrots and parsnips for the same reason. Wash your hands after picking fruit and vegetables, too.
- Cook all dishes containing meat, poultry, fish, game and egg thoroughly.

FOOD TO TAKE CARE OVER

Avoid unpasteurised milk, cream and cheese, mould-ripened or soft cheese such as Camembert, Brie and chèvre as well as 'blue' cheese such as Stilton and Gorgonzola as they can contain listeria bacteria, which can lead to miscarriage, still birth or severe illness in the newborn baby

Don't eat sheep and goat's milk or any food products made from them, such as cheeses and yogurts, because of the risk of harmful bacteria, including listeria

Beware of eating raw or partially cooked eggs as there is a risk of salmonella, so avoid mousses, soft-boiled eggs, mayonnaise and hollandaise sauce

Steer clear of pâtés made from meat, fish, seafood and even vegetables because of the risk of listeria

Avoid liver, liver sausage and liver pâté as they contain high amounts of vitamin A, which has been found to be linked to birth defects, though you would have to eat an awful lot

Don't eat raw meat, such as steak tartare or carpaccio, and undercooked meat, poultry or game. Ensure that meat is thoroughly cooked so that there is no trace of blood/pink juices. There is a risk of salmonella bacteria, e-coli and toxoplasma gondii, which can cause toxoplasmosis

Avoid raw or undercooked fish or shellfish such as oysters, mussels or scallops because of the risk of salmonella bacteria and e-coli – among others

Don't eat too much oily fish such as mackerel, salmon, pilchards, sardines and trout. Avoid swordfish, marlin and shark and limit the amount of tuna you eat to no more than one tuna steak a week (about 170 g/6 oz raw each) or two tins of tuna a week (about 140 g/5 oz when drained). These types of fish can contain high levels of mercury, which can cross the placenta and harm your baby's developing nervous system

It is also best to avoid ready-to-eat salads in bags as there is a risk of listeria. Always wash raw salad leaves, vegetables or fruit thoroughly under cold, running water

Take care with ready-prepared cooked foods that have been chilled for reheating as they can carry listeria. Make sure that they have been cooked through according to the manufacturer's instructions and are piping hot

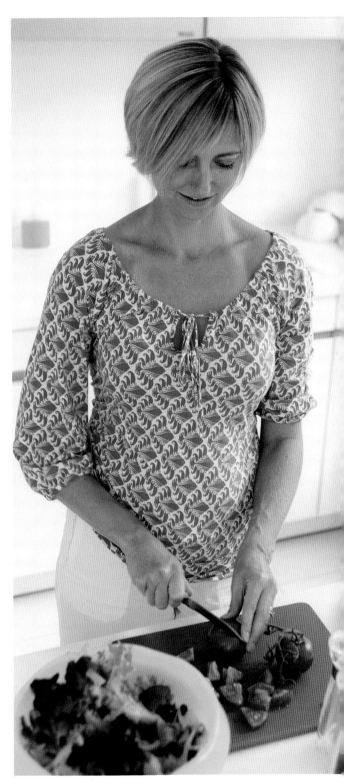

Use separate chopping boards for different types of food.

FOOD ADDITIVES TO AVOID

It is best to steer clear of any processed foods that contain additives. If you opt for fresh produce that you prepare and cook yourself, you can be pretty sure about what you are eating, but there may be occasions when you just fancy having a ready-meal, a take-away or a bag of crisps. But among these items you can still make good, informed choices. If you know what some of those mysterious 'E-numbers' are you can try to avoid them.

Aspartame (E951) One of the most common artificial sweeteners in fizzy drinks and ready-made desserts, it has been linked to birth defects in rodents and is suspected of causing damage to the foetal brain as it crosses the placenta

Saccharine (E954) Another widely used sweetener, this has been found to cause DNA damage and congenital abnormalities in animals

Sodium benzoate (E211) Used in baked goods such as cakes, ice lollies and soft drinks, this preservative has been linked to foetal abnormalities

Monosodium glutamate (E621) A flavour 'enhancer' that is often added to savoury foods. Check that your local take-away does not use it (or ask them to leave it out of your order). There is evidence that it causes DNA damage and abnormalities in animals

Sulphur dioxide (E220) This preservative is used in potato products (such as potato snacks – though not in ordinary crisps), and can be found in dried fruit as well as soft drinks. It is linked to foetal abnormalities and DNA damage in animals

Quinoline yellow (E104) and sunset yellow (E110) These are artificial food colourings that have both been linked to DNA damage in animals and are commonly used in ice cream, sweets, desserts and drinks

Note: You may notice that adverse effects are recorded in animals but not in humans. This is because it is illegal to carry out experiments on pregnant women and unborn babies, so it is impossible to know for sure what the effects might be on humans. However, if there are serious problems reported in animals, it seems wise for humans to avoid eating such things.

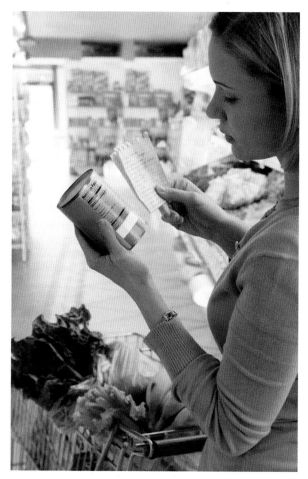

When you are shopping for food, check the labels carefully for useful information about ingredients and E-numbers.

What about drinks?

Keeping hydrated is important as it helps your kidneys filter everything else that goes into your body and stops muscle fatigue. Aim to drink at least 1 litre (2 pt) of fresh water every day, adding ice and a slice of lemon to perk it up, or a natural cordial such as elderflower or ginger.

Caffeine-containing drinks

Coffee, tea and soft drinks such as all the different types of cola contain caffeine, which in large quantities has been found to cause problems in pregnancy and an increased risk of miscarriage. So they need to be treated with caution – check the

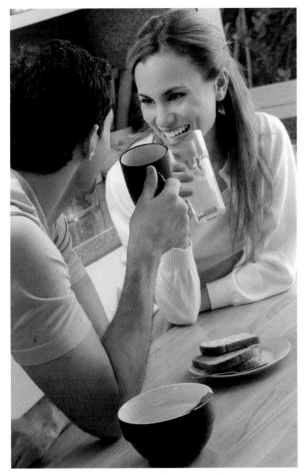

When you are eating and drinking socially, choose natural juices instead of coffee or alcohol.

contents of cola-style drinks to see whether they contain caffeine as it is all too easy to go over the limit. Consuming more than 200 mg of caffeine per day can interfere with your body's ability to absorb nutrients and raises the risk of not just miscarriage, but of your baby's birth weight being affected. A 'standard' cup of coffee contains around 80 mg of caffeine, but coffees served in coffee shops are generally larger than an average domestic cup and one standard latte may contain around 120 mg.

What about alcohol?

There is evidence to show that drinking even relatively small amounts of alcohol can increase the risk of miscarriage, so alcoholic drinks are to be avoided before and during pregnancy. In any event, abstinence is vital during the first three months of pregnancy, when your baby's major organs and body systems are being formed (see pages 62–5). After the birth, it is important, also, to realise that it is dangerous to handle a baby if you have consumed even a small quantity of alcohol.

Problems with alcohol

There is no doubt that drinking large quantities of alcohol (more than five units a day) causes serious foetal abnormalities such as foetal alcohol syndrome (FAS). This condition varies in severity, but the main effects are a failure to thrive after birth, poor growth and damage to the nervous system, which can manifest as mental retardation, difficulties with language and attention deficit disorder. Babies with FAS also exhibit a characteristic facial appearance of a flattened face and bridge of the nose (which can cause respiratory problems), a short upturned nose and thin upper lip. The problem is extremely common and thought to affect around one in every 1,000 babies. If you drink alcohol regularly or binge drink, you may need help with stopping, so talk to your doctor or midwife now. They need to be aware of your problem so that they can help you.

DON'T WORRY

Try not to be too anxious about food and drink during pregnancy. Although you need to be aware of potential hazards and avoid certain foods and drinks, the list of what you can enjoy (see pages 84–5) is so much longer than the one containing the risky items.

Most pregnant women actually find that they don't like the smell of items such as strong blue cheese, shellfish, coffee and alcohol anyway, so it may be easier to do without them than you imagine. Perhaps this is simply nature's way of keeping potentially harmful substances away from you and your baby.

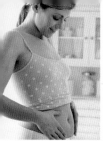

HEALTHY WEIGHT GAIN

By eating a balanced diet and exercising moderately during your pregnancy you should put on weight at a healthy rate. Exactly how much that should be depends on a number of factors.

There will be times during your pregnancy when you will gain weight at a faster rate than others. In the first trimester your weight will probably change very little, but the rate will increase through the second and third trimesters until the last fortnight, when you might gain a little more.

Assessing your weight

In an ideal world, of course, it would be good to be the 'perfect' weight before you even conceive, but often this is not realistic. Being overweight or underweight can have a huge impact on your pregnancy and developing baby, so you will need some extra help. If you are very overweight you will need to be monitored carefully and pregnancy is not the ideal time to be trying to lose significant amounts, but there are things that you can do to minimise the gain, while providing your baby with the nutrition she needs. Equally, if you are significantly underweight it is really important to your baby's health (and your own) that you change this pattern and eat enough to provide you both with what your bodies demand.

Taking a holistic approach

If your weight is a problem, it cannot be isolated from your diet and nutrition, exercise habits or your emotions, so you need to take a holistic approach and look at all aspects of your lifestyle to see how you can improve things.

It's good to keep it in mind that you are actually meant to put on weight in pregnancy. While it is best not to pile on pounds of excess fat, your pregnant body is quite different to your pre-pregnancy one and you should not feel pressurised to remain thin. It is quite normal to gain around 3 kg (6 lb) in fat over the 40 weeks of pregnancy, but if you breastfeed after your baby is born, you will probably lose most of your excess weight quite naturally and at a healthily steady pace.

RECOMMENDED WEIGHT GAIN

BMI	Ideal weight during pregnancy
Less than 19 (underweight)	You should be looking to gain more than average 12.5–18 kg (28–40 lb)
20–26 (normal weight)	You should be looking to gain 12–16 kg (25–35 lb)
27–30 (overweight)	You should be looking to gain 7–11.5 kg (15–25 lb)
Above 30 (obese)	You should be looking to gain no more than 7 kg (15 lb or less)

How the weight gain is made up

8 per cent	Breasts	11 per cent	Amniotic fluid
9 per cent	Placenta	22 per cent	Blood
11 per cent	Uterus	39 per cent	Baby

BODY MASS INDEX (BMI)

Read down the side bar to identify your pre-pregnancy weight, then read along the top bar until you find your height. Where the two figures intersect shows your BMI, which estimates how much fat you are, or are not, carrying. Use this to check how much weight you should gain over the full 40 weeks.

Remember that these are only guidelines, so don't worry too much if your pattern of weight gain is rather different. If you have suffered a great deal of nausea and sickness in the first trimester you may have gained very little weight or even lost some.

Your doctor or midwife will be keeping a close eye on your weight gain and if there is any cause for concern (if you are under- or overweight) you may be referred to a dietician for specific helpful advice.

If your BMI is:
Less than 19: you are underweight
Between 19–26: you are within the normal weight range
Between 27–30: you are overweight
Over 30: you are clinically obese

WEIGHT	HEIGHT									
	1.47 m (58 in)	1.52 m (60 in)	1.57 m (62 in)	1.62 m (64 in)	1.68 m (66 in)	1.73 m (68 in)	1.78 m (70 in)	1.83 m (72 in)	1.88 m (74 in)	1.93 m (76 in)
54 kg (120 lb)	25	24	22	21	19	18	17	16	15	15
57 kg (125 lb)	26	24	23	22	20	19	18	17	16	15
59 kg (130 lb)	27	25	24	22	21	20	19	18	17	16
61 kg (135 lb)	28	26	25	23	22	21	19	18	17	16
63 kg (140 lb)	29	27	26	24	23	21	20	19	18	17
66 kg (145 lb)	30	28	27	25	23	22	21	20	19	18
68 kg (150 lb)	31	29	28	26	24	23	22	20	19	18
70 kg (155 lb)	32	30	28	27	25	24	22	21	20	19
73 kg (160 lb)	34	31	29	28	26	24	23	22	21	20
75 kg (165 lb)	35	32	30	28	27	25	24	22	21	20
77 kg (170 lb)	36	33	31	29	28	26	24	23	22	21
79 kg (175 lb)	37	34	32	30	28	27	25	24	23	21
82 kg (180 lb)	38	35	33	31	29	27	26	24	23	22
84 kg (185 lb)	39	36	34	32	30	28	27	25	24	23
86 kg (190 lb)	40	37	35	33	31	29	27	26	24	23
88 kg (195 lb)	41	38	36	34	32	30	28	27	25	24
91 kg (200 lb)	42	39	37	34	32	30	29	27	26	24
93 kg (205 lb)	43	40	38	35	33	31	29	28	26	25
95 kg (210 lb)	44	41	39	36	34	32	30	29	27	26
98 kg (215 lb)	45	42	39	37	35	33	31	29	27	26
100 kg (220 lb)	46	43	40	38	36	34	32	30	28	27
102 kg (225 lb)	47	44	41	39	36	34	32	31	28	27
104 kg (230 lb)	48	45	42	40	37	35	33	31	29	28
107 kg (235 lb)	49	46	43	40	38	36	34	32	30	29
109 kg (240 lb)	50	47	44	41	39	36	35	33	31	29
111 kg (245 lb)	51	48	45	42	40	37	35	33	32	30

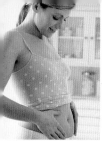

all about

KEEPING FIT

Exercise in pregnancy can bring all kinds of benefits to you and your growing baby. If you choose the right kind of activity, not only will you build stamina and suppleness, but you will feel fabulous, too.

Pregnancy is possibly not the time to embark on a campaign to get fit, but it is an ideal opportunity to take specially good care of yourself. Your aim should be to slowly but surely improve your posture, muscle tone and stamina. All these things will help you to face the challenges of pregnancy, labour and the demands of your newborn baby with far more energy and strength. Exercising will improve your heart and lung fitness, boost your circulation (and so deliver more oxygen and nutrients to your growing baby) and make you less prone to muscle aches and cramp. Physical activity also induces your body to release 'feel-good' chemicals such as endorphins, seratonin and dopamine, which will help to reduce mood swings

WHEN NOT TO EXERCISE

You should not do any exercise in the first 13 weeks if you:

Experience any bleeding or spotting

Have previously suffered a miscarriage or there is a chance that you might miscarry

Have had *in vitro* fertilisation (IVF) treatment

Are expecting twins or more

Have an incompetent cervix (see page 121)

Are suffering from an underlying medical condition: ask your doctor or midwife for advice before you begin a new exercise

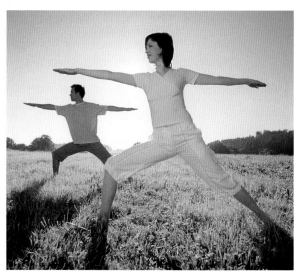

If you were doing yoga pre-pregnancy, then it's fine to continue during the first trimester and you may even want to encourage your partner to come to sessions with you.

and enable you to maintain a positive outlook.

It is important to take special care with any physical activity during pregnancy. If you have never exercised before or you have any kind of complicating factor in your pregnancy (see box left) you should consult your doctor or midwife before you attempt any exercise. Choose an activity that you enjoy and one that you can do with a friend or your partner. You are more likely exercise regularly if you enjoy it. Choose a cool time of day and stay out of direct sunshine, and wear loose clothes made from natural fibres. If it is chilly, wear layers so that you

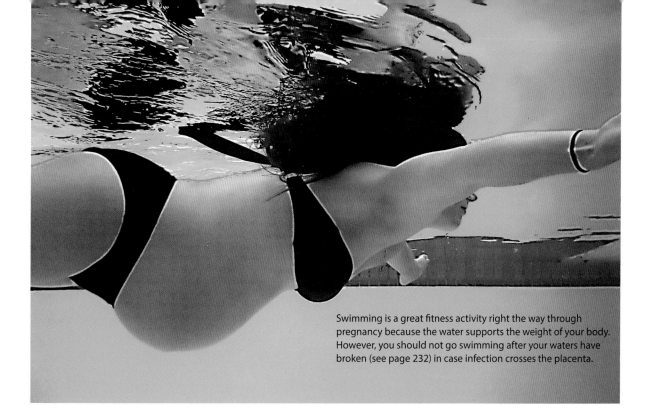

Swimming is a great fitness activity right the way through pregnancy because the water supports the weight of your body. However, you should not go swimming after your waters have broken (see page 232) in case infection crosses the placenta.

can shed items as you warm up. Make sure you wear a sports bra to fit your new shape and good-quality trainers to give your feet and ankles support.

What kind of activity?

The type of exercise that you choose is very important. Swimming is ideal throughout pregnancy (provided you have no complications) because the water supports some of your body weight, so it puts less strain on your joints. But you should make sure that the water is neither too chilly nor too hot (no warmer than 32°C/89°F). You may also like to try Pilates, yoga or cycling, among other activities (see pages 140–1). And whatever you do, one of the most vital things to practise during pregnancy is your pelvic floor exercises (see page 141).

Some activities are just too risky during pregnancy and these are: horse riding and eventing, skiing and snowboarding, water skiing, diving and scuba diving. Avoid any activity where you might get hit in the abdomen, such as netball or volleyball. If you are in doubt about any sport or activity, consult your doctor or midwife beforehand.

EXERCISE SAFETY

Whatever you do and whatever your fitness level, exercise safely using the following guidelines:

Never push yourself to the point where you have difficulty speaking or you experience any pain

Make sure that you keep properly hydrated before, during and after exercise – sip water frequently

Begin slowly and gently: 10–20 minutes three times a week is enough for beginners

Do not exercise for more than 45 minutes at a time

Avoid contact sports and very high-impact activities

Avoid all exercises lying on your front after 12 weeks

Avoid exercises lying on your back after 16 weeks

Take care when stretching – raised levels of the hormone relaxin will loosen your joints and ligaments in preparation for birth and make you more susceptible to strain and injury

Make sure you eat enough to sustain your level of activity

Take care to exercise on a stable base to minimise the risk of falling down

EXERCISE Q&AS

"How much exercise should I take?"

This very much depends on whether you were exercising regularly pre-pregnancy, on your current fitness levels and how you feel in the first 12 weeks. If you were exercising regularly pre-pregnancy and don't have any complications, you can carry on doing the same sort of activities as long as you listen to your body and follow the basic exercise guidelines (see opposite). Pregnancy is not the time to try to improve your fitness, but to maintain it. Have rest days between sessions to allow your body to recover. Be aware that in early pregnancy it is most important not to overheat the body, as it can be damaging to the foetus.

"What if I have had IVF?"

Avoid any exercise when you are going through IVF and during the first three months of pregnancy.

"What kind of exercise will give me the best work out?"

Having a 'work out' is not recommended in pregnancy. If you are normally fit and regularly do strenuous exercise, you could combine cardio with conditioning to keep you fit and toned throughout pregnancy. Not only does cardio work your heart and lungs, but it burns calories, so it can help to minimise fat gain, keep you supple, develop stamina and facilitate getting back into shape after the birth. Good cardio options in the first trimester are walking, jogging (as long as you were already jogging pre-pregnancy), cycling, cross-training and prenatal aerobics. Working with body weight is good for keeping toned. It is also important to include functional exercises that replicate activities in everyday life.

"Are abdominal exercises bad at this stage?"

No – you can continue your usual abdominal exercises in the first trimester as long as you feel comfortable. Avoid exercises lying on your back from 16 weeks as this can restrict blood flow to your baby. You can still train your abdominals by doing standing pelvic tilts, pulling your belly button in to your spine in an all-fours position or 'superman' – lifting your opposite arm and leg also in an all-fours position and holding for a few seconds before changing sides.

"I'm a bit overweight. How much exercise should I do?"

Pregnancy is not the time to try to 'go for the burn' or to try to lose weight. Remain as active as possible, however, and eat sensible amounts of fresh, unprocessed food (see page 78).

"What if I am underweight?"

If you are underweight you may need to limit the intensity and duration of your exercise sessions and ensure you are eating enough to sustain your level of activity.

"What about stretching exercises?"

When you are pregnant the hormone relaxin (see page 37) helps loosen your joints and ligaments in preparation for late pregnancy and birth. So you need to be careful during activity and while stretching during and after pregnancy. Never take a stretch to the point of discomfort and only hold it for a maximum of 10 seconds.

"Should I start pelvic floor exercises yet?"

Yes! Yes! Yes! Start them as soon as you are pregnant to build strength and stamina. They help you sustain the weight of your bump and limit stress incontinence (see page 141). Having a strong pelvic floor may also help you in the second stage of labour. If you have trained your pelvic floor throughout pregnancy it may recover faster after the birth.

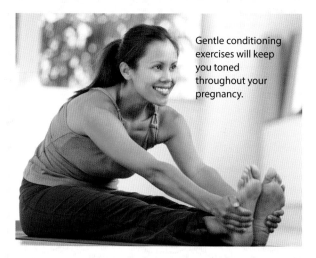

Gentle conditioning exercises will keep you toned throughout your pregnancy.

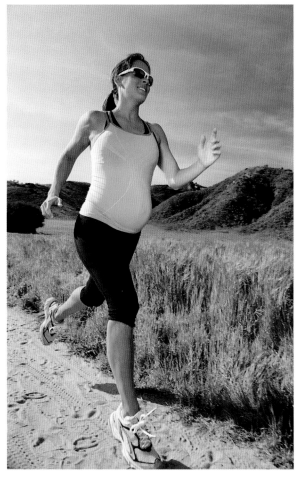

Jogging is fine as an exercise during pregnancy provided you were already doing it before you became pregnant. Don't start jogging for the first time during pregnancy.

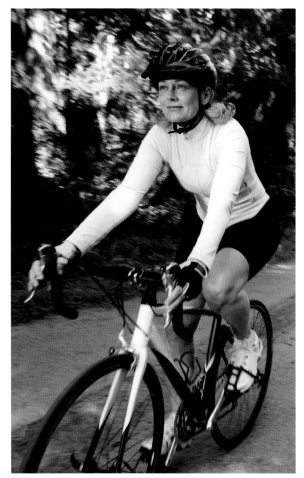

Cycling is a great cardio option throughout pregnancy, but it's best not to cycle outdoors after 20 weeks because of the risk of falling and hurting the baby. Indoor bikes are fine throughout.

WARNING SIGNS

Stop exercising immediately and seek medical advice if you suffer any of the following:

Excessive shortness of breath

Chest pain or palpitations

Dizziness

Painful uterine contractions

Leakage of amniotic fluid

Vaginal bleeding

Abdominal pain, particularly in the back or pubic area

Excessive fatigue

Pelvic girdle pain

Reduced foetal movement

Headache

Muscle weakness

Calf pain or swelling

Shortness of breath before exertion

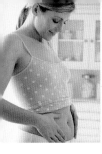

you & your

ENVIRONMENT

It is impossible to completely avoid contact with every environmental hazard, but at least if you are aware of which ones are potentially harmful you can take steps to keep your exposure to a minimum.

Your body does a remarkable job of filtering out many harmful materials that you may come into contact with, so that they cannot reach the baby in your uterus. However some substances have been found to cross the placenta, which means that there is a possible risk to your baby's health (see page 77). This is of particular concern in the first trimester, when the major organs are developing, so it is especially important that you should try to maintain a healthy environment, both in your home and at your place of work.

In the home

If you don't already use them, now is the ideal time to switch to environmentally friendly, natural cleaning products and avoid using strong chemicals such as bleach, spray polishes and oven cleaners. If you do use cleaning materials always make sure that the room is well ventilated and don't use insect spray, artificially scented air fresheners or candles. Take care with natural oils, too, as some are very powerful and unsuitable for you to use during pregnancy. If you are at all unsure about the safety of a product, it's probably best not to use it at all.

Redecorating & refurbishing

Many parents like to get a new nursery ready for their baby, which may involve redecorating – it's all part of the fun. If you are doing up and furnishing your baby's room, take care. Old carpets can harbour dust mites as well as dust and dirt and new carpets can contain powerful chemicals including formaldehyde so if you have to change the flooring, consider switching to a wooden finish that is easy to keep clean and dust-free. You could add a soft rug for extra comfort, but opt for one that is made from natural fibres such as cotton, wool or hemp. Choose furniture carefully, too. Wooden items are the safest,

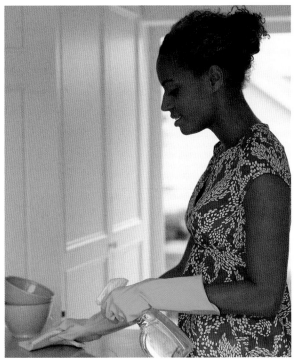

Be sure to take care that you use safe cleaning products during early pregnancy – and always wear rubber gloves.

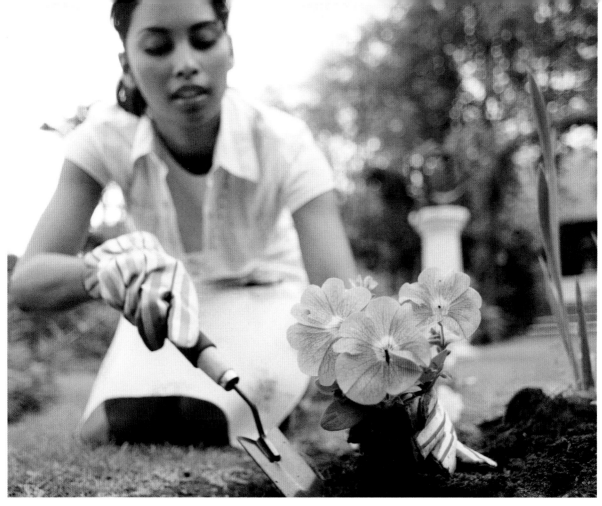

Enjoy your gardening, but wear sturdy gardening gloves and wash your hands carefully afterwards.

since those made from medium-density fibreboard (MDF) or veneers can release formaldehyde, a gas that has been linked to childhood asthma and a higher incidence of cancer among adults with a high level of exposure to it at work. Be careful, too, if you are planning to decorate the walls and paintwork.

Old houses, especially, may contain paint that has lead in it and you should try not to come into contact with it. So if you suspect that lead may be present, delegate the redecorating job to someone else. Water-based paints should be safe enough to use, but always check the label for contents because some latex-based paints contain mercury, which, again, should be avoided. If you do have to get involved with painting and decorating, ensure that the room is well ventilated and be sure to take regular breaks in the fresh air.

In the garden

Completely avoid contact with insecticides or pesticides and always wear tough, fit-for-purpose gloves when gardening because of the risk of bacteria in the soil and toxoplasmosis, a parasite found in cat faeces that can harm the developing foetus. Avoid changing cat litter for the same reasons and wash your hands thoroughly afterwards.

Out & about

Take care not to breathe in petrol fumes when filling up your car and try to keep the car windows closed if you happen to be stuck in traffic. Tobacco smoke is an obvious hazard to avoid (see page 103) and smoking is illegal in most public places now, but if people around you smoke, ask them not to. If that doesn't work, remove yourself from their vicinity.

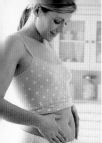

coping with

MINOR INFECTIONS

During early pregnancy your body has to suppress its natural immune system to prevent rejection of the growing baby. This means that you are slightly more vulnerable to infections and illness and you may take a little longer than normal to recover.

The two most serious viral infections that you should try to avoid during pregnancy are chickenpox and rubella (also known as German measles). Chickenpox can increase the risk of miscarriage in the first eight weeks of pregnancy and if it is caught between week 8 and week 20 it brings a small (1 to 2 per cent) risk of the baby developing congenital varicella syndrome. This can cause growth problems as well as abnormalities that can affect the brain, eyes, skin and limbs.

The rubella virus, if contracted for the first time

during early pregnancy, can increase the risk of miscarriage and if the pregnancy continues there may be severe problems for the foetus, including blindness, deafness, heart defects and mental retardation. Fortunately, it is rare in the UK because since 1970 there has been a national vaccination programme – you will be tested for rubella immunity in your first antenatal tests (see page 71).

It is impossible to avoid every illness, but if you know anyone with a high fever and a rash or spots, keep away. If you suspect that you have chickenpox or rubella, contact your doctor but do not go to the antenatal clinic in case you pass an infection on.

Coping with coughs, colds & flu

Colds won't harm your unborn baby, but check the labels of any cold or flu treatments carefully because as well as paracetamol they often contain antihistamines, caffeine and decongestants, which are not recommended in pregnancy. Try taking a paracetamol and making a hot lemon-and-honey drink instead. There may also be more unusual strains of viruses such as swine flu (H1N1) from time to time and you may need to be vaccinated against them, but seek advice from your doctor.

Dealing with headaches, aches & pains

Before the end of the first trimester (week 13) paracetamol is the only over-the-counter medication

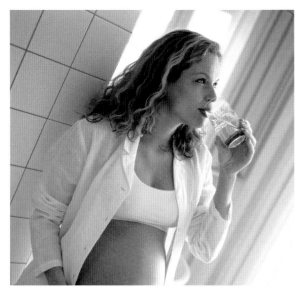

Drinking plenty of cool, fresh water will help your body deal with many minor ailment symptoms.

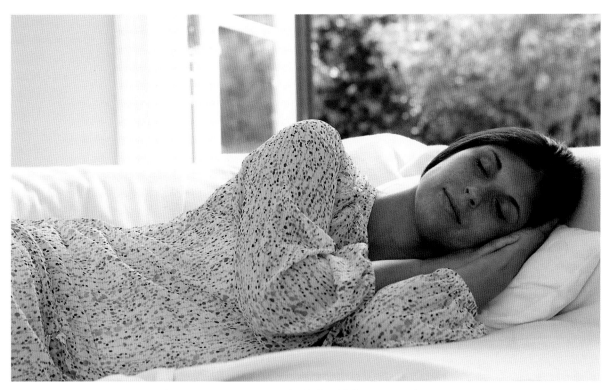

Resting as much as you can is one of the best ways you can help fend off and fight common ailments.

that is considered to be safe in small doses on a short-term basis. Aspirin and ibuprofen should be avoided throughout pregnancy. To recover from aches and pains, try taking a warm bath, drinking plenty of fresh, cold water and having short naps.

What about a fever?

If you are running a fever you need to reduce your body temperature – it can pose a threat to the baby, particularly during early pregnancy. Take paracetamol and drink plenty of cold water. You could also try bathing in tepid (not cold) water to help bring the fever down. If it persists, or if it is 38.9°C (102°F) or above, call your doctor or midwife for advice.

Tackling food poisoning

Severe food poisoning can cause serious problems, so take care to practise good kitchen hygiene (see pages 86–7). If you do get a stomach upset, with sickness and diarrhoea, try to keep drinking clear fluids and

rest as much as you can. If the situation continues for more than 24 hours contact your doctor or midwife.

All about urine infections

These can be quite common among pregnant women because the hormone progesterone relaxes the muscles in your body so that bacteria are able to make their way into the urethra (the tube leading to the bladder). If you find that you are urinating more frequently than usual, or feeling the urge to do so and have a burning sensation when you do go, you may have an infection. Other symptoms can include back or lower abdominal pain, nausea or even vomiting. Contact your doctor or midwife and they may prescribe antibiotics safe to take during pregnancy. To try to prevent an infection, drink plenty of water (at least 1 litre/2 pt per day) and have an occasional glass of cranberry juice because it is thought that the high vitamin C content acidifies the urine, making it harder for bacteria to multiply.

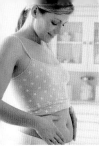

HOLIDAYS & TRAVEL

Of course, you will want to take good care of yourself when you are pregnant, but that doesn't mean that you have to stay at home for nine months. If your pregnancy is progressing well, there is no reason why you cannot travel abroad – just plan carefully.

If you are thinking of a holiday, do bear in mind that the normal discomforts of pregnancy may be exacerbated by extreme heat, high altitude or by staying in uncomfortable or unhygienic accommodation. Consider how long it will take to reach your destination and how you will get there. If you are thinking of flying, check that your chosen airline will take you – some will not carry pregnant women after week 34 of pregnancy. There is a risk that your body will find it difficult to cope with lower oxygen levels when you are flying at high altitude, and there is also the chance that you might go into premature labour in mid-flight.

Tummy bugs

During pregnancy your immune system is less efficient, so you are at greater risk of picking up infections, especially things like stomach upsets caused by contaminated water or food. There are a few simple precautions you can take to minimise the chances of illness (see right).

Diseases & immunisations

It is not advisable for pregnant women to travel to malarial-zone countries. Malaria is a serious disease and in pregnancy it can often be more severe and dangerous than normal. Although vaccines and anti-malarial drugs are not advisable during pregnancy, if a visit to a malarial zone is unavoidable

PLANNING A TRIP ABROAD

Take out valid medical insurance – you must inform your insurer that you are pregnant

If you are travelling to Europe you can apply for a free European Health Insurance Card (www.ehic.org.uk), which will entitle you to free medical care while you are there

Find out where you can get medical help while you are away and take a list of names and numbers to contact

Check the Foreign Office website or ask your doctor or midwife for information about the risk of endemic diseases

Take a note from your doctor or midwife stating your due date. You will also need their authorisation for travel if you are over 28 weeks pregnant. Pack your antenatal notes and any prescribed medication you are taking

If you have a 'high-risk' pregnancy (twins, IVF, history of miscarriage) think carefully about travelling abroad, especially during the first 12 weeks of pregnancy

it is much safer for you to take anti-malarial medication than to be unprotected, but ask your doctor or midwife for advice about which one is most suitable for you. Other vaccines, such as cholera, rabies, tetanus and polio, are thought to be safe, but pregnancy makes your body's response to them unpredictable. The safety of typhoid and yellow fever vaccinations is certainly unclear, so it is best to

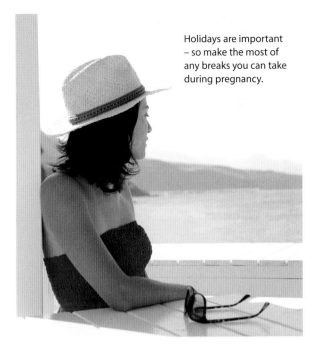

Holidays are important – so make the most of any breaks you can take during pregnancy.

avoid places where these diseases are present. Speak to your doctor or midwife and contact the Hospital for Tropical Diseases (see Resources) for more detailed information.

In the air

Book an aisle seat so that you can stretch your legs regularly and get up from your seat to walk around easily. You need to avoid sitting for long periods because of the risk of deep vein thrombosis (DVT). You could also try wearing compression stockings, which are available from most chemists. Air travel can easily make you dehydrated, so make sure that you have several bottles of water with you and keep sipping them throughout the flight.

Travelling by car

If you are making a long journey by car, ensure that you can take frequent stops to get out of your sitting position and walk around to stretch your legs. Push your seat as far back as possible to give yourself more leg room. It is important to wear a seat belt. A firmly secured belt will not harm your baby because she is already cushioned by the amniotic fluid. If you are unfortunately involved in an accident, your seat belt and airbag will protect you from severe injury. If you find the belt uncomfortable, adjust it so that the lap part of it stretches below your bump, but keep the shoulder strap in the usual position above it.

When to travel

The first trimester is when most women experience nausea and tiredness, so you may want to wait until the second trimester, when you are likely to feel at your best and the risk of miscarriage lessens considerably. After week 28 you may find that the size of your bump makes the prospect of travel much less appealing. You will need to consult your doctor or midwife if you are planning a foreign trip after 28 weeks, though, and you should check arrangements with the airline if you are flying.

KEEPING WELL ABROAD

Wash your hands thoroughly before you eat anything and after going to the toilet

Drink plenty of bottled water

Avoid eating any kind of shellfish or undercooked meat

Don't eat unpasteurised dairy products

Do not be tempted to buy food from street stalls – it may not have been cooked properly or been kept at the correct temperature to kill off any bacteria

Make sure that you know what you are eating and if in doubt, don't eat it

Avoid eating salad, as it may have been washed in contaminated water

Only eat fruit that you can peel yourself and don't eat watermelons as they are often injected with water (which may be contaminated) to make them bigger and juicier

Don't eat ice cream, sorbet or have ice in your drinks – all these may have been made with contaminated water

Use bottled water to brush your teeth

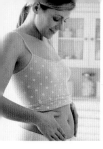

LIFESTYLE CHOICES

Now that you are pregnant, you need to take a critical look at your lifestyle. There may be aspects of it that could affect your developing baby and you may need to make a few sensible changes.

All about personal & beauty products

Deodorants, nail polish, hair dyes and especially hair spray should all be treated with caution. Many of these can contain organic solvents that cause other ingredients to give off fumes. Phthalates, parabens and formaldehyde are often found in toiletries and have been linked to health problems in babies, including hormone disorders and asthma. Read the labels carefully and try to switch to more natural products containing fewer chemicals. Plastic containers can also pose a possible risk to health, particularly if they are made from phthalates and bisphenol A (PBA). They are used in containers for cosmetics and toiletries, food packaging, toys and even babies' bottles. In the USA studies have found a link between these plastics and problems with pregnancy and foetal defects. As a result, since February 2009, several companies have stopped using them in the manufacture of toys and baby bottles. More research is needed, but if you want to avoid these substances altogether avoid buying a bottle or jar with the number '7' or the letters 'PC' (polycarbonate) in the triangle on the bottom.

The truth about sun beds

It's a good idea not to use sun beds during pregnancy, especially in the first 12 weeks, as there is evidence that the rays may break down folic acid, which is essential for the development of your baby's neural system. Sun beds may also damage your skin

because of its increased sensitivity and, perhaps most importantly, they can raise your body temperature, which can be extremely harmful to your pregnancy.

Stop using jacuzzis & saunas

If you have a jacuzzi, hot tub or sauna, or you use them at a gym or spa, stop doing so. Your pregnancy is especially vulnerable to extremes of temperature in the first eight weeks and women whose core body temperature rises above 38.9°C (102°F) for more than 10 minutes are at increased risk of miscarriage or having a baby with a neural tube defect.

Avoiding semi-surgical treatments

Doctors advise against having botox in pregnancy because although it is given as a localised injection the treatment is derived from botulinum, a toxic bacterium, and its effects on the unborn baby are as yet unknown. Chemical peels and collagen injections are advised against for the same reasons.

Going for a tattoo or body piercing?

You might fancy having a new tattoo or a fresh piercing to celebrate the forthcoming arrival, but this is not advised because you are at greater risk of infection while you are pregnant. If you already have piercings it may be a good idea to swap metal rings for flexible plastic retainers. If the piercing is in your tummy button, nipples or vulva, it is best to remove them, and certainly before your baby is born.

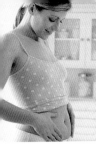

you & your

ENVIRONMENT

It is impossible to completely avoid contact with every environmental hazard, but at least if you are aware of which ones are potentially harmful you can take steps to keep your exposure to a minimum.

Your body does a remarkable job of filtering out many harmful materials that you may come into contact with, so that they cannot reach the baby in your uterus. However some substances have been found to cross the placenta, which means that there is a possible risk to your baby's health (see page 77). This is of particular concern in the first trimester, when the major organs are developing, so it is especially important that you should try to maintain a healthy environment, both in your home and at your place of work.

In the home

If you don't already use them, now is the ideal time to switch to environmentally friendly, natural cleaning products and avoid using strong chemicals such as bleach, spray polishes and oven cleaners. If you do use cleaning materials always make sure that the room is well ventilated and don't use insect spray, artificially scented air fresheners or candles. Take care with natural oils, too, as some are very powerful and unsuitable for you to use during pregnancy. If you are at all unsure about the safety of a product, it's probably best not to use it at all.

Redecorating & refurbishing

Many parents like to get a new nursery ready for their baby, which may involve redecorating – it's all part of the fun. If you are doing up and furnishing your baby's room, take care. Old carpets can harbour

dust mites as well as dust and dirt and new carpets can contain powerful chemicals including formaldehyde so if you have to change the flooring, consider switching to a wooden finish that is easy to keep clean and dust-free. You could add a soft rug for extra comfort, but opt for one that is made from natural fibres such as cotton, wool or hemp. Choose furniture carefully, too. Wooden items are the safest,

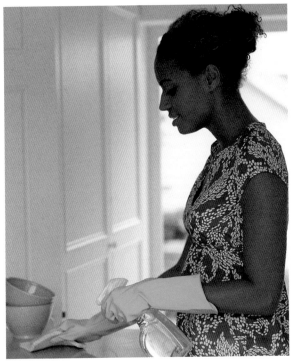

Be sure to take care that you use safe cleaning products during early pregnancy – and always wear rubber gloves.

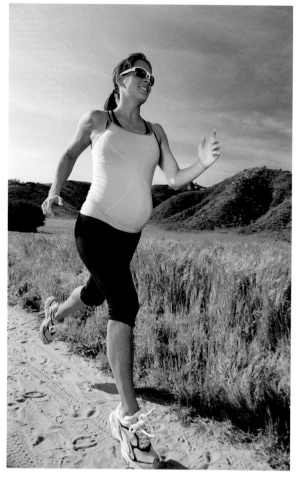

Jogging is fine as an exercise during pregnancy provided you were already doing it before you became pregnant. Don't start jogging for the first time during pregnancy.

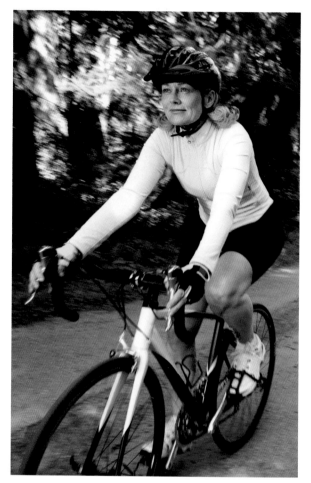

Cycling is a great cardio option throughout pregnancy, but it's best not to cycle outdoors after 20 weeks because of the risk of falling and hurting the baby. Indoor bikes are fine throughout.

WARNING SIGNS

Stop exercising immediately and seek medical advice if you suffer any of the following:

Excessive shortness of breath

Chest pain or palpitations

Dizziness

Painful uterine contractions

Leakage of amniotic fluid

Vaginal bleeding

Abdominal pain, particularly in the back or pubic area

Excessive fatigue

Pelvic girdle pain

Reduced foetal movement

Headache

Muscle weakness

Calf pain or swelling

Shortness of breath before exertion

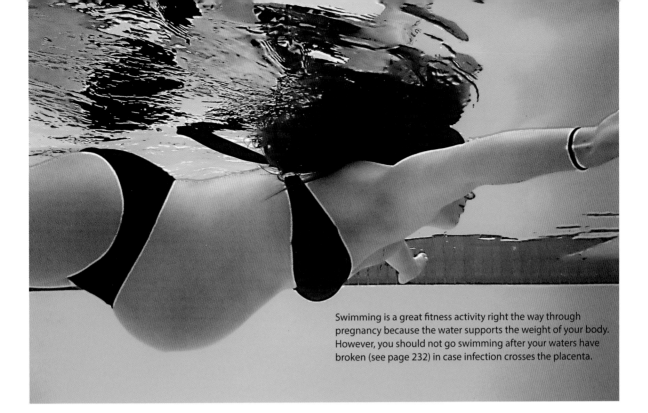

Swimming is a great fitness activity right the way through pregnancy because the water supports the weight of your body. However, you should not go swimming after your waters have broken (see page 232) in case infection crosses the placenta.

can shed items as you warm up. Make sure you wear a sports bra to fit your new shape and good-quality trainers to give your feet and ankles support.

What kind of activity?

The type of exercise that you choose is very important. Swimming is ideal throughout pregnancy (provided you have no complications) because the water supports some of your body weight, so it puts less strain on your joints. But you should make sure that the water is neither too chilly nor too hot (no warmer than 32°C/89°F). You may also like to try Pilates, yoga or cycling, among other activities (see pages 140–1). And whatever you do, one of the most vital things to practise during pregnancy is your pelvic floor exercises (see page 141).

Some activities are just too risky during pregnancy and these are: horse riding and eventing, skiing and snowboarding, water skiing, diving and scuba diving. Avoid any activity where you might get hit in the abdomen, such as netball or volleyball. If you are in doubt about any sport or activity, consult your doctor or midwife beforehand.

EXERCISE SAFETY

Whatever you do and whatever your fitness level, exercise safely using the following guidelines:

Never push yourself to the point where you have difficulty speaking or you experience any pain

Make sure that you keep properly hydrated before, during and after exercise – sip water frequently

Begin slowly and gently: 10–20 minutes three times a week is enough for beginners

Do not exercise for more than 45 minutes at a time

Avoid contact sports and very high-impact activities

Avoid all exercises lying on your front after 12 weeks

Avoid exercises lying on your back after 16 weeks

Take care when stretching – raised levels of the hormone relaxin will loosen your joints and ligaments in preparation for birth and make you more susceptible to strain and injury

Make sure you eat enough to sustain your level of activity

Take care to exercise on a stable base to minimise the risk of falling down

EXERCISE Q&AS

"How much exercise should I take?"

This very much depends on whether you were exercising regularly pre-pregnancy, on your current fitness levels and how you feel in the first 12 weeks. If you were exercising regularly pre-pregnancy and don't have any complications, you can carry on doing the same sort of activities as long as you listen to your body and follow the basic exercise guidelines (see opposite). Pregnancy is not the time to try to improve your fitness, but to maintain it. Have rest days between sessions to allow your body to recover. Be aware that in early pregnancy it is most important not to overheat the body, as it can be damaging to the foetus.

"What if I have had IVF?"

Avoid any exercise when you are going through IVF and during the first three months of pregnancy.

"What kind of exercise will give me the best work out?"

Having a 'work out' is not recommended in pregnancy. If you are normally fit and regularly do strenuous exercise, you could combine cardio with conditioning to keep you fit and toned throughout pregnancy. Not only does cardio work your heart and lungs, but it burns calories, so it can help to minimise fat gain, keep you supple, develop stamina and facilitate getting back into shape after the birth. Good cardio options in the first trimester are walking, jogging (as long as you were already jogging pre-pregnancy), cycling, cross-training and prenatal aerobics. Working with body weight is good for keeping toned. It is also important to include functional exercises that replicate activities in everyday life.

"Are abdominal exercises bad at this stage?"

No – you can continue your usual abdominal exercises in the first trimester as long as you feel comfortable. Avoid exercises lying on your back from 16 weeks as this can restrict blood flow to your baby. You can still train your abdominals by doing standing pelvic tilts, pulling your belly button in to your spine in an all-fours position or 'superman' – lifting your opposite arm and leg also in an all-fours position and holding for a few seconds before changing sides.

"I'm a bit overweight. How much exercise should I do?"

Pregnancy is not the time to try to 'go for the burn' or to try to lose weight. Remain as active as possible, however, and eat sensible amounts of fresh, unprocessed food (see page 78).

"What if I am underweight?"

If you are underweight you may need to limit the intensity and duration of your exercise sessions and ensure you are eating enough to sustain your level of activity.

"What about stretching exercises?"

When you are pregnant the hormone relaxin (see page 37) helps loosen your joints and ligaments in preparation for late pregnancy and birth. So you need to be careful during activity and while stretching during and after pregnancy. Never take a stretch to the point of discomfort and only hold it for a maximum of 10 seconds.

"Should I start pelvic floor exercises yet?"

Yes! Yes! Yes! Start them as soon as you are pregnant to build strength and stamina. They help you sustain the weight of your bump and limit stress incontinence (see page 141). Having a strong pelvic floor may also help you in the second stage of labour. If you have trained your pelvic floor throughout pregnancy it may recover faster after the birth.

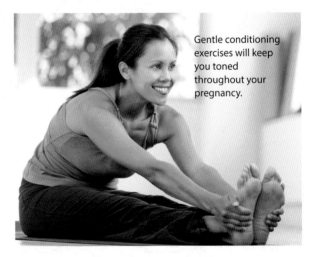

Gentle conditioning exercises will keep you toned throughout your pregnancy.

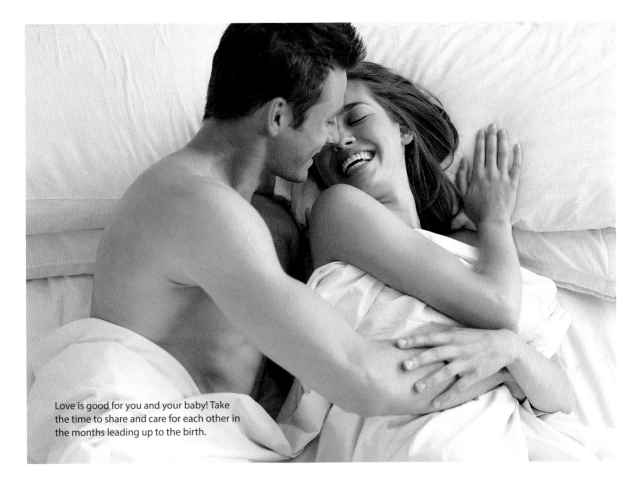

Love is good for you and your baby! Take the time to share and care for each other in the months leading up to the birth.

you has a sexually transmitted disease, there is no risk of an infection because the baby is safely encased in the amniotic sac and further protected by the mucous plug that seals the cervix. Do remember, though, that after around week 16 it is best not to lie on your back for too long and that your partner should not lie or press on your abdomen.

The love hormone

You may be keen, but your partner may worry about hurting you or the baby. He might also feel a little daunted by your unfamiliar shape, or he might just feel rather conscious of the baby being 'with' you both during such an intimate time. Try to remain patient with each other if you are not having sex (whatever the reason may be) and remember that intimacy is really the key factor in your relationship

as a couple. There may be times during your pregnancy, particularly at the beginning and at the end, when your bump is very large and you may have heartburn or indigestion, when you may not want to have intercourse, but try to keep showing each other affection. Kisses, cuddles, baths together and massages are ways that you can express your feelings and by talking about your emotions, too, you can maintain your closeness. When you are able to share intimate moments and you feel loved, your body releases oxytocin, a powerful hormone that also circulates in your body after you give birth and promotes emotional bonding with your baby. Some studies have shown a link between low levels of oxytocin during pregnancy and an increased risk of postnatal depression, so any gentle, positive physical contact between you will do you both good.

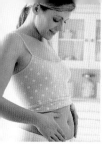

MANAGING STRESS

From as early as the seventh week of pregnancy your baby may be receiving pleasure-inducing chemicals from your bloodstream – but if you are unduly stressed she may be getting high levels of stress chemicals, so you need to know how to deal with such problems.

Learning to control stress early on in your pregnancy will not only help you to get through the nine months with ease, but will give you vital tools for the years of parenting to come. If you are under stress you may feel almost powerless in the face of problems – but you can control your stress response by changing your reaction to it. We are all wired differently to deal with stress and so what might be a challenge to one is a dreaded source of anxiety in another. Many factors are stressors on the body and they prevent it from

MANAGE YOUR MIND

Identify the major stresses in your life

Which area of your life do you most need to change?

Think about who can help and support you

How can you change your reaction to a problem?

Implement changes: 20 minutes a day of sitting quietly, visualising or meditating will help and if you practise it regularly it will give you a greater sense of control

Improve your breathing (see page 147)

Try some gentle exercise (see pages 92–3)

Protect yourself, where possible, from stressful situations (and people who make you feel anxious)

Nourish and nurture yourself

being at its best. Stressors can range from food additives and chemicals to emotional turbulence. Most stress is manageable and a little is beneficial, but if the balance is upset, stress becomes a problem and you may feel overwhelmed. Knowing how to manage stress by learning simple techniques early in pregnancy can be empowering. So instead of worrying about the effect stress is having on your baby, perhaps you can learn to manage it.

Emotions

We all experience a host of emotions daily, but as a pregnant woman your emotions may be heightened by the fact that you are carrying your growing baby and because the hormones rushing around your body intensify your feelings and responses. We are all also sensitive to the emotions of others – if they are positive it helps us feel happy; if they are negative it can make us fearful or angry. So emotions trigger different reactions in the body.

It is impossible to avoid all stress, but long-term exposure to it during pregnancy is to be avoided. Some stressful scenarios can feel overwhelming, such as job pressures, tiredness or rows with a partner. The common factor in these situations is a lack of control. Calm parenting can do a lot to make things go better and the baby's ability to cope is much improved, but of course it is best to try to avoid the stressful situation getting out of hand in the first place.

TACKLING ANTENATAL DEPRESSION

Although most people seem to have heard of postnatal depression, the antenatal form is much less commonly known about. It is thought that up to one in every ten pregnant women may have some form of depression while pregnant, but it often goes undiagnosed. This is partly because it is natural to feel low from time to time during pregnancy. However, it may also be due to the unfamiliar nature of the problem as there is an expectation that you should feel 'elated' during pregnancy and it may be hard to admit that you are finding things difficult. This may make you feel guilty and isolated. With luck, you will be unaffected, but it is useful to be aware of the symptoms. You may be suffering from antenatal depression if you notice that you feel low, anxious or stressed without relief for more than a fortnight or experience some of the following symptoms:

Symptoms

Crying regularly or for prolonged periods

Changes to, or loss of, appetite

Difficulty sleeping or perhaps wanting to sleep all the time

Lack of energy

Restlessness or irritability and lack of concentration

Sadness or powerlessness

Feeling isolated and extremely depressed

Withdrawing from family, friends or partner

Feeling guilty or worthless

Losing interest or enthusiasm for things you usually enjoy

The causes may include:

A chemical or hormonal imbalance due to pregnancy

A fear of losing the baby

Worries about a relationship, work or finances

A past history of depression

Anxieties about your rapidly changing shape or weight gain

Uncertainty about the future

If your pregnancy is unplanned/unexpected

What you can do

Talk to your doctor or midwife. They are there to help you.

Find a relaxation technique that works for you (see pages 110–11)

Join a local network or antenatal group

Try to improve your sleep patterns/quality (see pages 206–7)

Try to take gentle exercise in the fresh air (see pages 92–3)

Look at ways to improve your diet (see pages 78–85)

Keep a journal – this can help put problems into perspective

DEPRESSION Q&A

"I'm three months pregnant and I've been taking antidepressants, but I'm worried about the effect they might have on my baby. Should I stop taking them?"

You may need to stop taking antidepressants during pregnancy, however, do not reduce your medication without your doctor's supervision (however, be aware that St John's wort, though a natural antidepressant, works in the same way as antidepressant medications and should not be taken while trying to conceive, in pregnancy or during breastfeeding).

Antenatal depression is not yet well known about, but it is common and you need professional counselling. After talking to your doctor, you may be referred to a perinatal psychiatrist. This expertise is especially important for women taking antidepressants.

The process of having a baby is profoundly life-changing. From taking that first step to start trying for a baby, right through to after the birth, the experience places intense pressure on your body and on your mind, too, which can affect your ability to cope with day-to-day tasks.

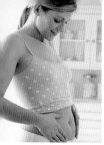

MIND-BODY-BABY

Connecting up the three elements of mind, body and baby during pregnancy is an important consideration, as your thoughts and emotions and how you manage them can have an impact not only on your own well-being but on your baby's, too.

When you are having a baby it's all too easy to focus on practical aspects, but it's vital not to ignore the more mental considerations – bonding with your baby coming at the top of the list. So how do you connect with your baby at such an early stage? By using relaxation and visualisation techniques (see right), you can send 'happy hormones' to your baby, which will help to establish bonding. Spend 20 minutes a day on these techniques – they'll help with a positive pregnancy.

Trying out visualisation

Visualisation is not as mysterious as it sounds and you are probably already doing it subconsciously. This happens, for example, as you lie in bed thinking about your baby. You will find that visualisation doesn't require unusual skills and that there are no right or wrong ways to do it. You will know when it is working because of your increased sense of well-being and you produce 'happy hormones' as a result, to pass on to your baby. Even at this early stage your baby is making a connection with you. The changes you feel as a result of being pregnant, such as nausea or tiredness, are coming from the hormones that your baby's placenta is producing.

Turning negative thoughts around

The mind is a powerful tool, the subconscious part particularly so. If you imagine an iceberg, the tip is

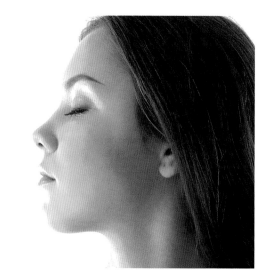

Visualisation can help you establish a positive mental bond with your baby. Spend a little time every day trying this out.

the 5 per cent you see, like the part of the mind that is your conscious awareness. Below the surface is the more powerful subconscious, where fears, anxieties and patterns of behaviour reside.

So how do you challenge negative thought patterns? Visualisation techniques, breathing techniques and relaxation are beneficial, and there can be an 'eureka' moment of release, when there is a sudden understanding of why you are feeling as you do. Once you have been through this, you can start to manage your feelings about your pregnancy in a highly positive way.

Visualisation – practice makes perfect

Very early pregnancy is a good time to start to try visualisation. It doesn't matter exactly how you do it as long as you feel that it is right for you. Yoga and meditation techniques will help you, too. Experiment with the following exercise:

- Make yourself comfortable – perhaps lie on a bed.
- Place your hands in a heart-shaped position, with your thumbs to your tummy button and your fingers to your pubic bone. This helps you make a connection – with your fingers and with your baby.
- Close your eyes and breathe slowly. Thoughts will enter your mind. Let them drift in and out.
- Imagine a stream of light passing through the top of your head to your forehead and down through your cheekbones. Feel yourself relaxing as the light reaches your jawbone.
- Release the tension, allowing your lips to part a little and your tongue to relax in your mouth.
- Send the light down through your neck and shoulders; feel the muscles relax and loosen as it continues down through your arms and hands.
- Now imagine the light flowing down through an imaginary line in the centre of your body. This is an acupuncture meridian called the 'conception vessel'.
- Imagine the place between your breasts where you connect with the heart, where you feel love, warmth and deep relaxation. The hormones you produce when you are happy are the 'love hormones', including oxytocin, which is sent through your body after the birth to help you to bond with your baby.
- Allow the light to continue in a straight line until you reach the uterus. Feel the light flow through your hands to your baby. Talk to the baby. Tell her how much you want her. See her developing in a calm environment, every heartbeat and pulse bringing her nourishment to thrive.
- Stay with this for a while and then allow the stream of light to pass on down to your knees and lower legs, letting you feel calm and relaxed.

CALM YOU, CALM BABY

Hormones cross the placenta – and that means not just the 'happy' hormones, but stress hormones, too. So practising calming techniques for just 20 minutes a day will help you to create a tranquil environment for your baby.

WHEN YOU FIND THINGS DIFFICULT

Bonding with your unborn baby can be hard if you have had difficulty conceiving or have suffered miscarriages in the past. You may lose belief in your ability to carry a baby successfully, so the first 12 weeks can be a testing time – you have to wait for that first scan, so this can seem like a period of limbo. Fear can be a crippling emotion, so this is where the mind-body-baby connection can really help.

In Traditional Chinese Medicine (TCM) the heart and uterus lie on the same meridian, the channel through which qi energy flows and the heart is considered the seat of the emotions. The emotions you are experiencing – fear, worry or grief – are inherently connected to the uterus through that channel, bringing qi to the developing baby.

WRITING POSITIVE AFFIRMATIONS

Try writing affirmations down. List the things that may be worrying you and then write down positive responses that you can offer instead. Find out by experimenting what form of wording works best. Pregnancy may bring discomforts and worries, but stay focused on the end result – your lovely baby. So, for example, you might say:

"I'm frightened of telling my boss about my pregnancy."
Your response could be:
"My boss has to be fine with this – this stage will pass."
or
"I feel so sick, I don't know how I am going to get through this business meeting."
Your response could be:
"I will start to feel better very soon – this phase will soon pass."

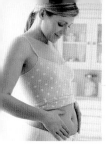

PARENTHOOD

Think your baby won't change your lives? Don't fool yourself! She will – in so many wonderful ways – and it's never too early to start considering how you will all fit together as a family.

Until now, you and your partner may have put each other first. If you both work, you are probably used to having a double income and sharing household tasks. In spare time perhaps you are used to deciding activities on the spur of the moment. Having a baby doesn't mean you have to abandon all social life, but there'll be adjustments to make. You may feel that things are already changing. Perhaps you are spending more time at home and are less able to cope with physically demanding tasks. This could mean that chores are divided along more traditional lines. You might find this an enjoyable novelty or you may have difficulty adjusting. The best way to deal with any problems is to face them together. By sharing feelings, hopes and fears you can build trust and understanding that will establish a firm foundation for your new family life as a family.

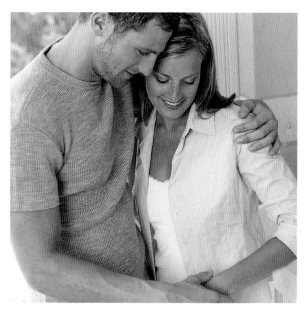

Having a baby together is a joint journey of exploration and discovery – a little careful thought now will help you prepare.

PARENTING ISSUES TO CONSIDER

Pregnancy and becoming a parent for the first time challenges any relationship. Why not redefine it in terms of your new role? Consider:

What works well for you now? What might change?

What are your weaknesses as a couple? How can you strengthen them?

Worried about financial pressures? Can you resolve them?

Are you concerned about being emotionally torn between your partner and your child?

How do you feel about your work–life balance now and how it might be after the baby is born?

How do you think intimacy with your partner might be affected by the arrival of your new baby?

How much fun do you have in your life at the moment and how do you see this being affected by the baby?

PRACTICALITIES TO CONSIDER

Sleeping, crying and feeding issues

How will you cope with night-time feeds?

Will you get up to attend to your baby on your own or will your partner share this with you?

Must your partner be up and out early for work – if so, perhaps he/she should sleep undisturbed in the spare room – at least sometimes.

The Department of Health recommends that babies should sleep in their parents' room for at least the first six months of life. Are you able to do this and have you made plans for it?

What do you feel about co-sleeping?

How well will you cope with a crying baby?

Are you planning to breastfeed (see pages 328–9)?

What can your partner do to support you?

Maternity leave and returning to work

If you have the option to take extended (half-pay or unpaid) maternity leave, can you afford to take it (see pages 202–3)?

Is returning to work full time important? If so, would your partner want to become a stay-at-home parent or are there other childcare options?

Would you prefer to be a full-time parent or work part time?

If you are on your own

The prospect of having a baby on your own can feel a little daunting. Do you have a close friend or relative who can be there in an emergency?

Have you found out about joining local support groups?

Are you entitled to any financial support?

Making a will

No one likes to think about the worst-case scenario, but with a baby on the way, it is sensible to consider whether you need to make, or alter, your wills. If something should happen to either of you, you would want to be able to focus on your child rather than having to worry about bureaucratic details.

EMOTIONAL ISSUES TO EXPLORE

New roles

In the first few weeks after birth, with so much feeding, comforting and nappy-changing to do, mothers and babies are almost inseparable. It's very common and natural for fathers/partners to feel left out. Are there ways that you can both be involved with your baby's care (see pages 350–1)?

Your upbringing

What was good about the care you received from your parents? What would you do differently?

Your parents and parents-in-law

How can you involve your parents and your partner's family (see page 151)?

Have you thought about how you will cope with receiving 'advice' and how you can gently turn it down if you disagree with it?

Other children

If you already have other children, how can you prepare them for the arrival of a new brother or sister (see page 151)?

Is there anything that might be worrying them? For example, some children think that the new baby will absorb all the parents' love and attention.

How can you make your other kids feel involved?

Have you thought about who will look after them when you go into labour?

If you are same-sex parents

You will probably have been through a long process in order to have your baby and you will have thought through many of the issues and implications already, but have you decided what you would like your baby to call you both?

How will you handle other people's questions?

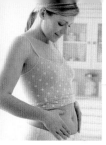

COMMON COMPLAINTS

Complementary therapies are very useful in treating the ordinary complaints of pregnancy. Although they are generally safe, check with your doctor first and always consult a qualified practitioner.

Nausea & sickness

Almost half of all pregnant women experience some nausea and sickness. It is thought to be caused by the rising hormone levels in your bloodstream (see pages 36–7), but it is also associated with some vitamin and mineral deficiencies.

Symptoms

The common symptoms are nausea and perhaps even vomiting, excessive amounts of saliva in the mouth and feelings of dragging fatigue and dehydration.

Nutrition

Choose foods that appeal to you and eat small amounts of them, often, to keep your blood-sugar levels stable (see page 147). In pregnancy, your need for vitamins B_6 and B_{12}, folic acid, iron and zinc increases and morning sickness is especially linked with deficiencies in vitamin B_6 and zinc.

If you have actually been vomiting you may also have become deficient in magnesium. If you feel very sick it is not easy to swallow vitamin and mineral supplements and real foods will be better for you as they will also provide other nutrients and fibre.

- B_6: wholemeal bread, raisins, chickpeas, hazelnuts and seeds.
- B_{12}: white fish, milk and yogurt.
- Iron: apricots, broccoli and fortified breakfast cereals.
- Folic acid: leafy green vegetables, asparagus, pulses, nuts and fortified breakfast cereals.
- Zinc: lean meat, poultry, wholemeal bread, sunflower seeds.
- Magnesium: apricots, tofu, wholegrains, nuts.

Complementary therapies for nausea & sickness

Consult your doctor or midwife before you try any complementary therapies and make sure that any practitioners you go to are qualified and accredited.

Acupressure This therapy is based on the same traditional Chinese principles as acupuncture –

SELF-HELP TIPS FOR NAUSEA

Try breathing deeply before each meal and focus on your stomach – put one hand on your stomach and the other on your chest

Rest as much as you can

Eat small, simple meals frequently

Avoid fatty or spicy foods

Try sucking lemon drops if too much saliva in your mouth makes you feel nauseous

Drink plenty of water

Keep a snack (such as ginger biscuits or plain crackers) by your bed so that you can have something to eat just before getting up

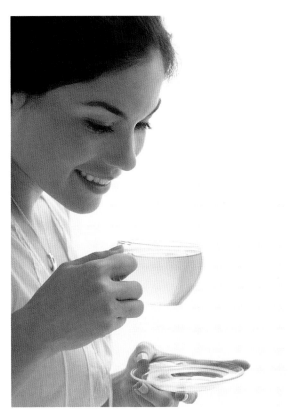

Try a refreshing cup of ginger tea to combat feelings of nausea during early pregnancy.

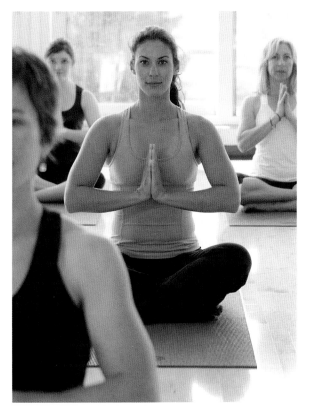

Regular, relaxing yoga and meditation may help you get over nausea more easily.

the belief that illness is caused by a blockage of qi or energy (see pages 38–9).

The aim of the practitioner is to balance the qi points by stimulating acupoints on your body. For a do-it-yourself approach, you could also try acupressure wristbands, which you can purchase from pharmacies and health-food shops.

Acupuncture Fine needles are inserted into acupoints on your body. Sessions for this form of treatment may take 40 to 60 minutes.

Homeopathy Follow the manufacturer's dosage instructions, however remedies are best prescribed by a professional homeopath to match your precise symptoms. Contact a registered homeopath.

- For sickness in the morning and irritability: nux vomica 30c
- For evening sickness and crying: pulsatilla 30c
- For vomiting: ipecac 30c

Reflexology This therapy works on the principle that there are reflex points on the feet that are nerve receptors for the body's organs. A reflexologist may gently massage the part of the foot that corresponds to the solar plexus.

Western herbalism Ginger is rich in zinc and is one of the best and easiest remedies for nausea and sickness. Try it in ginger biscuits, or slice or grate fresh ginger root into stir-fries or over steamed vegetables or fish. You can also nibble on chunks of crystallised ginger.

To make ginger 'tea' infuse 5 g (1 tsp) grated fresh ginger in a cup of freshly boiled water for five minutes. Sip slowly and drink a cup two or three times a day.

Yoga and meditation Relaxing the diaphragm, breathing deeply and improving posture may help with feelings of nausea.

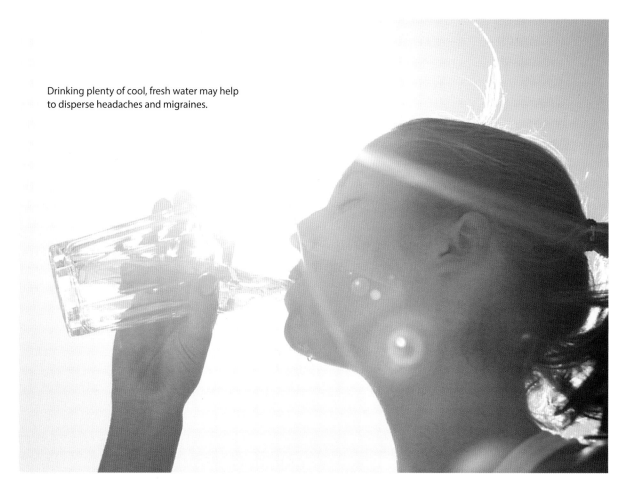

Drinking plenty of cool, fresh water may help to disperse headaches and migraines.

Headaches & migraines

Headaches are all too common in pregnancy and around one in ten pregnant women suffer from migraines, too. These headaches can be particularly painful and debilitating and are thought to be caused by the dramatic hormonal changes of pregnancy, tension in the muscles of the head and neck and in the case of migraine, by the too-rapid dilation of blood vessels in the brain.

If you were not pregnant you might normally try strong analgesics to deal with a bad headache or migraine, but in pregnancy the only painkiller that may be safe to take (and then only in small and infrequent doses) is paracetamol, so complementary treatments can be especially useful. You may need to try one or two before you find one that suits you.

Symptoms

You may experience a heavy, dull pain in the head, which gets worse when you move. You may also have a pain on one side of the head, behind the eye or in your temples. You may suffer from nausea, vomiting, numbness and visual disturbances and have the side-effects of fatigue and dehydration.

SELF-HELP TIPS FOR HEADACHES

Get as much fresh air as possible daily

Try to take 20 minutes of gentle exercise every day

Sleep and rest as much as you can

Drink at least 1 litre (2 pt) of fresh water every day

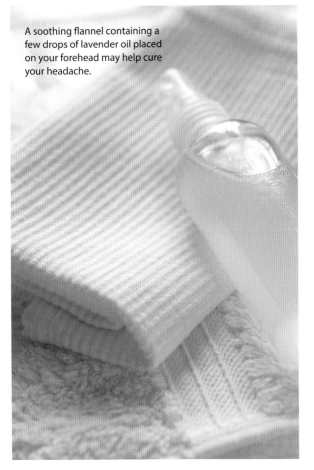

A soothing flannel containing a few drops of lavender oil placed on your forehead may help cure your headache.

Nutrition

Headaches are often the result of dehydration or low blood-sugar levels (see page 147). Drink plenty of water (at least 1 litre/2 pt per day) and eat small amounts of food at regular intervals to keep your blood sugar levels stable.

- Opt for slow-release carbohydrates such as porridge, wholemeal bread and root vegetables.
- Avoid common triggers such as chocolate, coffee, citrus fruits and cheese.

Complementary therapies for headaches & migraines

Consult your doctor or midwife before you try any complementary therapies and make sure that your practitioners are fully qualified and accredited.

Acupressure Traditional Chinese Medicine (TCM) sees headaches as the result of a blockage of liver and gallbladder meridians. This prevents the smooth flow of qi or energy (see pages 38–9). An acupressure practitioner will seek to restore the flow by stimulating acupoints on the head. Also try massaging the point between your eyebrows, just above your nose, with a circular movement of your thumb.

Acupuncture Using the same principle as acupressure, the gallbladder meridian may be treated by an acupuncturist, but the precise siting of the acupuncture needles will depend on your individual symptoms.

Aromatherapy Lavender oil can be particularly soothing and is perfectly safe to use in pregnancy. Try having a warm bath with four drops of lavender oil diluted in carrier oil or a small cup of milk. Or try using four drops of lavender oil on a lukewarm flannel and place it across your forehead and temples.

Homeopathy Take care to follow the manufacturer's dosage instructions, but remedies are best prescribed by a professional homeopath to match your precise symptoms. Contact a registered homeopath.

- For sudden pain that feels like a tight band around your head: aconite 30c
- For sudden, acute headache: belladonna 30c
- For pain that is unrelenting and made worse by movement: bryonia 30c

Reflexology A reflexologist may gently massage the tips of your big toes to help relieve a migraine. Take care to find a qualified practitioner, though, as the site of the massage must be accurately pinpointed.

Western herbalism Try chamomile or ginger tea (see page 115).

Yoga, massage and meditation A relaxing shoulder and neck massage can help to ease muscle tension and improve your circulation. If you suffer from frequent headaches or migraines they may be caused by poor posture or pressure on the nerves as your bump expands. A qualified chiropractor or cranial osteopath can help to gently realign your vertebrae.

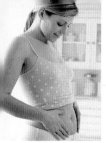

OVER- & UNDERWEIGHT

Being either over- or underweight can cause problems for you and your baby. You will need help from your doctor or midwife, but you can begin to change things with a few simple steps.

If you are overweight

If your body mass index (BMI) is 25–30 (see page 91) you will be classified as 'overweight', or 'obese' if it is above 30. This means you are at greater risk of miscarriage or from problems such as diabetes (see page 72) and pre-eclampsia (see page 208). You are also more likely to have a larger baby and a difficult labour and may be more prone to thrombosis.

Getting help

This may make depressing reading, but habit and emotional factors play a big part in being overweight and it is important that you try to get the help you need. Nobody advocates dieting in pregnancy: it can be detrimental to your developing baby. But if you are overweight you should be closely monitored. You will be advised to take extra folic acid and for the first 12 weeks you should probably be taking extra vitamin D as well. Discuss the exact amounts with your doctor. As your pregnancy progresses you may be tested for diabetes and your options for labour will need to be explored. You may be referred to a dietician to help you with your weight, but you can also try some of the tips below:

TIPS FOR LOSING WEIGHT

Keep a three-day food diary and be honest with yourself about what you are eating, especially any 'unhealthy' foods

Don't eat pre-prepared 'low-fat' foods as they can contain artificial ingredients and additives

Limit your portion size – if it helps, use smaller plates

What are the triggers that make you eat? Can you try to change them?

Be organised and plan your meals, rather than being tempted to snack

Take more exercise than usual (check with your doctor first)

Cut out, or at least cut down on, sugar (see page 78)

Try alternative therapies such as hypnotherapy (see page 41)

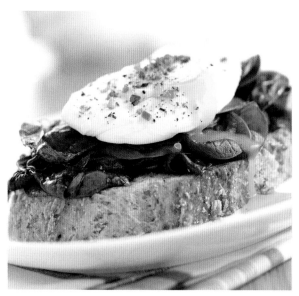

If you are trying to keep weight gain within safe limits, using small plates might help you limit the size of your portions.

If you are underweight

If your body mass index (BMI) is below 20, you are classified as 'underweight' (see BMI chart, page 91). Many women routinely worry about their size and shape and once they are pregnant they may be terrified of putting on weight and being unable to control their bodies. Women following very low-fat diets increase the chance of being malnourished because many of our most essential nutrients for fertility are actually fat-soluble and so they must be accompanied by fat in the diet. Even if they eat sensibly, some women try to counteract the natural weight gain and the swelling of their abdomen and breasts by over-exercising. This can raise the risk of miscarriage, or restricted growth and brain development in the foetus, and may lead to problems such as pre-eclampsia later on in the pregnancy or even to a premature birth.

Your underweight baby

An underweight baby faces a greater risk of ill health, so if you are seriously underweight you need to tackle the problem urgently. Your midwife may refer you to a dietician, who will advise you, but don't feel that you have to eat fatty, stodgy food to gain weight. There are plenty of appealing and healthy foods that can help you to build yourself up and give your baby the vital nourishment that she needs.

FOODS FOR WEIGHT GAIN

Avocados

Bananas

Butter – use plenty on wholemeal toast and on baked potatoes

Cheese (but not soft, mould-ripened or blue cheeses – see page 87)

Coconut milk – add this to Thai and Indian curries. Also add it to fruit smoothies

Dried fruit

Full-fat, natural yogurt

Hummus (not low-fat)

Nuts – especially peanut butter (unless you have a history of allergy to nuts)

Olive oil – have it with grilled or steamed vegetables and crusty bread. Use it liberally in your cooking and add a tablespoon to tomato-based pasta sauces. Mix it with walnut oil for salads and sesame oil for oriental stir-fries

Oily fish such as salmon, mackerel or sardines (restrict your intake of all oily fish, however – see page 87)

Pesto sauce

Seeds such as sunflower and sesame

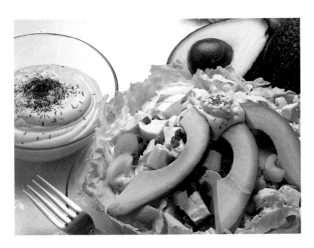

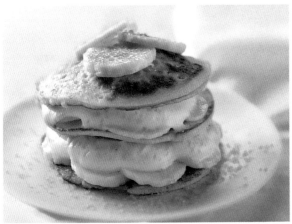

If you are trying to gain a little weight during your pregnancy, you can afford to eat healthy, calorific foods such as avocado (top) and/or banana pancakes (above).

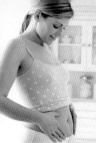

WHEN THINGS GO AWRY

The loss of a baby before 24 weeks is classified as a miscarriage and is a very distressing experience. As many as 3 in every 10 pregnancies may end this way, so it is by no means uncommon.

There are many reasons why a miscarriage may occur (they are often linked to the mother's age), but in the early stages of pregnancy at least half are caused by chromosomal abnormalities in the foetus and so you can think of miscarriage as nature's way of dealing with a pregnancy that is unable to develop. Occasionally miscarriage is caused by something happening because of an existing medical condition or because your blood type is rhesus negative and your baby is rhesus positive (see page 33). It is important that you should never feel guilty about miscarriage since you cannot control how your body behaves. Miscarriage is a common occurrence, but if you suffer from repeated miscarriages, the cause should be investigated because you may require treatment.

Signs & symptoms

Symptoms of a threatened miscarriage may include vaginal bleeding (anything from light spotting to expelling large clots), abdominal and/or back pain similar to period pain or a cessation of typical first-trimester pregnancy symptoms such as nausea. If you experience any of these problems you should contact your doctor or midwife immediately, but even with these symptoms a miscarriage will not necessarily follow, so it is vital that you ask for help. If you go on to expel tissue, bleed heavily and the pain is more severe, however, your cervix will have opened and your pregnancy will not then continue.

Proper checks

If you do experience any of the warning symptoms, you will be given an ultrasound examination to find out whether your pregnancy is continuing. A pelvic examination will also confirm whether your cervix is still closed or not.

A complete miscarriage

If your body has expelled all the pregnancy tissue and blood it is known as a 'complete miscarriage'. The pain will subside and an ultrasound scan will show that your uterus is empty.

An incomplete miscarriage

If all the pregnancy material has not been spontaneously expelled, you may be offered an evacuation of retained products of conception (ERPC), which is a minor procedure carried out under anaesthetic. Its purpose is to clean your uterus and it is done by widening the cervix and removing any remaining tissue from the endometrium (lining of the uterus). If you are not bleeding too heavily and are fit enough to cope, you may be advised to wait a few days before having an ERPC, to see if your body will expel the rest of the tissue naturally or with the aid of some medication.

Other kinds of miscarriage

Occasionally you may experience no symptoms at all, or just a little brownish spotting. An ultrasound scan

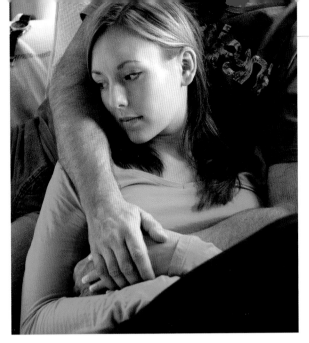

Look to your partner and family for loving support after suffering a miscarriage – they will want to help you.

HOW TO COPE WITH MISCARRIAGE

If you suffer a miscarriage, you will need time to grieve for your loss, no matter how early on in your pregnancy it has occurred. Hospitals are not always able to offer a great deal of support, though some do offer grief counselling. Your partner will be grieving, too, but you will both need emotional and physical support.

Get plenty of rest and eat lots of nutritious food, continuing to take your folic acid supplement. Concentrate on rebuilding strength and energy and remember that there is an excellent chance that your next pregnancy will be successful. Usually there will be no reason why you should not try to conceive again as soon as you and your partner feel ready. But check with your doctor or midwife.

may then reveal what is called a 'blighted ovum'. This is when there is an amniotic sac inside the uterus, but no foetus, because it has failed to develop. The doctor may carry out another scan in seven days' time to see whether a foetus has developed in the meantime, or to be sure that there is no viable pregnancy. At other times, the ultrasound scan may show there to be a foetus in the sac, but that its heart is not beating. You will then be offered the option of waiting for your body to complete the miscarriage or to have an ERPC straight away.

Problems with the cervix

In the second trimester, the most common cause of miscarriage is due to what is rather unfortunately called an 'incompetent' cervix. The name makes it sound as if your body is not up to doing its job properly. However, if this happens to you, you should not feel that you are to blame. The problem is that the cervix opens under the pressure and weight of the growing uterus and baby. This may be caused by a genetic weakness, damage caused during a previous delivery or treatment for a cervical disease or abnormality. If you are diagnosed early, your pregnancy has a good chance of being saved because

you can be offered a cervical cerclage. This is a minor procedure carried out under local anaesthetic or epidural (see pages 246–7) at around 12 to 16 weeks of pregnancy and where the cervix is sutured to keep it closed. The sutures are then removed a few weeks before your expected delivery date, although they may be kept in place until early labour has begun.

Ectopic pregnancies

An ectopic pregnancy is where the fertilised egg becomes established in the fallopian tube rather than the uterus. Sadly, the pregnancy will not be able to continue and does pose a serious threat, so it requires urgent medical treatment. If you have a negative pregnancy test that is followed by a positive one and you experience any of the following symptoms, there is a possibility that the pregnancy is an ectopic one. Take note if you: have one-sided pain in your abdomen; pain on urinating or painful bowel movements; dark, watery or light bleeding that is unusual for your periods; pain in your shoulder. If you think you are pregnant and have any of these problems you should contact your doctor or midwife immediately or go to the accident and emergency department of your nearest hospital.

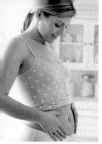

WORK–LIFE BALANCE

No matter how fit and energetic you may feel, it is important to recognise that you will need to make some adjustments to your life at work during your pregnancy and to find a healthy balance between your career and life at home.

A part from a few high-risk jobs (see opposite) most women can continue working when pregnant and many find it helpful to have a distraction from some pregnancy's discomforts. However, it is well worth looking at what you can do to make work life more comfortable.

Speak to your employer once you have confirmed that you are pregnant (though you might want to wait until you have had your booking appointment, so that you have a clearer idea of your expected delivery date – see page 31). You are legally entitled to time off from work for your antenatal appointments, but you will need to let your employer know so that plans can be made. It may also be possible to negotiate more flexible hours if, for instance, you are suffering from nausea or sickness. If your job involves very long hours or prolonged periods of standing up you have a right to ask your employer to give you some alternative tasks.

Workplace stress

Remember that you now have your baby to consider and if your job is very stressful you will need to make a few adjustments. Although you probably still have deadlines to meet, see if it is possible to delegate some of your work. Think carefully about taking work home, if that is your usual habit. If you are struggling to get everything done, it is best to discuss this with your employer, but be careful to negotiate a compromise and not to demand special treatment.

Find out about your maternity rights and benefits (see pages 202–3) so that you know what your rights and responsibilities are. Think about when you want to start maternity leave. Many women work up until the last minute so that they can take maximum time off later. However, in the last stages of pregnancy, it is vital to have time to rest, relax, eat and sleep so you have energy to cope with labour and birth and enjoy your baby once she arrives.

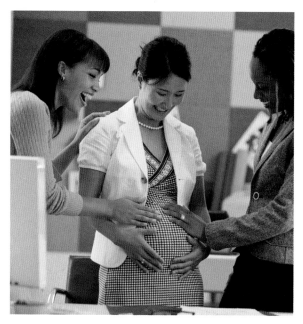

Colleagues will want to share the excitement of your pregnancy.

COMFORT AT WORK

Keep a supply of healthy snacks and drinks by you while you work – to keep your energy levels up

Eat a nutritious breakfast and make time for a proper lunch

Keep a comfortable pair of shoes under your desk if your workplace is quite 'dressy'. Wear them to travel to/from work

Make sure that your chair is positioned at the correct angle for your desk, so that your back is supported. Perhaps keep your feet raised on a footstool

While you sit at your desk you can do a few leg-stretching exercises to prevent your ankles and feet from swelling

Take regular, short breaks from your sitting position (and from working in front of a computer)

If there is a smoking area at work, make sure that you avoid it

If there is a spare, empty office, meeting room or first-aid room you may be able to arrange to take a short nap at lunchtime – if you are feeling particularly tired

Keep an easily accessible record of your ongoing projects so that your colleagues can take over from you more easily if you are unable to get to work

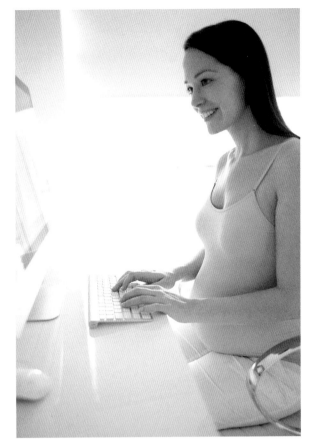

There are a lot of things you can do to alter your physical environment at work to make things more comfortable.

SAFETY IN THE WORKPLACE

Most jobs can be safely carried out by pregnant women, but certain occupations may mean exposure to potential hazards. If you work in a factory, pharmacy, laboratory, garage, dry-cleaners, hairdressers, funeral parlour or carpentry workshop, or with paints, plaster or pesticides you may be at risk from a range of solvents that can cross the placenta and cause harm to the growing baby (see page 77). For the same reason, you should also avoid handling your partner's work clothes if he/she works with any of these substances. You can contact the Health and Safety Executive (HSE) for more information. You should also tell your midwife about your occupation at your booking appointment so that you can discuss any possible problems you may have.

If you work with X-rays, you will already be aware of the dangers of radiation and be following stringent safety rules, but if you are at all concerned, you may be able to transfer to other duties within the department for the duration of your pregnancy.

There is no evidence that working at a computer or VDU causes harm to you or your baby, but it is important that you take regular breaks and get up from a sitting position to move around freely. If you use a mobile phone, keep it in your bag and away from your abdomen. More research is needed on the long-term effects of mobiles, so it is sensible to try to limit your exposure to them.

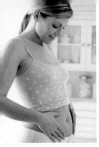

considering new challenges

BECOMING A DAD

You are embarking on an incredible journey of discovery that will change you for ever. Fatherhood will bring you exciting new challenges and responsibilities, but also a love that is unlike anything that you have ever felt before.

A s the news of your impending fatherhood sinks in you may find that you experience strong, conflicting emotions. You may have been waiting a long time for this baby, or it may have come as a surprise. Either way, it is normal to need a bit of time to adjust to that positive pregnancy result.

Taking second place?

You might be shocked to find that you feel a little jealous of your baby before she has even been born, but don't worry, this is quite common and all part of the process of adjusting to parenthood. With so much attention focused on your pregnant partner, it can be easy to start to feel as though you are taking second place in your partner's life and that friends, family or even her midwife or doctor know more about what is happening to her than you do. Try not to withdraw, but talk about your feelings – your partner may interpret your quietness as a lack of enthusiasm for the pregnancy.

Talking & sharing

Once you begin to talk you may find that your partner shares some of your anxieties, but she might also find it difficult to give you a great deal of support. She is going through momentous emotional and physical changes and in the first trimester, especially, she may find it hard to do anything much beyond working, eating and sleeping. Your sex life

may suffer during these early months, too, either because your partner has lost her libido for a while, or perhaps because you find her changing body off-putting. This can also contribute to you feeling alienated, but try to remember that you both need time to adjust and that if you keep talking you can remain close. Although sex may be off the agenda for now, you can still show affection and be intimate in other ways (see pages 106–7). If you are finding it really difficult not to feel left out, try talking to a close friend, your doctor or perhaps a counsellor.

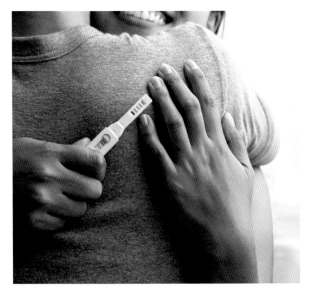

A positive pregnancy test may be what you both wanted, but it may surprise you by bringing with it some conflicting emotions.

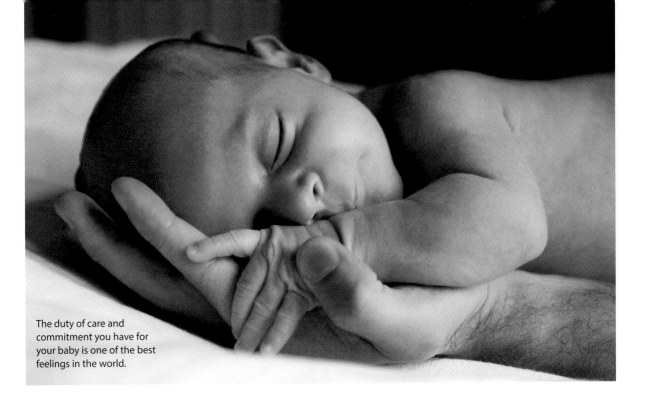

The duty of care and commitment you have for your baby is one of the best feelings in the world.

MALE & FEMALE BRAINS IN PREGNANCY

The early weeks of pregnancy for a woman are hormonally driven. She is flooded with new hormones and the levels go up and down every day. She can go from being elated and happy, to biting your head off or crying miserably. But don't worry – this is completely normal.

It is useful to know that even early on in pregnancy, the woman's brain is being prepared for the huge adjustment to motherhood. There are up to a hundred times more oestrogen and progesterone coursing through the body than before and this increase helps the mother's brain to prepare for giving birth, bonding with the new baby and for breastfeeding. Very soon after the baby has been born, a mum can distinguish her own baby's cry.

However, recent studies have shown that the brain of an expectant father also goes through a major transformation. The pheromones made in the woman's sweat glands during these high-oestrogen and progesterone states release pheromones that the prospective father picks up, helping his brain to change into a 'daddy' brain.

Being there for the scan

If you cannot make it to any other appointments, try to be there for the first ultrasound scan. Up until the moment when you see your baby moving on the screen, your partner's pregnancy may have seemed slightly unreal to you. She will have been 'feeling' pregnant for some time, with so many hormones rushing around her system (see pages 36–7) and perhaps some typical pregnancy symptoms (see pages 26–7). For you, though, it may be harder to believe until you have the tangible proof.

Parenting classes

Classes can really help fathers to get involved (see pages 158–9). Some run special sessions for dads-to-be, where you may be able to air your hopes and fears with other partners. By attending these classes you will learn more about what is happening to your partner and your growing baby and this will help you feel more in control. You may also find you and your partner build lasting friendships there. All the couples will be going through the same experiences and once your babies have been born, they will have the benefit of ready-made playmates as they grow up.

There are lots of ways in which you can be involved in your partner's pregnancy.

• Try to go to at least one antenatal appointment with your partner. You'll find out a lot more about what is happening to her and your baby (see page 69).
• Attend the scans – you'll see your baby move and be able to track her growth (see pages 74–5).
• From about week 30 you will be able to hear your baby's heartbeat by putting your ear to your partner's tummy.
• Talk and sing to your baby. She'll be able to hear you and will recognise your voice after her birth.
• From around week 20 you may be able to feel your baby move. Stroke your partner's tummy and you may be rewarded with a kick. Later you may be able to identify a hand or a foot.
• You could start finding out about parenting classes. Discuss the options with your partner to select the type that suits you both best.

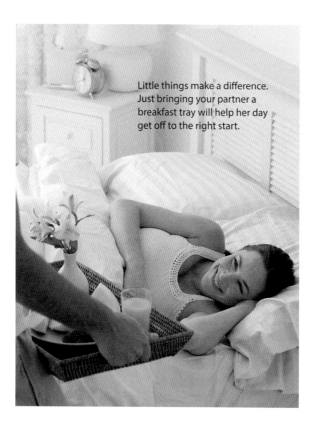

Little things make a difference. Just bringing your partner a breakfast tray will help her day get off to the right start.

Practical ways you can get involved

The role of partners and fathers and the level of their involvement in pregnancy, birth and childcare has changed enormously in the last 50 years or so. It is very likely that you already do some of the shopping, cooking and household chores anyway, but if you don't, now is the time to get involved in them.

By working as a team and sharing practical tasks as well as your feelings, you will build a stronger bond as a couple that will stand you in good stead for parenthood. There are lots of ways to help to make things run more smoothly, and by thinking of your partner's needs you can help her to have a more relaxed pregnancy. Research shows that a supportive relationship may also make labour and birth less stressful and postnatal depression less likely. It should also help you all to settle into family life more easily.

• Find out how your partner's body is changing (see pages 44–9) and what is happening to your baby week by week (see pages 50–5).
• Go for regular walks together. You'll benefit from the fresh air and exercise and it will give you both a break – to think and talk.
• As the pregnancy progresses and your baby increases in size and weight, your partner may have backache, and swollen feet and legs. Gentle massage can really help.
• Help with food shopping and cooking. Your partner should avoid carrying heavy bags anyway, especially towards the end of pregnancy. But this is a great chance for you to get involved in the food shopping – you both need to eat healthily.
• Go on breakfast duty – especially in the first trimester when your partner may be feeling tired and nauseous in the mornings. Encourage her to have breakfast in bed. Wholemeal toast and a warm drink may help with pregnancy sickness.
• Get your finances in order and draw up a budget to help you cope with extra expenses. If you are concerned about how you will cope, seek advice and discuss things calmly with your partner. You

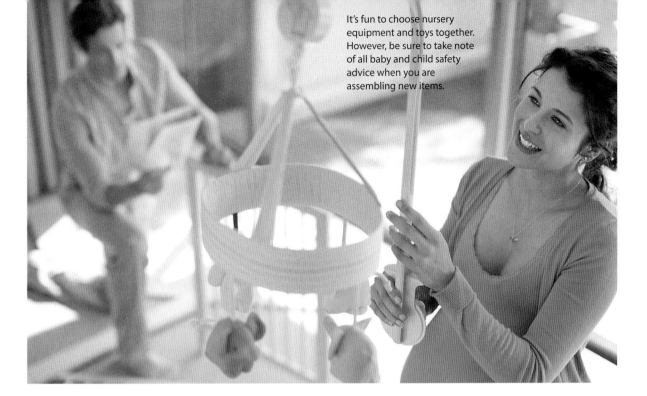

It's fun to choose nursery equipment and toys together. However, be sure to take note of all baby and child safety advice when you are assembling new items.

may need to make a few adjustments to your standard of living, but discuss it properly first.

- Encourage family and friends to get involved. You will both need extra support and your child will benefit from having other close relationships later.
- Later in the pregnancy you could start getting your baby's room ready. Discuss the colour scheme and get on with the painting and decorating (see pages 96–7). Also start thinking about ways of making sure your home is a safe environment for your baby.

Looking ahead

If you are present at your baby's birth (though this is not compulsory – only attend if you feel you really want to), you will have a vital role in supporting your partner and you will need to be properly prepared (see pages 260–5). However, if you are not going to be the primary birth partner, there are still plenty of things that you can do to help your partner to prepare herself and cope with the challenges of labour and birth (see page 263)

It's never too early to start thinking about parenthood and you and your partner can perhaps begin by discussing your experiences of your own parents. There may be things you will want to do very differently, or you may be anxious about the kind of father that you will be (see pages 112–13). Talk over your ideas. You will have lots of decisions to make once your baby arrives and as she grows up, so it makes sense to start working together now.

UNEXPECTED FATHERHOOD

If this pregnancy was unplanned, you may be feeling a bit overwhelmed. If your contraception failed you (and your partner) you might feel frustrated, or even angry, about this situation, especially if you were not in a long-term relationship. If you and the baby's mother are not going to stay together, you will need to sort out practical arrangements between you.

But whether you are couple or not, you will be a father and you have the opportunity to form a lifelong bond with your child that will reward you in ways that you cannot yet imagine. Try to take some time to adjust and find ways to be involved in the pregnancy, so that you begin building a good relationship with your son or daughter.

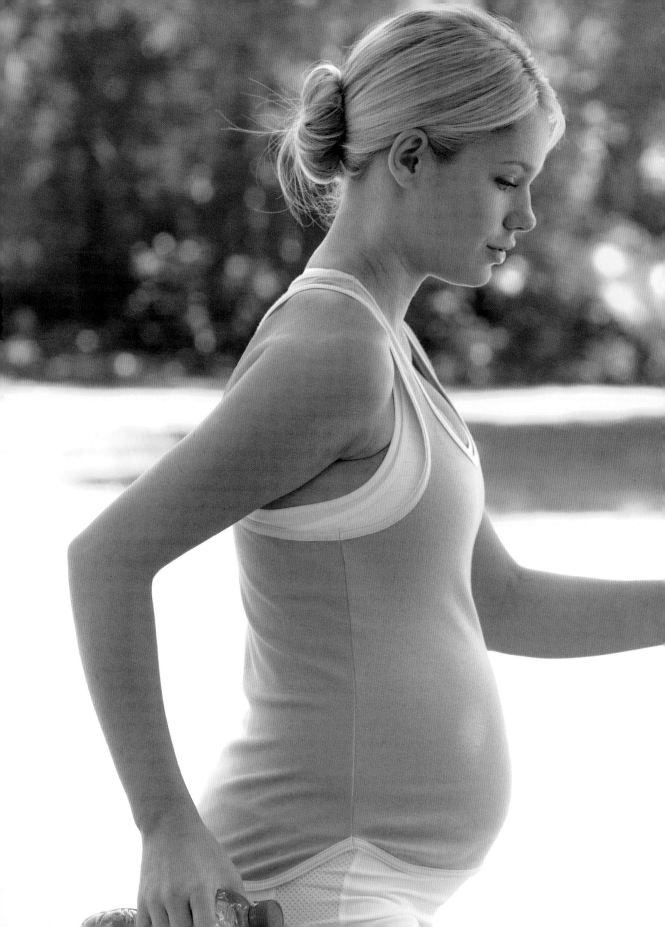

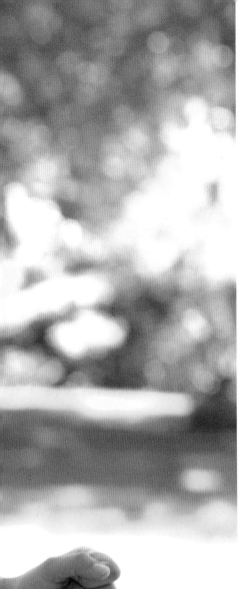

chapter 4

your second
TRIMESTER

This is the time in pregnancy when you start to feel much better – you can focus on your fitness and general health and really start to enjoy this phase.

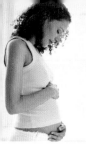

during the second trimester

YOUR CHANGING BODY

Your pregnancy is by now becoming quite noticeable and you will probably feel a surge of renewed energy, good health and a relaxed sense of well-being.

Week 14

Your waist will have become noticeably thicker now, while your tummy will be looking rounder. The size and shape of your bump will be individual to you, partly depending on whether this is your first baby or your second, or more.

Week 15

Your uterus is now about the size of a small melon and you will probably feel it rising above your pubic bone. From now on, your midwife will be able to assess its size quite easily, simply by palpating it gently with her hands.

Week 16

Your hair may seem thicker, as you shed fewer hairs during pregnancy. You may also find that your skin looks and feels softer and that your lips look plumper. As any nausea subsides, your appetite may increase and you might notice that you have sudden enthusiasms for particular foods (see page 79).

Week 17

Before you were pregnant, just 2 per cent of your blood flow was sent to your uterus. Now it is 25 per cent. In the first trimester the water content of your blood increased, but by now the number of red cells in it is much greater, and the amount of blood that is pumped through your heart continues to increase. All this might be expected to result in dramatically raised

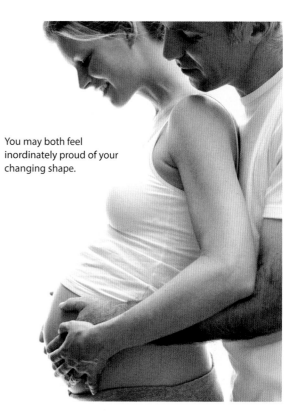

You may both feel inordinately proud of your changing shape.

blood pressure, but the hormone progesterone has prepared your body to cope, by relaxing and dilating your blood vessels so that they can accommodate the increased blood flow.

Have you felt a slight fluttering in your abdomen? You might feel your baby's first movements this week, but if this is your first baby, you may not be fully aware of movement until week 20 or so.

Week 18

Your centre of gravity will be changing now that your bump is becoming heavier. Make sure that you maintain good posture and when you are at home walk around barefoot as often as you can, to flex your feet and ankles.

Week 19

The pigmentation of your skin will continue to darken on your nipples, areola and genitalia. You may also notice changes in your libido as more blood is pumped around the pelvic area, and your breasts and nipples become more sensitive, making you more easily and quickly aroused (see pages 106–7). You will tan more easily – any freckles or moles will probably look darker and you may get dark patches called 'chloasma' on your skin (especially your face). Most of these patches will fade once your baby has been born, but always protect your skin from sun damage by using a good sunscreen or sunblock.

Week 20

If you haven't already been aware of your baby moving, you may now realise that the gentle, bubble-like sensations in your tummy are not wind. It might feel like a tiny fish flipping about or it may just be a very definite kick. Try sitting still and very gently pressing on your abdomen (you won't hurt your baby) – you and your partner may be rewarded with an answering thump.

Week 21

Your uterus will probably be level with, or just below, your navel now. You will probably gain around 5.4 kg (12 lb) during this trimester and you will generally feel much warmer, so you may have a rosy 'glow'. You will also perspire more easily, so wear layers of clothes that you can peel off, if necessary.

Week 22

As your uterus continues to rise and expand within your abdominal cavity your ribcage will move upwards and your lower ribs will spread outwards. You may experience some discomfort and breathlessness as a result.

Week 23

Your abdominal organs and digestive system are being compressed by your growing uterus and baby, so you will probably have some heartburn, indigestion, trapped wind and constipation. Drink plenty of water and try to eat small amounts of food at more frequent intervals.

Week 24

You may feel a little dizzy, especially when you get up suddenly from a sitting or lying-down position. This is perfectly normal, but if it is accompanied by shortness of breath and extreme tiredness, you may be anaemic, so consult your doctor or midwife.

Week 25

Are you bumping into things? You can probably blame it on the hormone relaxin, which is making your joints loosen in preparation for birth. Your extra weight may also put you off balance, so take care, especially when you lean forwards.

Week 26

The weight of your bump and the increased blood flow may also have caused haemorrhoids, which are dilated veins in and around your anus. They can be itchy and sore and may bleed, but are not dangerous to your health or your baby. Try to prevent becoming constipated as this can make things worse. There are a number of things that may help (see pages 161–3).

Week 27

This is the end of the second trimester and you may find that sleeping is becoming more difficult (see pages 206–7). Just as you lie down to relax your baby may become more active and his somersaults may keep you awake. You may find that you have some very vivid dreams.

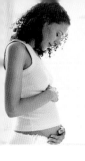

STAGE BY STAGE

In these next few months all your baby's organs, systems and structures that were laid down in the first trimester will grow and develop at an astonishing rate. He will be making his presence known, too, at first with tiny, fluttering movements, but soon with more definite and recognisable kicks.

Week 14

Your baby can roll from side to side and perform a somersault. He sometimes stretches and yawns. He is swallowing small amounts of amniotic fluid (see page 53) and occasionally hiccups. His neck is elongating and the thyroid gland is using iodine from your bloodstream to produce thyroxine, a hormone that helps regulate growth and metabolism.

Week 15

By now, your baby is able to use fat as a source of energy, although most of what he needs is still supplied by glucose that is converted from what you eat (see page 79). Your body is also supplying essential fatty acids that are used in your baby's organs and for the myelin sheaths that enclose and insulate his nerves (see page 64).

Week 16

Your baby has almost reached a peak in his activity levels. He looks more like a newborn now – albeit a miniature version. He often touches his face with his hands and may alter his position in the uterus as often as twenty times in an hour. He makes a wide variety of fluid and quite graceful movements because he has plenty of space and is still incredibly light, so he is almost floating in the amniotic sac.

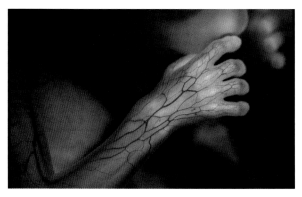

A foetus at the age of 16 weeks. The network of blood vessels for the arm and hand are clearly visible through the thin skin.

Week 17

Your baby's respiratory system is continuing to develop. The trachea (windpipe) is in place and from it bronchi (the lungs' larger air passages) are branching into bronchioles (air passages), which in turn will lead to the alveoli (smallest air passages).

Week 18

Your baby's hands and feet look quite large in relation to the rest of his body – rather as if he is yet to 'grow into' them. Until now, the skin on his feet and hands has been smooth and wrinkle-free, but now ridge patterns begin to emerge on the fingertips and toes. These will appear first on the hands, are genetically determined and will be his unique fingerprints. His skin colour will be determined by the amount of melanin or pigment that his melanocytes (skin cells) produce. Melanin protects the human skin from sunburn and your baby will not produce his full complement until much later in his childhood. This is one of the reasons why young babies should be carefully protected from strong sunshine (they should always wear a hat and be placed under a sunshade).

Week 19

Gradually, your baby is becoming slightly less flexible because the cartilage that has formed his joints is slowly calcifying into bone. His tooth buds (both 'milk' teeth and adult teeth) are already in place in the jaw bones and are collecting calcium. The first teeth to harden will be the front incisors (which will probably be the first ones to appear when he is about six to eight months old).

Week 20

Your baby is now heavier than the placenta. The umbilical cord has grown stronger and thicker and continues to supply your baby with nutrients and blood. It is forming coils, which help to ensure a continuous flow of blood between you and your baby and prevent kinks forming that could put pressure on the umbilical vein and arteries. The abdominal organs, including the stomach, intestines and liver, should now be enclosed behind the abdominal wall.

Week 21

By now your baby will be able to recognise your voice. He will also startle or 'jump' at a sudden loud noise. His brain is picking up electrical signals from his nerves, so he reacts to sensations such as touching his own face. Most of his movements will be unconscious reflex actions, but as the neural pathways develop and mature he will gain greater control of his movements.

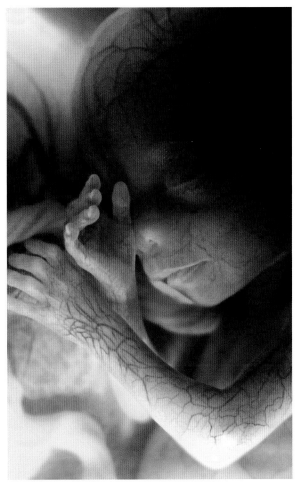

The foetus at 20 weeks.

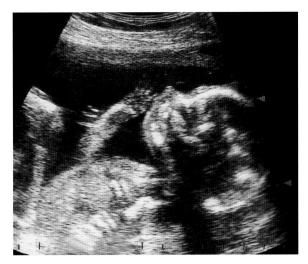

An ultrasound of the foetus at 20 weeks.

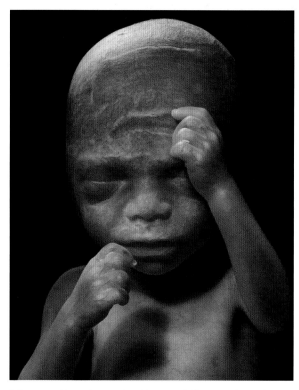

A foetus at about six months old, covered all over in downy hair called 'lanugo' and a waxy vernix, which protects the skin.

COMPARING SIZE

At 16 weeks the foetus is about 108–116 mm (4⅓–4⅔ in) long, or about the size of your palm. At 24 weeks he is about 21 cm (8½ in) long, or about the same length as your elbow to your wrist.

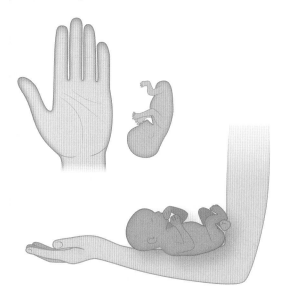

Week 22

Although blood vessels are still visible, your baby's skin is gradually becoming less transparent and is beginning to lay down tiny amounts of fat. His eyelids are still shut to protect his developing eyes from his own fingers and toes.

Within his brain vital connections are being made that will link up with the sense of sight, hearing, touch, taste and smell, to process the information that his body will send back.

Week 23

Most babies who are monitored at this stage of pregnancy show very few differences in their levels of activity in relation to what time of day or night it is, but in the next month or so, there will be more distinct periods of activity or rest taking place. Your baby's eyes are now sometimes moving from side to side, but they are still protected by fused eyelids.

Week 24

By now, your baby's lungs have developed just enough for him to have a one-in-four chance of survival (though, of course, with the help of professional neonatal care) were he to be born now (see pages 298–301).

His anal sphincter muscle is now functioning, so this should help to prevent any meconium (semi-solid waste matter) from being passed into the amniotic fluid.

Meconium is mainly formed from the baby's own discarded cells that were contained in the amniotic fluid he has swallowed (see page 76). This begins to form at around 12 weeks and it passes down into the large bowel at about 16 weeks. Because there are no foreign organisms present in your baby's gut, the meconium is actually sterile. It will be passed by your baby as soft, greenish-black faeces around 24 hours after his birth.

Week 25

By now, every bone in your baby's body contains marrow and stem cells that are capable of producing red and white blood cells and platelets. Once he has been born the platelets will give your baby's body the ability to form a blood clot and so stem the bleeding, should he suffer from a minor injury.

Red blood cells are replaced approximately every 80 days. This is a faster turnover than your own adult body, in which your red blood cells are changed after 120 days.

The white blood cells will help to protect your baby against infection once he has been born. If you breastfeed him, he will also be protected by the antibodies in your colostrum and breast milk. This is partly why breastfed babies have a lower risk of developing asthma or an intolerance of cow's milk and food allergies.

Week 26

Your baby's external ears have been developed for some time and gradually the inner ear is maturing. In order for him to hear properly, the three tiny bones will need to harden. These are the malleus (also known as the 'hammer'), the incus ('anvil') and the stapes ('stirrup').

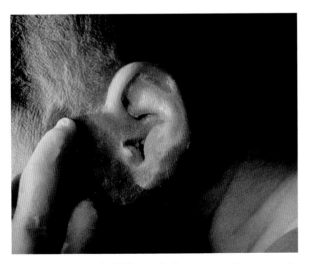

The ear of an 18-week-old foetus; the inner ear won't mature until the age of 26 weeks.

The bones have been initially formed from soft cartilage and protected by connective tissue, but as the soft tissue gradually dissolves and the bones harden, the eardrum can vibrate on the hammer, which then passes the vibrations on to the anvil and the stirrup. The vibrations then travel to a cavity in the inner ear called the cochlea, where they are changed into nerve impulses that are transmitted to the brain.

The inner ear will not only enable your baby to hear a wide range of sounds at varying frequencies, but it will also control his sense of balance.

Week 27

The proportions of your baby's body now become much closer to what they will be when the baby is newly born. Until the third month of pregnancy, his head was as long as the rest of his body, but now his head, trunk and legs each comprise about one-third of his overall length.

Until this point, too, most babies grow at more or less the same rate as each other. However, from this stage on his genetic inheritance and the various environmental factors will kick in and have a much greater influence on what his size and weight will be when he is born.

PLAYING IN THE WOMB

Babies in the womb have been observed to spend some of their time 'playing'. They will often reach out and grab their umbilical cord or get close to the membrane that forms the amniotic sac. Your baby will often bring his hands to his face and may already have a preference for using his left or right hand. Twins seem to begin their interaction as early as after 12 weeks of pregnancy, beginning with one reacting to the touch of the other. More complex movements between them have been observed from week 14 onwards and twins in adjacent amniotic sacs have been seen to take it in turns to 'bat' at each other by pushing against the membrane between them.

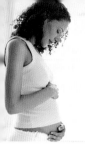

BUILDING BONES

The second trimester is a crucial time for the development of your baby's skeleton. He will be growing and developing 300 bones, so it makes sense for you to do everything you can to help them to grow to their full potential.

In the next three months your baby will go through several rapid growth spurts and to ensure a steady supply of nutrients you need to maintain your balanced diet (see page 78). However, you also need to focus on calcium, magnesium, phosphorus, manganese and vitamin D for strong bones (see pages 138–9). By week 16 all his limbs have formed and his joints can move. His legs have grown tremendously and are now longer than his arms.

Ossification

Apart from his skull, all your baby's bones have soft cartilage at their core that will gradually be reabsorbed and converted into bone (see box right). This process is known as 'ossification' and begins as early as five weeks into pregnancy. At this first stage, the bones have 'primary' ossification centres that are filled with specialised cells producing spongy bone that will later harden as mineralisation takes place.

Mineralisation

Mineralisation is the process, whereby calcium and phosphorus salts start filling in the honeycomb-like chambers of the spongy bone, gradually causing it to harden. This hardening continues all the way into early adulthood, so the process of ossification needs to happen at just the right rate or the bones will be soft and weak. Within this hard bone is the red bone marrow that will later be responsible for the

BONE TURNOVER

Bone turnover is a lifelong process whereby mature bone tissue is removed from the skeleton by cells known as 'osteoclasts' in a process called 'bone resorption'. New bone tissue is then formed (or replaced) by cells called 'osteoblasts'. This is how bone heals itself after damage.

In the first year of your child's life, almost 100 per cent of his skeleton will be renewed and replaced. It is this process of regular renewal that gives bones their thickness and strength, so that by early adulthood they will have reached their optimum condition. After that, around only 10 per cent of an adult's bones are renewed each year and gradually, in middle and old age, bone density decreases, which is why elderly people are at greater risk of suffering from bone fractures. An imbalance of the two processes of removal and formation may result in bone diseases such as osteoporosis. To achieve the right balance requires an adequate supply of calcium, which in turn requires sufficient levels of vitamin D and minerals such as magnesium, manganese and phosphorus (see page 139) to be present, too.

production of red blood cells. In the second trimester, 'secondary' ossification centres form at each end of the bones and it is the part in between (the 'growth plate') that continues to grow and lengthen.

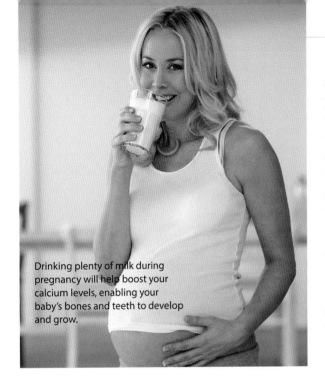

Drinking plenty of milk during pregnancy will help boost your calcium levels, enabling your baby's bones and teeth to develop and grow.

D – the vital vitamin

The crucial importance of vitamin D in bone formation has been overlooked recently. A survey of over 1,000 women, who were either pregnant or trying for a baby, found that around 70 per cent of them were deficient in vitamin D. The problem is especially pronounced in dark-skinned women because vitamin D is absorbed from sunlight and stored under the surface of the skin. Darker skin is better protected from ultraviolet rays (UV), but that also means that it requires greater amounts of sunshine to be able to absorb enough vitamin D.

Drop in exposure to sunlight

In recent decades, with the dangers of skin cancer in mind, sunbathing has been seen as a risky activity and as we have lessened the amount of time spent in the sun, the chances of absorbing enough vitamin D from this source have also dropped. We may think of rickets as a disease associated with poverty and poor nutrition, but in the 21st century there is an increasing number of mothers with low levels of vitamin D in their breast milk. Low levels of sunshine mean that it is advisable to take a supplement during the winter, and it is not easy to get adequate amounts

from food. Current recommendation across the population is 400 iu (10 mcg), but pregnant women need more. If you have entered pregnancy with diabetes, polycystic ovary syndrome or an autoimmune problem, or if you have had IVF and are taking medications such as heparin and steroids, you might request a vitamin D blood test. You may then be advised to take a supplement. However, taking overly high doses of vitamin D can be toxic. If you have not been tested, take it as part of a supplement, but be guided by your doctor or midwife.

SUN FOR VITAMIN D – DO'S & DON'TS

Vitamin D is found in a small number of foods (see page 84), but exposure to sun is one of the best ways to get your quota. These tips for staying safe in the sun are based on Oliver Gillie's recommendations in *Sunlight Robbery:*

Do expose your skin (especially arms and legs) when you can In the UK, the middle of the day is a good time for sunbathing because UVB, which generates vitamin D in skin, is most intense at this time, but expose your skin for short periods only (see below). Make sure that you drink plenty of water to stay well hydrated and never get too hot

Do remove as many clothes as you can in the sun. Begin by exposing your skin for just two to three minutes on your back or front (sit, or lie propped up), then increase from day to day to a maximum of half an hour in the UK, or less abroad

Do be cautious. Remember that the sun's intensity varies with the season, the time of day and amount of cloud. Allow for differences in skin tone, so only do what suits your skin

Don't use sunscreen creams while aiming to boost vitamin D

If you feel hot or uncomfortable, expose a different area of your body, cover up or move into the shade. If you cannot avoid continued exposure, use a sunscreen

The face is easily over-exposed and pregnant women are prone to chloasma (see page 105), so wear a hat

If you are in very strong sun abroad, expose your body for much shorter periods than you would in the UK

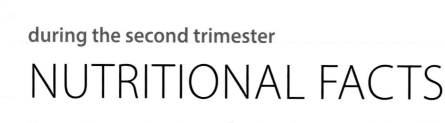

NUTRITIONAL FACTS

Key nutrients, vitamins and minerals are needed at this stage of your pregnancy to ensure the good health of your baby's bones and teeth – and the maintenance of your own, too.

The placenta is now growing at an even faster rate than your baby: and the larger and healthier it is the more nutrients pass across it. Continue to choose foods from each of the major food groups (see page 78), but help your baby's skeleton to develop to its full potential, with good sources of calcium, magnesium, phosphorus, manganese and vitamin D (see opposite).

During the next twelve weeks aim to eat around 200–300 extra calories per day of nutrient-rich foods. Really good nutrition in the first and second trimesters will determine your baby's growth and birth weight (see pages 18–19). If you cut back on what you eat and slow the supply of nutrients because you are nervous of gaining weight, you could deprive your baby of vital elements and the result may be growth restriction (see page 192).

A varied diet

Magnesium, phosphorus and manganese are also needed as part of the delicate balance of vitamins and minerals that help your baby's bones and teeth to develop to their full potential. You should be able to get all the magnesium, manganese and phosphorus you need via a varied diet (see pages 78–85). Consult a doctor or nutrionist before taking supplements. Besides making sure you have a good supply of these vitamins and minerals in the second trimester, make sure that you eat foods that contain plenty of iron, zinc and essential fatty acids (EFAs) (see page 43).

WHY YOU NEED PLENTY OF VITAMIN D

It is well known that calcium is vital for strong bones and teeth, where about about 99 per cent of the body's stores are found, but it is also needed for other parts of the body, including brain-cell development, blood clotting and muscle contraction. Over the course of your pregnancy you will need to transfer about a 30 g (1 oz) of calcium to your baby. Your body can become very efficient at making this available, but if you are not eating foods that supply the extra amount you need for your baby (see pages 136–7) it will be drawn from your body's own reserves. If your levels of vitamin D are deficient, calcium absorption will be affected and low levels will have negative effects on you and your baby's health. Vitamin D is also needed in a number of other important ways:

Aids the development of babies' brain cells

Linked with optimal health and a reduced risk of cancer

The babies of mothers with higher vitamin D levels seem to have a lower incidence of respiratory infections

During pregnancy adequate levels are associated with healthy bone mass and body weight

May help to prevent miscarriage and pre-eclampsia (see pages 120–1 and 208–9)

Strengthens babies' heart muscles and helps to prevent heart failure

Studies have shown that infants given vitamin D supplements have a reduced risk of type 1 diabetes

MAGNESIUM, PHOSPHORUS & MANGANESE

Mineral	Best sources	Benefits
Magnesium	Green, leafy vegetables such as spinach and kale, nuts, wholemeal bread, fish, meat and dairy products	Magnesium is a crucial part of many enzymes involved in the respiration system. It aids the transmission of nerve impulses, is necessary to help muscle relaxation, helps to regulate body temperature and maintain a healthy pH balance in the body, assists the absorption and utilisation of calcium, phosphorus, sodium, potassium and vitamins C, E and D
Phosphorus	Bread, dairy products, fish, oats, poultry, red meat and rice	Helps to release energy from the food you eat, builds strong teeth and bones
Manganese	Bread, cereals, nuts, tea and green vegetables such as runner beans and peas	Helps to turn the food you eat into energy and enables the normal function of the parathyroid glands, which produce hormones important for bone health

MEAL IDEAS FOR THE SECOND TRIMESTER

Choose from the following (organic options if possible):

Breakfast

Fortified cereal (cornflakes with semi-skimmed milk topped with sliced banana and sunflower seeds)

Homemade muesli (oats, fortified wheatgerm, sliced or grated Brazil nuts, dried or fresh fruit and seeds) with semi-skimmed milk

Wholemeal toast with butter and yeast extract and slices of hard cheese

Natural yogurt with figs, dried apricots, or fruit purée, topped with sliced almonds

Scrambled egg on wholemeal toast and orange juice

Lunch

Wholemeal bread or pitta sandwich filled with salad and sunflower seeds and hummus or avocado

Baked potato with grated cheese and a mixed salad topped with sunflower seeds and/or pine nuts

Broccoli soup, wholemeal bread and cheese

Baked cheese, spinach and tomato omelette with salad

Grilled sardines on wholemeal toast spread with butter/polyunsaturated margarine, served with crunchy seed/nut-topped salad

Supper

Baked fish cooked on a bed of vegetables such as peppers, courgettes, carrots and fennel

Tofu, baby corn, mangetout and cashew nut stir-fry served with brown rice

Grilled mackerel with gooseberry sauce, potatoes steamed or baked in their jackets and curly kale

Chicken baked with lemon and thyme and served with lightly cooked green beans, curly kale and peas served with rice or steamed potatoes

Grilled, thinly sliced beef or whole salmon steak with sweetcorn, baked potatoes and runner beans

Puddings and desserts

Baked bananas with lemon juice and honey

Vanilla panna cotta served with fresh figs

Natural yogurt with dried apricot purée, crushed nectarines and bananas, sprinkled with sliced or grated Brazil nuts

Snacks

Raw vegetable sticks and hummus

Nuts and grapes or prunes

Celery sticks with cottage cheese, walnuts and apple

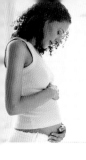

POSTURE & EXERCISES

During this second trimester, you will undergo some dramatic physical changes and your bump will become larger and heavier. Stretching and strengthening exercises will help your body to cope.

Perfect posture

As your baby grows, your pelvis tends to tilt forwards, creating a deeper curve in your lower back. This can lead to back pain and other related aches and pains in your neck, shoulders, hips and even arms. One of the best ways to counteract this is to pull your tummy button in towards your spine at all times. This activates a band of muscle around your abdomen called your transverse abdominus, which helps support your growing bump and takes the pressure off your back.

Good stretches

The pull of your growing bump can lead to the tightening of certain muscle groups, while others are being stretched and weakened. Muscles that can become tight tend to be in your lower back, chest, hip flexors and quads (thighs) and the muscles that are most often stretched are your abdominals, upper and middle back, bottom and hamstrings. So your aim in any exercise is to gently work the stretched, weakened muscles using light weights, resistance bands or your own body weight and to gradually stretch muscles that have a tendency to tighten.

It's also a good idea to stretch through your chest muscles as these are likely to get tighter as your breasts grow. Do not hold any stretches for too long, though. Ten seconds should be the maximum because the hormone relaxin will have altered the elasticity of your joints.

BASIC POSTURE TIPS

Try to 'stand tall' and loosen and push your shoulders back so that you open out your chest. Make sure that you don't lean too far back to try to compensate for the forward pull of your bump and keep your knees soft, so that they are not 'locked'. At first, you will probably find that you have to make a special effort to correct your posture, but with practice you will gradually find that a well-balanced stance comes more naturally to you. Wear flat shoes and try tilting your pelvis up and under slightly when you are standing. If you do have to wear heels, limit the amount of time that you spend in them as this can increase the pressure on your lower back.

Push your shoulders back

Don't lean too far back

Pull your tummy button in towards your spine at all times

Tilt your pelvis up and under slightly when you are standing

Wear flat shoes or just have bare feet when you are at home

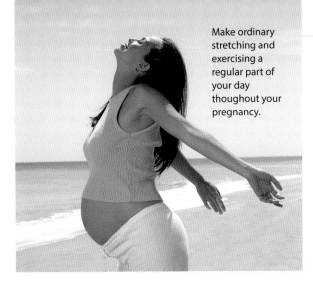

Make ordinary stretching and exercising a regular part of your day throughout your pregnancy.

CURL-DOWNS FOR FLEXIBILITY

Curl-downs are one of the best and simplest ways to maintain flexibility and mobility in your spine:

Stand with your feet comfortably apart, keep your knees 'soft' and curl your neck and back, one vertebra at a time, down towards the floor, starting with your head, all the way down to your lower back

After a deep breath in that position, reverse the movement so that you are coming back up to a standing position, stacking your vertebra on your tail bone, one at a time, from your lower back to your head

Pelvic floor exercises

Start pelvic floor exercises as soon as you know you are pregnant, to begin building strength and stamina. The muscles that support your urethra and rectum will have to work extra hard to support the weight of your growing baby and having a strong pelvic floor will also limit stress incontinence. This is important for avoiding leaking urine every time you cough or lift something heavy. Strong pelvic floor muscles may also help you in the second stage of labour. Practise them regularly – 50 times a day is ideal. Set aside special time to focus on your pelvic floor exercises – that way you'll make sure you do them properly without getting distracted. Try doing them lying down, with your knees bent and back supported.

DOING PELVIC FLOOR EXERCISES

It is tricky, but try not to hold your breath, pull your tummy in or tense your buttocks while doing these pelvic floor exercises. These muscles tire quite quickly at first, so don't be disheartened if you cannot 'hold' the positions for as long as is recommended to start with. Keep practising and your strength and stamina will increase.

In each session make sure that you use at least one of the 'slow' exercises combined with the 'fast' one, so that you are toning all your pelvic floor muscles:

'Slow' exercises

Squeeze and hold Tighten all the muscles around your vagina and anus and try to draw them upwards and inwards. Try to hold for 5–10 seconds and repeat 10 times.

Pyramid Think of your pelvic floor as being the four corners of a pyramid – the front of the pyramid is your pubic bone, the two sides of the pyramid are your 'sitting bones' and the back of the pyramid is your back bone/coccyx. Focus on pulling in the muscles from the front, the sides and the back to the top point of the 'pyramid' – you are essentially pulling in all the four corners together and then up inside you. Hold for 5–10 seconds and repeat 10 times.

Lift to fifth floor Repeat the same action as the 'pyramid', except this time focus on pulling the muscles up inside you, imagining a lift going up to the first floor, higher again to the second floor, third, fourth and fifth floor and then releasing all the way down to the 'basement' before returning to the ground floor and repeating. Try 5–10 repetitions.

'Fast' exercise

Squeeze and release Because you have different types of muscle fibres in your pelvic floor, you also need to perform quicker repetitions – pull all four 'corners' of your pelvic floor in as firmly and as quickly as possible and then immediately release. Repeat 20 times.

Note: Go to the bathroom before you start. Don't try to stop urination mid-stream. It may lead to urine going back into the bladder and causing infection.

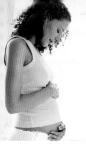

thinking about your

MATERNITY WEAR

Fortunately, the coy Peter Pan collars and girlish florals of yesteryear's maternity wear has been replaced by much more glamorous, style-conscious clothes. There is a great selection to choose from, but if resources are limited, you can get away with a few key pieces.

There's no need to rush out to buy maternity clothes straight away. You will certainly be able to make do with your existing clothes for a few months, at least. Perhaps, for example, you could cover slightly open trouser zips with longer shirts or tops. But by about week 20, or slightly earlier if this is not your first pregnancy, you may need to invest in a few items of proper maternity wear.

Designed to fit

Maternity clothes are designed to drape over your expanding bump without riding up in front or at the back. Tucks and darts will be in the right places, too, so that your clothes hang well without bunching up or puckering. If you carry on wearing ordinary clothes but in larger sizes you may find that they are too tight and too loose in the wrong places and that hemlines pull up higher at the front than the back.

Build up gradually

Begin with a few items and add more as you get bigger. Choose long, loosely fitting dresses, tops or soft, stretchy T-shirts. Think about whether you'll be wearing the items for work or at home. If you need

USEFUL MATERNITY ITEMS

Maternity briefs can fit under your bump if they are of the mini variety, or over it if they are more generously cut. Choose whatever style is most comfortable for you. If you are expecting more than one baby and you suffer from backache, you may find that maternity support briefs are a real plus

Maternity tights and leggings have waistbands that will sit above your bump and so they are far more comfortable than the ordinary variety. Although they won't restrict your bump, hold-up hose are less suitable in pregnancy because they can restrict the blood flow to your legs and possibly cause varicose veins. Maternity support tights are available, offering light, medium or firm support and they can be very useful if your job demands periods of standing

Abdominal bump support belts may be helpful at the end of your pregnancy (especially if you are expecting twins or more) and after the birth too, but don't wear them all the time as they could cause abdominal muscles to weaken

Belly bands are a real boon for providing that little extra support.

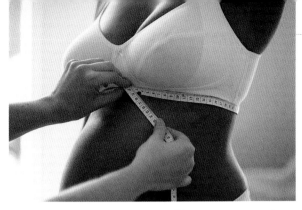

When finding out your bra size, start off by measuring around your ribcage underneath your bust.

to look smart, try a maternity suit of either trousers or skirt and add a variety of tops. Maternity trousers and jeans can be useful for weekends and they have stretchy panels or extra buttons so that they can be adjusted as your bump expands.

You can buy maternity clothes from specialised maternity wear retailers either on the high street or online. Some online companies offer a capsule pregnancy wardrobe that can be a good basic foundation on which to build. If you are planning to breastfeed and want your clothes to be useful after the birth, too, you might want to choose clothes that allow you to feed your baby without pulling your top up or taking things off, and many maternity tops have panels that allow quick and discreet access.

Accept offers of cast-off maternity clothes; they will expand your repertoire, but always buy new maternity underwear. Bras need to fit properly to give you the support you need (see box right).

Shoes are important

High heels are not recommended during pregnancy. They may be uncomfortable and, combined with the weight of your bump, may throw your posture forwards, resulting in backache. Ballet pumps, loafers or low-heeled court shoes may suit smart occasions and trainers will give you soft support at other times. Your feet may swell by the end of your pregnancy and you may need to buy an inexpensive pair of pumps in a larger size than normal. At home, try to walk around in bare feet as much as possible. This will give all parts of your feet a natural flex.

THE IMPORTANCE OF MATERNITY BRAS

Perhaps your most essential maternity garments will be your bras. Breasts have no muscles of their own and so are held up by the muscles of the chest wall. As your pregnancy progresses, your breasts will enlarge (possibly by several cup sizes) and become much heavier. A properly fitting bra will help to prevent them from sagging and may also make stretch marks less likely to develop. It is best to go to a specialist maternity-wear retailer or the lingerie department of a big store and be professionally measured. You may need to do this several times during your pregnancy and as soon as your bra feels tight, you should buy a new one. If your breasts feel particularly heavy, you could also buy a sleep bra that will give you soft support while you sleep. When buying a maternity bra look for:

A style that is mostly made from cotton This will allow your skin to breathe more easily (remember that your body temperature is slightly higher than normal when you are pregnant, so you may perspire more easily)

Broad shoulder straps Wide adjustable straps will distribute the weight of your breasts more evenly and are less likely to dig in or chafe

An adjustable back strap Several fastenings will allow you to alter the back strap as your ribcage expands to accommodate your growing baby. When you buy your bra, make sure that it can be comfortably worn it on the tightest fastening, so that you can expand from there

A wide band of elastic under the cups This will help to support your breasts and stop the bra from riding up

A maternity/nursing bra From around week 36 you could opt for a nursing bra to see you through the last stages of pregnancy and the weeks after the birth. Nursing bras are very similar to maternity bras, but enable you to feed your baby without taking it off. You can choose from drop cups (where each cup unhooks from the shoulder strap), zip cups (that usually unzip from under the breast) or front-opening designs. Try on each type to see what suits you best and practise opening and closing the cup fastening with one hand – this is what you will have to do when you are holding your wriggling baby

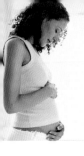

MIND-BODY-BABY

By now you have probably got into the swing of being pregnant and you may be in the 'honeymoon' period, with lots more energy plus a renewed sense of well-being. Now is the time to start communicating with your baby on a much deeper level.

Hopefully, in your first trimester you practised the visualisation techniques for that first stage of pregnancy (see page 110). Now you can move on to the next phase. Screening tests should now be out of the way (see pages 154–5) and you will probably be feeling much more confident about the health of your baby. Ultrasound scans will have given you those first precious glimpses of what he looks like (see pages 74–5). If you have had a 3-D scan you will have seen your baby's face quite clearly, but whatever image you have in your mind, you can now use it to deepen your emotional bond.

All of your baby's organs are now formed and will gradually be maturing in the months to come. In fact, so much will happen in the next twelve weeks – your pregnancy will really begin to show and you will feel those magical first movements.

Introduce your baby to some of your favourite music. Sing to him and talk. You can tell him how

HYPNOBIRTHING

Hypnobirthing is a birth education programme that teaches simple but specific self-hypnosis, relaxation and breathing techniques. Classes are available to help you to manage your labour and to be able to cope with the pain more easily. Classes usually start from between 25 and 29 weeks, which may sound rather early, but it is important to be able to practise the techniques on a daily basis, and you may find them useful for dealing with other fears and anxieties, too.

Hypnobirthing doesn't involve you being in a trance or asleep. Rather, you should be relaxed and calm, but in control. This enables you to cope with the pain and encourages your body to release endorphins (the feel-good hormones) to replace the stress hormones that make your body more tense. At the classes you will learn how to:

Use self-hypnosis and relaxation techniques to gain confidence and remain calm

Find comfortable and productive positions to use during labour and birth

Understand the way that the neuromuscular system functions in your body – and work with it

Use breathing (not panting), massage and visualisation techniques

You can take your parter along, too. One benefit is that if he or she intends to be present at the labour, they can really help to keep you focused and so play a much more active role. And while hypnobirthing cannot guarantee you a completely pain-free labour, many studies have shown that it can really help.

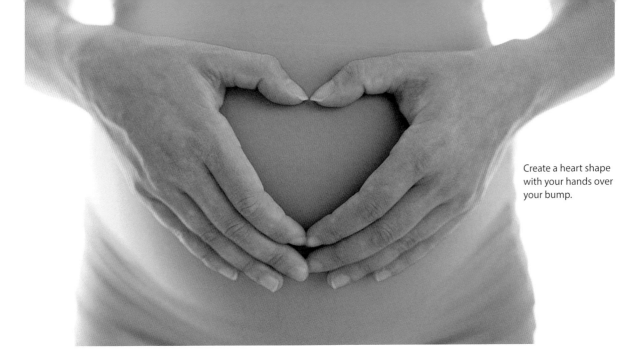

Create a heart shape with your hands over your bump.

much you are looking forward to holding him, what the rest of his family is like, how much you long for him – the point is that you are making a connection on a very deep, personal level. Choose a quiet time and find privacy, where no one can overhear you – then spend some quality time with your baby.

Bonding visualisation

Try this visualisation technique:

- Make yourself comfortable – perhaps by lying down on your bed or on a couch.
- Place your hands in a heart-shaped position with your thumbs to your tummy button and your fingers pointing to your pubic bone. This helps you to make a connection with your baby.
- Close your eyes and begin to breathe slowly. Let thoughts drift in and out of your mind.
- Imagine a stream of light passing down through the top of your head to your forehead and down through your cheekbones. Feel yourself relaxing as the light reaches your jawbone.
- Release any tension, allowing your lips to part a little and your tongue to relax in your mouth.
- Send the light down through your neck and shoulders; feel your muscles relax one by one, as it continues down through your arms and hands.

- Now imagine the light flowing down through an imaginary line in the centre of your body. This is an acupuncture meridian called the Conception Vessel.
- Just imagine, for a minute or so, that place between your breasts, where you have that connection with the heart, where you feel love, warmth and deep relaxation. The hormones you produce when you are content are the 'love hormones', including oxytocin, which is sent through your body after the birth to help you bond with your baby.
- Allow the light to travel down into your uterus and picture your baby's little body. His fingers and toes may be curled up or wriggling. He is snug, safe and secure. He is responding to your calm, relaxed state with your heartbeat slowly beating as his backdrop. He is thriving and growing at an amazing rate.
- Visualise the umbilical cord allowing all the nourishment that you are taking in to pass through to your baby. You are also sending all those wonderful 'happy hormones' and the amazing love, warmth and emotion that you feel for him.
- Think of how your baby is connecting to you, that he is conscious and becoming aware of your love.
- Stay with this for a while and then allow the stream of light to pass on down to your knees and lower legs, feeling calm and relaxed.

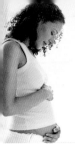

you & your baby
COPING WITH STRESS

Pregnancy is one of the most challenging experiences in a woman's life and some stress is inevitable. If it is prolonged, it can affect both you and your baby, so it is important that you understand what causes it and how to cope with it.

How the brain reacts to stress

Depending on the stress or stressors, the pituitary gland in the brain and the adrenal glands, which sit at the top of the kidneys, determine the amount of the stress hormone cortisol to release.

The effects of cortisol

Research has shown that having high levels of cortisol in an expectant mother's body over a long period of time is detrimental to the developing baby as it can cross the placenta. Unborn babies who are repeatedly exposed to high levels of stress chemicals can then have their own stress response system distorted, so that it becomes unable to regulate itself. Therefore, the baby, child and later the adult will overreact to stress and his response to quite minor stressors may be overwhelming fear, anxiety or rage.

It is easy to see, then, why a baby who has been severely stressed before his birth may be difficult to settle and comfort once he has been born. Gentle, calm parenting can do a lot to make the situation better and the baby's ability to cope can be much improved, but of course it is better to try to avoid the stressful situation in the first place.

How your body responds

In a stressful situation, the brain sends a signal to the adrenals to produce adrenalin and cortisol. These compounds increase your blood pressure, heart rate and breathing, and raise your blood sugar levels, preparing the body for a 'fight or flight' predicament. Adrenalin kicks in quickly, but cortisol tends to stay in the system for longer.

This reaction is perfectly normal when it happens occasionally, but if you become stuck in a more continuous stress response, the reaction can become chronic. The constant presence of cortisol in your body also uses up B and C vitamins, so you can easily become depleted of these vital nutrients – you may therefore need to boost these.

NEUROTRANSMITTERS

The brain communicates with the rest of the body and body systems via neurotransmitters (chemicals made from proteins). They are produced in varying amounts in response to the different situations that you encounter (such as feeling in danger when you are crossing a busy road). The key neurotransmitters for stress are:

Adrenalin	Endorphins
Cortisol	Serotonin
Dopamine	Acetylcholine

Many of these are also involved in giving us 'feel-good' chemicals. Whether we feel 'good' or 'bad' depends on how they are balanced.

BLOOD SUGAR BLUES

The levels of 'sugar' (glucose) in your blood are affected by stimulants, sugar and additives in your diet, and by stress. Blood glucose needs to be properly balanced for your body to function properly. If it is too low (hypoglycaemia) you will feel shaky, sweaty and hungry. If it is too high, hyperglycaemia will result. Both conditions are associated with diabetes (see page 72), but everyone experiences the symptoms on a mild level when they have the sudden 'high' of too much sugar in the blood. After this sugar 'hit' (which may be caused by stress rather than food), the blood-sugar level falls abruptly and as a result, you can feel tired, anxious and irritable. To relieve the discomfort you may then reach for sources of sugar, perpetuating a vicious cycle. We probably all feel the 'mid-afternoon slump' from time to time: this is why. The answer is to regulate your food and drink intake more carefully and eat slow-release carbohydrates (see page 79) and to practise managing your stress levels (see pages 108–9).

The effect of stress on you

Effects may include:

• Suppression of your immune system
• Depletion of your vital nutrients
• Slowing down of your metabolism
• Slowing down of your body's ability to repair itself

The effect of stress on your baby

The developing unborn baby is particularly susceptible to stress chemicals and hormones from the mother in the third trimester, when his brain is developing rapidly (see pages 182–3). A certain level of cortisol is good for the baby and levels naturally rise towards the end of pregnancy to help his organs, such as the lungs, to mature. However, if the levels are continually high, your baby will be in an anxious state, his own levels of stress hormone will rise and it may not only influence his response to stress (see opposite) but also affect his cognitive function. The cortisol in your adult body has physical effects on both of you and speeds up the heartbeat and constricts the blood vessels. So for your baby, this can mean that stress restricts the flow of oxygen and nutrients that he needs to grow in the womb.

WHAT YOU CAN DO

There are a number of things that you can do to ease stress and anxiety in your life. Start by looking at your lifestyle and identifying what causes you the most stress (see pages 108–9). Then you can try to make any necessary changes to alleviate them. An improvement in your diet and some relaxation techniques such as visualisation (see pages 110–11) and deep breathing will also help.

Avoid eating highly refined or sugary foods and opt for complex carbohydrates that release energy slowly and steadily (see page 79)

Boost your intake of B vitamins, which are essential for the smooth running of the nervous system and for adrenal production. Vitamins B_1, B_2, B_3, B_6, B_{12}, calcium, magnesium and omega-3 are all important and can be found in a range of foods (see pages 43 and 84–5).

Eat plenty of zinc-rich foods (see page 85)

Avoid stimulants such as caffeine

Try this deep-breathing exercise. Lie (propped up) or sit comfortably. Place one hand with the palm flat on your chest just below your collarbones. Place the other on your abdomen, over your tummy button. Breathe in through your nose deeply and slowly. Then breathe out in the same way. You should aim for around 12 to 15 breaths per minute. You may also find that listening to music as you do this increases your level of relaxation

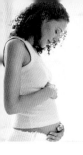

how to deal with

'DAD ISSUES'

Now that your partner is in the second trimester of her pregnancy, there will be plenty of practical things for you to do and help with, but have you also begun to make emotional preparations for your new role, too?

If you have an image of fatherhood in your head, perhaps you are looking forward to being able to kick a football around or have a game of rough-and-tumble with your child. The idea of a helpless baby in your arms may seem almost impossible to imagine – but try.

Your relationship with your child can begin as soon as you know about the pregnancy. How you interact with your partner affects not just her, but sets the tone for your relationship with your baby, too. You will soon be a family and that will require all sorts of adjustments to be made.

Strengthening bonds

The birth of a baby brings untold rewards, but also some acute stressors. However good your relationship is with your partner, there will be areas of division and the challenges of parenthood will test it out to the full. Pregnancy is a great opportunity to strengthen the bonds between you and to find ways of settling differences that do not upset the equilibrium of the family unit.

Addressing differences

It is estimated that around 80 per cent of conflicts in close relationships are unresolved and if they are not too serious you can probably learn to live with them. However, major differences do need to be addressed, but the key to a harmonious emotional life is

empathy. Empathy does not require a solution – only understanding. It is often mismatched expectations that can cause resentments, so if you talk about 'sharing' the care of your baby, look at what you really mean. As the father, do you plan to work part time? Or do you hope to get home early from work to feed and bathe your baby before you cook the evening meal? Both these scenarios are difficult to achieve in our competitive modern world, but your partner may be hoping that late-night working and evenings in the bar will be a thing of the past for you once your baby is born.

Making space

It is hard for expectant parents to think about the reality of life with a baby. During pregnancy, you are both so focused on the nine months of gestation and the D-Day of your baby's birth that it's all too easy to forget that the real challenges and pleasures come after the baby is born.

If you can discuss vital issues such as the division of practical tasks before you actually have to cope with them, then you have a better chance of parenting your baby as a team and remaining close as a couple (see pages 350–1). Acquiring the necessary baby equipment and making space in your home for your baby is very important, but more essential is the space that you make in your life and the feelings that you have for your child.

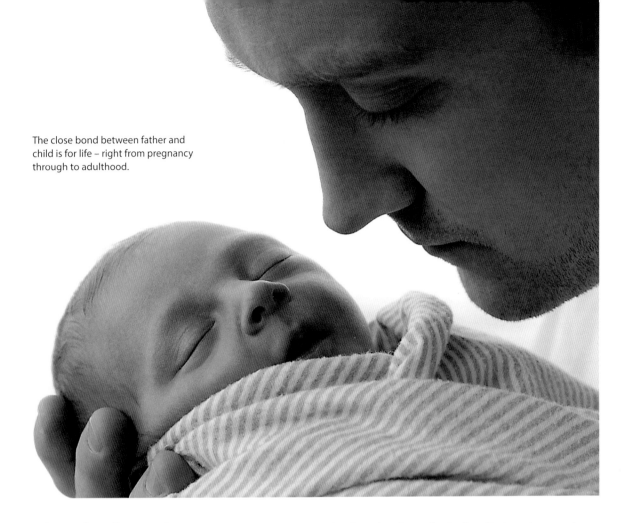

The close bond between father and child is for life – right from pregnancy through to adulthood.

How do you handle stress?

When you are tired and under pressure, do you find it easy to talk about the tension that you are feeling or do you find yourself becoming withdrawn or even angry and argumentative?

Up until now, when you have felt stressed, you might have slumped in front of the television, had a heated discussion with your partner or gone to the pub, but once you have a baby in your home, you will have to put your baby's needs first.

Studies have shown that babies less than six months old experience significant physiological changes, such as a markedly increased heart rate, raised blood pressure and a surge of stress hormones if they hear or see their parents arguing. Babies brought up in emotionally unstable homes have been found to be far less able to deal with stress and regulate their emotions, which of course in turn make them harder to look after. So it makes good sense to try to find some strategies for dealing with conflict – and most importantly to find ways of averting it. This doesn't mean that you should bottle up any negative feelings for the sake of peace and quiet, but there are ways of expressing them without causing hurt and distress.

A rewarding mission

There is no point in pretending that life as a new parent is easy, but becoming a father may be the most rewarding and worthwhile thing you will ever do. In the first year of parenthood there will be tough challenges: a lack of sleep, perhaps a strain on finances, an unequal workload, a reduced sex life and perhaps feelings of isolation. But life with your baby will also provide you with fun, laughter, fascination, pride as well as deep and lasting love.

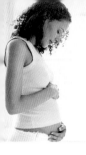

RELATIONSHIPS

Now that you have moved on into the second trimester, you will probably be sharing your news with more of those closest to you. Your baby will be having a relationship with them in the future, too, so it's a good idea to build some firm foundations.

If you already have one or more other children you may be feeling anxious about telling them about the new baby and seeing how they react. If your pregnancy has complications that have required you to be absent (perhaps in hospital) then you might have decided to tell your children about it sooner than the second trimester. The sudden disappearance of a parent can be very worrying for younger ones especially, so explanations and reassurance are surely better than trying to 'protect' young children from such things through ignorance.

If all is going smoothly, you may have delayed telling your children until the second trimester. As your pregnancy progresses it will become more obvious, and it is much better that they should hear the news from you than from someone else, so now may be a good time to start the discussion.

Making adjustments

Your children will need time to adjust to the news. Most are thrilled at the idea of a new sibling, but some are less enthusiastic. Young children take time to process information, so don't force the issue. They may come back to it later. If so, continue the discussion and reassure them that all will be well.

It is difficult for young children to grasp the concept of time and so they may find months of waiting rather frustrating. Whether they are keen on the idea of the new arrival or not, you can use this time to get them involved (see right). They may worry that you might not love them as much as the new baby. You may also be feeling anxious about having 'enough' love to go around. This is a common fear and can seem a shameful one. However parental love is limitless and you will find that you love all your children with the same intensity. Keep reassuring them that your love is without bounds and always will be.

IF YOU ARE ON YOUR OWN

If you are pregnant and on your own, it can be hard, whatever your circumstances, and it is not a sign of weakness to ask for help. Having sole responsibility for your baby can feel overwhelming at times (especially when you are coping with fluctuating hormones, too). It will make life much easier if you can enlist some help. Think about close family and friends and their different strengths. Some may be able to help in practical ways, while you can rely on others for emotional support.

If your family are not available, perhaps your closest friends could help. Not all your friends may be ready to take on a significant role in your child's life, but some may and you and your baby will be all the richer for it. If your friends really aren't cut out to share your pregnancy on a deeper level, ask your midwife about local support groups or contact single parent organisations (see Resources).

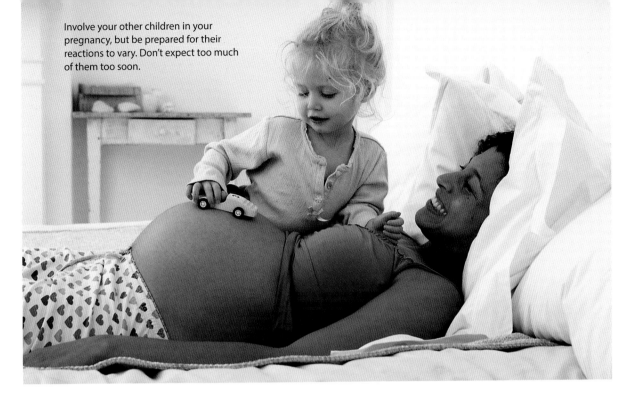

Involve your other children in your pregnancy, but be prepared for their reactions to vary. Don't expect too much of them too soon.

Ways to involve & reassure other children

- Explain that although the new baby will be unable to play for a while, he will be ready to give love to his big sister or brother, too.
- Encourage your child to talk to, gently pat and stroke your bump. She may feel a kick.
- Set aside time to give your child undivided attention. Cuddle up and read a book, do some drawing together or go for a walk.
- Encourage your older child to ask questions and to talk about her feelings. If you know what's worrying her, you can do something about it.
- Go clothes shopping with your child and let them choose a few items for the baby.
- Try not to discuss pregnancy symptoms in front of your child. If you seem unwell it may worry her.
- Explain that the new baby will need a lot of attention, but that you will still have time for your child. If they know what to expect, they are less likely to feel resentful.
- Involve your older one in some of the preparations. Explain what things like changing mats and nappy bins are for. Let her look at everything and suggest that she might like to help when the baby arrives.

Involving the older generation

While the news of your pregnancy brings excitement and joy to parents and in-laws, it can also alter your relationship with them. If your parents are available, you may find their love and support more valuable now. If you are finding it hard to cope with tiredness, they may be able to offer practical help. You may just want to find out more about your own birth and babyhood. However, if your parents are no longer around, their absence can feel more pronounced, but perhaps an older friend can step into the role. You may find that your relationship with your parents or in-laws becomes more difficult. They may offer 'advice' more often than you would like and you may also find that you have rather different ideas (see page 351). Try to talk to your partner and make sure that you back each other up. If you show you are making decisions together you may find that 'suggestions' are a little more sensitively put.

You, your partner and your baby will all benefit from the extended family. And as your baby grows, his relationship with them can help to give him love, security and the benefit of accumulated wisdom on everything from table manners to family history.

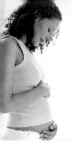

ANTENATAL CARE

Now that you have reached the second trimester of your pregnancy it is time for another antenatal appointment. This will reassure you that you and your baby are progressing well.

A t around 16 weeks, you will probably have your second antenatal appointment. If you haven't already received them, you will be given the results of any tests you had at your first booking appointment (see pages 70–1). Depending on these and other factors, such as your age, you may then be offered further tests (see pages 154–5).

Routine checks

You will have your blood pressure taken and your urine will be tested for sugar and protein. Almost 50 per cent of women have some sugar in their urine at their booking appointment and if the level is high, they may be advised to cut back on sweet foods. If this applies to you and your urine still shows significant levels of sugar at the second appointment, you may be offered a glucose-tolerance test check for developing gestational diabetes (see page 72).

What protein presence indicates

Normally, your kidneys filter out all the protein from your urine, but in pregnancy increased blood flow can place an extra burden on them. If protein is detected, it will need to be investigated. It may indicate that you have a urine infection, which you are more prone to in pregnancy because the tubes that connect your urethra with your bladder and your kidneys is relaxed by pregnancy hormones (see pages 36–7). If there is an infection, you will need prompt treatment in the form of antibiotics

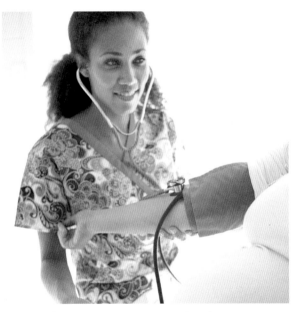

Your midwife will keep a close eye on your blood pressure throughout your pregnancy.

because if the problem reaches your kidneys it can irritate the uterus and there is risk of miscarriage. In later pregnancy, protein in the urine can be a sign of pre-eclampsia (see pages 208–9), so expect to have your urine tested at further appointments, too.

Supplements

If previous blood tests revealed low levels of haemoglobin, you may be offered an iron supplement. Your midwife may also listen to your baby's heartbeat.

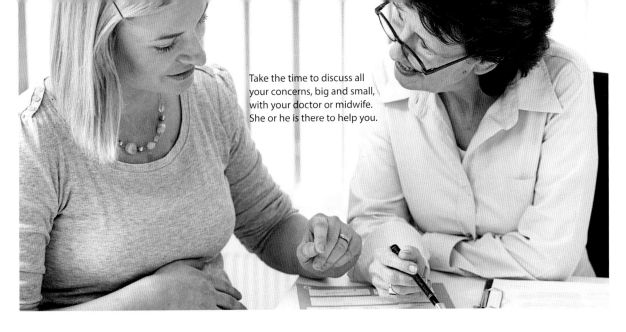

Take the time to discuss all your concerns, big and small, with your doctor or midwife. She or he is there to help you.

HOW TO DECODE YOUR ANTENATAL NOTES

Now that you will be keeping a copy of your notes with you at all times, it may be useful to understand some of the abbreviations that are used in your records. Do take care, though, because not all hospitals and midwives use the same terms, so if in doubt, ask for an explanation:

Primagravida First pregnancy

Multigravida Subsequent pregnancy

Hb Haemoglobin levels

BP Blood pressure – the average blood pressure for adult women is around 120/70. A persistent increase of 20 or more in either figure at the next reading may indicate a higher risk of pre-eclampsia (see pages 208–9)

Length of pregnancy For example: 16+4 (16 weeks and four days pregnant)

FHH Foetal heart heard

FHHR Foetal heart heard and regular

FHNR Foetal heart not heard (don't panic if you see this – your baby may just have been lying in an awkward position)

FMF Foetal movements felt

FMNF Foetal movements not felt (don't worry if you see this – your baby may have been sleeping)

Urine tests NAD means Nothing Abnormal Detected; Nil means none found (normal); Tr (trace) means that a small

amount of protein or glucose has been found; +, ++, +++ indicate that greater amounts have been found

Oed Swelling or oedema – recorded as +, ++, +++

Your baby's position in the uterus This is usually recorded as the presenting part or 'lie' and there are several abbreviations used for the different positions. (see pages 212–15). 'Occiput' refers to the back of your baby's head

Ceph or C or Vx Cephalic or vertex and means 'head down'

Br Breech or 'bottom down'

Long Longitudinal or vertical

Tr Transverse, or across, your body

Obl Oblique, or diagonally across, your body

OA Occipito-anterior (head down, facing your back)

OP Occipito-posterior (head down, facing your front)

OL Occipito-lateral (head down, facing your side)

How far your baby's head is engaged in the pelvis NE, NEng, Not Eng: not engaged or 'free' means that your baby's head is above your pelvis. 1/5, 2/5, 3/5, 4/5 refer either to how much of the head can be felt above your pelvis or to how much of it is in your pelvis (ask your midwife which form she uses)

E or Eng Engaged. Your baby is considered to be engaged once 3/5 of the head is in your pelvis

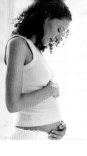

FURTHER SCREENING

The risk of your baby having an abnormality may be hard to contemplate, but it is important to know about the tests you may be offered so that you can make properly informed decisions.

There are two important types of antenatal tests available to you: 'screening', which tell you the level of possible risk of abnormality and 'diagnostic', which tell you whether your baby has an inherited disorder or a chromosomal abnormality.

Screening tests are non-invasive and carry no risk to your baby, but they cannot tell you for certain whether or not your baby has a particular problem. Diagnostic tests are invasive and there is a small risk of miscarriage, but they are far more accurate.

Screening

You may have had a nuchal translucency scan (NTS) between 11 and 14 weeks (ideally at week 13) of

WHAT IS DOWN'S SYNDROME?

Down's syndrome is caused by an abnormal number of chromosomes and affects around one in every 1,000 babies in the UK. People with Down's syndrome have learning difficulties, but the degree of severity varies. There is no cure at present, but there are treatments and support that can help people who have the syndrome to lead an active and independent life. Down's syndrome is also linked to heart problems and impaired hearing and sight. Many problems can be treated, though, and frequent health checks can detect them early on in life. Most people with Down's syndrome have a life expectancy of around 60 years and some will live beyond 70.

your pregnancy (see pages 74–5) that measures the amount of fluid under the skin behind the foetus's neck. This figure, along with the results of blood tests and your age are then combined to give you an individual risk assessment.

The combined test can only give you an indication of the possible risk of Down's syndrome, and it is only if your risk is deemed to be one in 150, or less, that you may need further investigations.

Weighing everything up

It is important to remember that although the combined screening test has an accuracy of around 85 per cent, it is possible that it will give a 'false-positive' result, which means that although the screening test may have indicated a high risk of Down's, further diagnostic tests reveal that there is no such problem.

Most women given a high risk (one in 150 or less) will go on to have a baby who does not have Down's syndrome and even with a risk as high as one in five, your baby has four out of five chances of not having Down's.

Because diagnostic tests are invasive and carry risks of their own, you need to discuss the issues with your partner and decide whether or not you should go ahead with them. If you both feel that you will continue with your pregnancy whatever the result, then it may not be necessary for you to undergo further testing.

Diagnostic tests

If you are offered diagnostic tests they are likely to be amniocentesis, chorionic villus sampling (CVS) or foetal blood sampling.

Amniocentesis

This test is most commonly carried out at around weeks 15 to 20. It tests for genetic abnormalities, so it is used to check that all 23 pairs of chromosomes are present and normal. It is offered if Down's syndrome is particularly suspected and it may also be used to look for spina bifida and sickle cell anaemia as well as disease-specific genetic disorders that may be an inherited risk.

Chorionic villus sampling (CVS)

The CVS test can be carried out earlier than amniocentesis (at around 11 weeks), so it can give you an earlier diagnosis if you think you are at risk of having a child with an inherited disorder, such as cystic fibrosis, sickle cell anaemia, thalassaemia or muscular dystrophy.

The procedure takes around 10 to 20 minutes and may cause a little discomfort. As with amniocentesis, ultrasound is used to guide the insertion of a fine needle that is passed through the abdomen and into the uterus. Sometimes a fine tube may be passed through the vagina and cervix into the uterus instead. A tiny sample of the developing placenta, known as 'chorionic tissue', is then taken. The chromosomes in the cells of this tissue will then be examined. As with amniocentesis, a rapid and quite accurate result can be obtained if the laboratory is looking for a specific problem, but if all the chromosomes are checked the results can take a fortnight or more to come through. Whether the procedure is carried out through the abdomen or cervix depends on where the placenta is lying and neither is more risky than the other, but CVS does carry a 1 to 2 per cent risk of miscarriage and there is also a slight risk of infection. Some vaginal bleeding is common after CVS, but if it persists for more than three days or if you have a fever, you should contact your doctor or midwife.

Foetal blood sampling

Foetal blood sampling is more rarely used, but it may be done at a later stage of pregnancy, when a result is needed urgently. The procedure is similar to amniocentesis, but the needle is inserted into the umbilical cord, where some of the blood can be extracted. Although the results are thought to be accurate, the risk of miscarriage is higher than amniocentesis, and there is also a possibility of infection or ruptured membranes.

AMNIOCENTESIS – HOW IT'S DONE

Using an ultrasound scan as a guide, a thin needle is inserted through your abdomen and the wall of the uterus into the amniotic sac. A small amount of amniotic fluid (see page 76) is then extracted for testing. The procedure is usually carried out by an obstetrician and once the needle has been inserted, it will probably take a few minutes. You may be given a mild local anaesthetic to numb your skin for the penetration of the needle, but you will feel some discomfort as it enters the uterus. Afterwards you should rest for a few days and avoid sex or any form of exercise. The results are usually available within three working days.

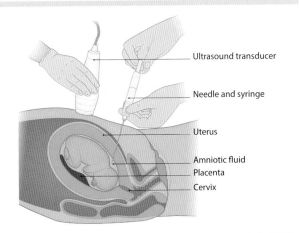

Ultrasound transducer

Needle and syringe

Uterus

Amniotic fluid
Placenta
Cervix

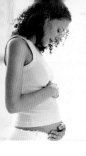

when you are having

MORE THAN ONE BABY

Every pregnancy is special, but if you are expecting twins, or even triplets, or more, you will be in the high-risk category – but don't worry, your care will be extra special, too.

You may not know that you are expecting twins (or more) until you have your dating scan (see pages 74–5), so you might need a little time to get used to the idea of having more than one baby. If there are already twins in your family, you are more likely to have them yourself and if you have had fertility treatment (such as IVF), you are also more likely to have a multiple pregnancy.

Getting used to the idea

You might have experienced pregnancy symptoms that seemed particularly severe, so if you have been pregnant before, you may have had a few clues that something was different. Seeing more than one embryo on screen at the scanning appointment can still come as a bit of a shock, and if you are first-time parents, you may be a little nervous.

Finding out that you'll have to cope with more than one baby can seem a little overwhelming at first. It would be foolish to pretend that it won't be hard work, but you will find a way to make things work. Talk to other parents of twins if you can as they'll have useful tips to pass on. They will probably also tell you just how much work is involved, but that you will be able to give and receive 'double the love', too. Contact the Twins and Multiple Births Association (TAMBA) for advice/information (see Resources).

You will also need extra equipment – cots, car seats, nappies, clothes and later, high chairs and beds. Make a list and see if you can either borrow some

items or buy second hand. Take care, though, as it is not a good idea to buy used car seats since cracks or faults can make them less safe. Cots, too, need to be thoroughly cleaned and you should buy new mattresses for them (see pages 164–5).

Your antenatal care

As soon as you know that you are expecting more than one baby, your antenatal team will plan a specially tailored programme of care. Multiple pregnancies are more complicated and so you will have more frequent check-ups, blood tests and scans. Blood tests will check that your haemoglobin levels are high enough and if not, you may be given a supplement to boost it. Your blood pressure will be monitored more closely, too, because pre-eclampsia (see pages 208–9) is more common in women expecting multiple babies.

More scans

You will also have more ultrasound scans to monitor your babies' growth and development. If you are expecting identical twins who were created from the same group of genes they may share a placenta, and one may manage to obtain more nutrition that the other. It is not unusual for identical twins to be born with the same features, therefore, but to be quite different in size. Small differences do not matter too much, but your midwife will want to keep a close eye on such things. If you are having non-identical

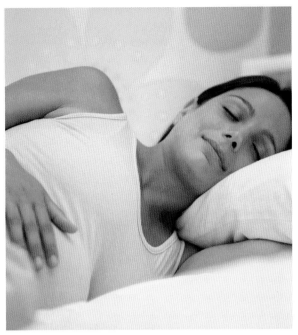

Rest as much as you can if you are expecting twins or more. Even if you can't take a restful nap, just putting your feet up for a few minutes whenever you can will help.

twins you can probably expect to have a scan every four weeks and with identical twins (see page 24) it is more likely to be every two.

Your options for delivery

If you were planning a home birth before you knew about your multiple pregnancy, you will have to rethink your plans because the hospital really is the safest option. Try not to feel disappointed. The most important thing about labour and birth is not the way that it occurs, but the end result: that you and your babies should be safe and healthy. It is common for twins to be lying head to toe in the uterus, so while one baby will be head first, the other is likely to be in the breech position (see pages 212–15), which may present complications. So for this reason, among others, it is common for twins and multiples to be delivered by a scheduled Caesarean section (see pages 286–9). Twins also often arrive early (50 per cent in week 37), so you will need to be prepared and be flexible in your approach to their birth.

DOUBLING UP ON YOUR CARE

Here are a few things that you can do to make your pregnancy with twins more comfortable:

Eat a little and often, but eat more With twins on board you will need extra fuel, so you should be consuming around 2,700 calories per day. Eat plenty of fresh wholefoods taken from the main food groups (see pages 78–81)

Take plenty of naps Your body is nourishing two (or more) babies at once and that probably means two placentas and extra amniotic fluid, so you may also feel doubly tired. Put your feet up – backache, leg and feet swelling is common

Improve your posture You will be carrying extra weight, so you need to stand and sit up straight. Invest in a 'pregnancy pillow' to support your lower back

Go swimming You will find the water relaxing and supportive, as it helps to reduce the effect of gravity on your bump. Try to use a flotation aid for relaxation and swim using crawl or backstroke rather than breaststroke, so that you don't have to arch your back

Slow down Get up and out of bed slowly by rolling on to your side first and rise from a sitting position gently, too. Your blood vessels are dilated (open) and the blood will rush to your feet as you stand up, so you are extremely prone to dizziness. This, combined with your extra-heavy bump, can make you vulnerable to falls, so take care

Enlist support Get some regular help with chores (especially any strenuous ones) and take care not to lift anything heavy

Prop yourself up Try not to lie flat when you go to bed, to avoid putting too much pressure on the major blood vessels that supply the placenta. Use a 'pregnancy pillow' or place a soft pillow under your bump (when you lie on your side) and a few more arranged around your back, so that your head and chest are slightly elevated

Make contact Get in touch with other parents of twins and find out how they manage the practicalities of life with more than one baby (see page 326)

Be prepared You may need to rethink your maternity leave plans. Many multiple babies are delivered early, so you may need to stop working sooner than you had anticipated

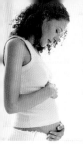

what to expect when you attend

ANTENATAL CLASSES

Antenatal classes help you and your partner to prepare for labour, birth and early parenthood. Besides being a good source of information, they can also be a great way to form networks of friendship that may last long after your baby's birth.

Pregnancy and birth are natural aspects of life, so you may feel that you don't need to be taught how to do things. However the more information that you have about the process of labour and giving birth, the easier it is to make informed decisions about how you will do it. Antenatal classes can give you the chance to explore issues such as options for pain relief in greater detail and, importantly, they give you and your partner an invaluable chance to prepare for parenthood together.

Courses usually begin at around week 28 of your pregnancy and you can either sign up for a series of classes, a weekend 'workshop' or just a one-off session. Ask your midwife and friends for recommendations. Classes are usually held once a week for between four and six weeks, in the evenings or at weekends, so that partners can come too, but find out what is available as soon as you can, because spaces often fill quickly.

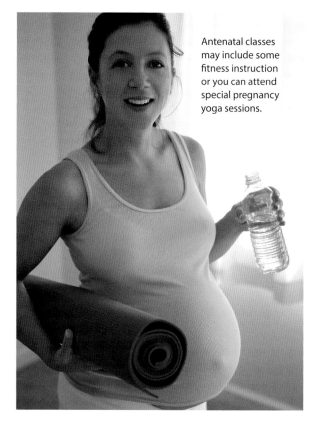

Antenatal classes may include some fitness instruction or you can attend special pregnancy yoga sessions.

What will be taught?

Although the emphasis may vary, all antenatal classes cover the essentials: what happens during labour and birth; breathing and relaxation; pain-relief options; what happens if you need to have assisted labour (e.g. ventouse delivery or a Caesarean section); and how to take care of your newborn. The information that you receive is important, but perhaps even more valuable are the friendships and support that you

may find for you, your partner and later, your child. Once your baby arrives your social life will inevitably change and you may find that you have less in common (at least for a while) with some of your existing friends. All the prospective parents at antenatal classes will be going through the same sorts

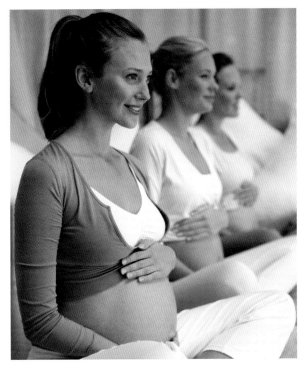

It's good to get together with other prospective parents who are all going through the same thing as you.

of experiences with their babies at roughly the same time and in those early days of parenthood it can be really helpful to have a ready-made social network of people who understand exactly why you feel so tired, haven't had time to go to the hairdresser's, or have to drop everything to feed a hungry baby. And if all goes well, by the time your baby becomes more aware of the world around him, he too will have a group of baby friends who are all at roughly the same stage as him – and will be throughout his childhood.

A choice of options

Apart from financial or time considerations, there is no reason why you can't attend more than one type of class. NHS classes (sometimes called 'parentcraft' classes) are free and welcome partners, but although they are informal, they sometimes comprise quite large groups, so while you receive plenty of information, you might not have so much time to get to know people. The National Childbirth Trust

(NCT) is the second-largest provider of classes in the UK and tends to have smaller groups, where it is easier to get to know other couples, but there is a charge. Don't be discouraged if money is tight – the NCT is a charity and so, depending on your circumstances, you may be able to get a concession.

Active birth classes

Besides the information-based classes for couples, you may want to sign up to an exercise class for pregnant mums. Sometimes called 'active birth' classes, they teach yoga, breathing and relaxation techniques as well as exercises suitable for pregnancy designed to improve your fitness and strength in preparation for labour and birth. You may also be able to attend an aqua aerobics class for pregnancy. Swimming is an ideal form of exercise when you are expecting, enabling you to improve your flexibility, muscle tone and stamina. The water supports your whole body, so there is less pressure on your muscles and joints, but take care that the pool is not too cold or too hot (over 32°C/89°F). Whichever form of exercise you choose (see pages 92–3), make sure that it is suitable for pregnancy and inform your instructor that you are expecting a baby.

SINGLE PARENT AT CLASSES?

If you are a lone parent, you don't have to attend classes on your own. You could ask a friend or relative to go with you – it makes most sense to ask the person who you would like to be your birth partner. If this is not possible, or you would prefer to attend by yourself, ask your midwife whether there are any classes for single expectant mothers – it may be helpful to meet other women also having their baby on their own and you may be able to form a support network extending beyond the birth of your babies. Whatever happens, try to find a class that suits you, they really are an important way to learn about pregnancy, labour and parenting and studies have shown that, on average, the better informed you are, the shorter and more positive your birth experience will be.

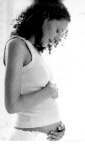

complementary therapies for the second trimester

COMMON COMPLAINTS

As your uterus expands and gets heavier you may find that you have a few problems associated with your digestive and circulatory systems. Don't despair – there are some simple, safe, complementary remedies that may help.

Heartburn

Heartburn is caused by acidic gastric juices and fluids from the stomach coming up into the oesophagus and you may experience a burning feeling in the chest and throat. Your pregnancy hormones are probably to blame (see pages 36–7) because as the abdominal muscles are relaxed by the action of progesterone and relaxin, the valve at the entrance to your stomach fails to close properly. As your pregnancy progresses and your growing uterus presses more on your stomach, the problem can worsen and feel more uncomfortable.

Symptoms

You may have a burning sensation in your throat, nausea and an unpleasant taste in your mouth acccompanied by bad breath.

Nutrition

Eating large meals can make the problem worse, so eat small amounts at a time and avoid rich, fatty, greasy, spicy or very acidic foods.

Complementary therapies for heartburn

Consult your midwife or doctor before you try any complementary therapies and make sure that your practitioners are fully qualified and accredited.
Acupressure Place four fingers at the midway point between your tummy button and the lowest part of

SELF-HELP TIPS FOR HEARTBURN

Eat small, simple meals, frequently, and chew slowly. Avoid having just one or two large meals per day

Avoid certain 'trigger' foods

Try to eat a light, simple meal early in the evening (at about 6 pm) and don't eat late at night before you go to bed (heartburn occurs when you lie down)

Sleep with pillows ranged around and under your upper body so that it is slightly raised

Drink plenty of water at all times, but limit your fluid intake at mealtimes

Avoid bending over

your breastbone. Press here for ten seconds at a time, during a period of five to 10 minutes.
Acupuncture Traditional Chinese Medicine (TCM) (see pages 38–9) sees heartburn as a problem associated with excessive 'heat' in the stomach. By treating certain acupoints on your arms or feet, an acupuncturist will aim to restore balance to your digestive system. She may examine the tip of your tongue (which is often red) and is linked with the heart, and the middle of the tongue, which is linked with the stomach.
Homeopathy Take care to follow the manufacturer's dosage instructions, but remedies are best prescribed

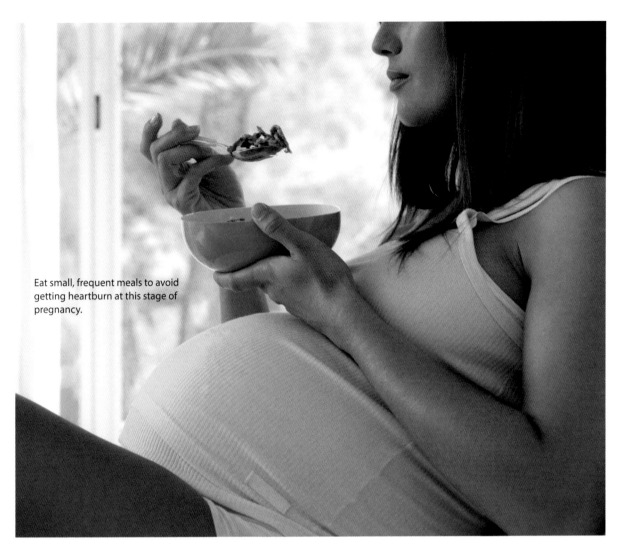

Eat small, frequent meals to avoid getting heartburn at this stage of pregnancy.

by a professional homeopath to match your precise symptoms. Contact a registered homeopath.

• For flatulence and bloating: carbo veg 30c
• For a heavy, overly full stomach: nux vomica 30c
• For a gurgling stomach: pulsatilla 30c

Reflexology A reflexologist may gently massage the part of the foot that corresponds to the stomach and intestines.

Western herbalism Caraway, dill and fennel seeds may help. Try grinding them up and adding them to your food, or chewing them whole after a meal. Also try two or three cups a day of fennel, peppermint, lemon balm or chamomile tea, sipped slowly.

Constipation, haemorrhoids & varicose veins

During pregnancy, your bowel movements are slowed down by the action of the hormone progesterone (see pages 36–7), and this means that you may find that you can easily become constipated. You may also develop haemorrhoids because the constipation, combined with your increasingly heavy uterus, causes the veins in the lining of your anus to swell. Your increased overall weight and extra blood volume may make the blood vessels in your legs enlarge, too, and this may result in the appearance of varicose veins.

Symptoms

You may find it difficult or painful to pass faeces and have a heavy feeling in your lower abdomen and anus. There may be painful or itching protruding veins in your anus, possibly with some bleeding. You may have large, distorted, raised veins on your legs.

Nutrition

To strengthen your veins and blood vessels:
• Eat foods that are rich in vitamin C (see page 84) and bioflavonoids such as onions, garlic and parsley.
To ease constipation:
• Drink plenty of water (at least 1 litre/2 pt) every day) and watered-down fruit juice.
• Eat plenty of fruit, vegetables and wholegrain cereals that provide lots of fibre (bran, oats, dried fruit, cabbage, kale, peas, figs, plums and prunes).
• Avoid processed foods such as white bread.

Complementary therapies for constipation, haemorrhoids & varicose veins

Consult your midwife or doctor before you try any complementary therapies and make sure that your practitioners are fully qualified and accredited.
Acupressure To ease constipation, stimulate the acupoint that is halfway along between your pubic bone and your tummy button. Press your finger there intermittently for ten seconds.
Acupuncture An acupuncturist may examine the back of your tongue (a yellow coating may indicate constipation) because in Traditional Chinese

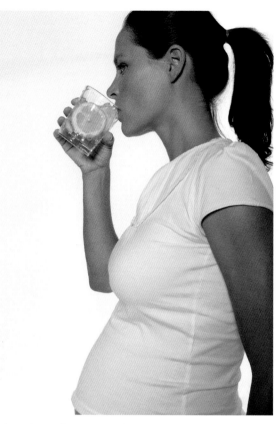

Drinking plenty of water every day is important throughout pregnancy and it can help a range of common ailments.

Medicine (TCM – see pages 38–9) this part of the tongue is linked with the bowels. If so, she may stimulate the large intestine meridian. For haemorrhoids, she may stimulate the bladder meridian on the back of the calf. Varicose veins may be treated with needles inserted around the vein.

SELF-HELP TIPS FOR CONSTIPATION, HAEMORRHOIDS & VARICOSE VEINS

To ease constipation drink plenty of water and eat foods containing fibre and that are naturally fermented such as live yogurt, sauerkraut or vegetable pickles. They contain 'good' bacteria and enzymes that help your body to digest food more easily. To stimulate your bowels, stroke your lower abdomen in clockwise direction. Take some regular exercise as this encourages the bowels to become more active.

To help haemorrhoids, avoid tea, coffee and spicy foods and drink plenty of water. Avoid getting constipated. Get plenty of rest and gentle exercise. Do pelvic floor exercises.

To relieve varicose veins avoid standing for long periods. Sit with feet elevated and flex them. Take some exercise and try wearing support tights. Don't massage areas over varicose veins as there is a risk of prompting thrombosis.

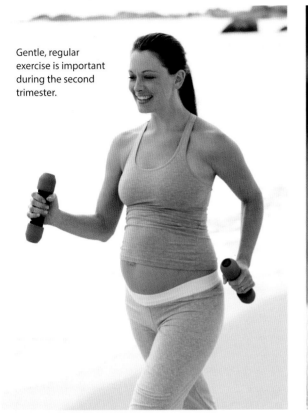

Gentle, regular exercise is important during the second trimester.

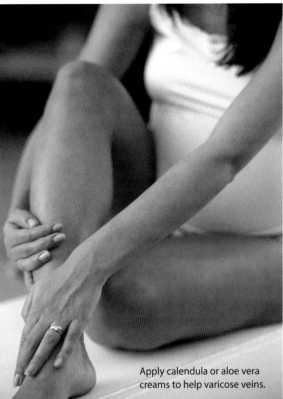

Apply calendula or aloe vera creams to help varicose veins.

Aromatherapy Gentle abdominal massage may help, but check which oils are safe (see pages 40–1).

Homeopathy Take care to follow the manufacturer's dosage instructions, but remedies are best prescribed by a professional homeopath to match your precise symptoms. Contact a registered homeopath.

You may be able to ease haemorrhoids with one of the following remedies. Select the one that most closely matches your symptoms:

- For protruding, itching, bleeding haemorrhoids that seem better for bathing in cool water: nux. vomica 30c.
- For internal, bleeding, painful haemorrhoids that seem better when bathed in warm water: arsen. alb 30c.
- For oozing, protruding, painful haemorrhoids: sepia 30c
- For large, sore, bleeding, painful haemorrhoids: hamamelis 30c

Hydrotherapy To temporarily relieve and reduce varicose veins use a shower head to spray your leg with hot water, then cold, for two minutes each.

Western herbalism Try drinking a cup of hot water before breakfast to help constipation. For haemorrhoids, apply St John's wort ointment that has been kept cold in the refrigerator or cold witch hazel or nettle tea compresses. Varicose veins can be helped by applying calendula or aloe vera creams or a cold witch hazel compress.

Yoga Lie with your feet and legs raised against a wall for around 15–30 minutes twice a day.

WARNING

If you have a feeling of heaviness in your calf or deep, niggling pain, contact your doctor without delay as this could be a sign of deep-vein thrombosis.

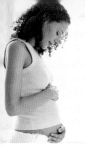

buying baby items

EQUIPMENT & SAFETY

It's exciting to buy equipment, bedding and clothes in preparation for your baby's arrival, but try to resist the temptation to purchase everything you see. Safety should be the priority and it is best to start with the basics and add more items as and when you need them.

During this trimester you are probably feeling reasonably energetic, so you could take advantage of this and prepare for your baby's arrival. Later, in the third trimester, you may be feeling less enthusiastic about shopping, and you need to give yourself time to get some rest and gather your physical and mental resources before the birth. Don't leave everything to the last minute or you may end up feeling tired before the birth and for the first few days with your new baby.

Baskets & cots

While furnishing your baby's nursery is a good way for you to get ready to welcome him into your home, remember that what he needs most is simply for you to be there. For the first six months of his life it is recommended that your baby should sleep in your room with you (see pages 340–1). In the first few weeks of his life, a Moses basket is easily transported from the living area to your bedside and may seem more snug than a cot for one so tiny.

WHAT TO BUY BEFORE YOUR BABY ARRIVES

Nursery basics

A Moses basket, cot, cradle or co-sleeper bedside cot

Bedding and clothes (see page 167)

A plastic, wipe-clean changing mat

A baby monitor

A night light

A comfortable chair for night-time feeds, settling your baby or reading bedtime stories

A soft rug made from natural fibres for play and 'tummy time' (see page 352)

A baby rocker or bouncy chair

Bathing and changing basics

A baby bath (see pages 344–5)

Flannels and soft towels

Gentle baby toiletries

Bowls for 'topping and tailing' (see page 345)

Disposable nappies – begin with one pack of newborn size and one pack of a larger size

Towelling nappies – you will need 24 nappies, nappy liners, some plastic/rubber overpants, safety pins or clips, two nappy buckets and sterilising fluid (see pages 346–7)

Unscented wipes and barrier cream

Nappy disposal bags

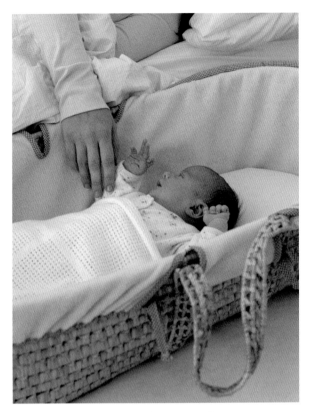

A Moses basket keeps your newborn snug and cosy next to your own bed – it is also convenient for carrying around.

Remember, though, that your baby will grow very rapidly, so you will need a sturdy cot for him before long. Cots may have adjustable mattress heights and drop sides that make it easier for you to pick him up and put him down to sleep. Before you buy, try using the drop-side mechanisms of several types to see which is easiest for you. Check that all the parts have smooth, rounded edges and that the gaps between the side rails are no more than 8 cm (3 in) apart so that your baby cannot get his head stuck. Mattresses (like car seats) should always be purchased new and you should make sure that they conform to the latest safety standards (see Resources). You can choose either foam or sprung types and look for ventilated sections at the top and in the middle. You will also need some simple bedding such as sheets and blankets, but you should never use duvets or pillows for a new baby (see pages 340–1).

BABY SAFETY IN THE HOME

It may seem a long way off now, but once your baby is born, it's only a matter of weeks before he's on the move (first rolling over and then crawling before grasping on to things), so you need to start looking hard at how safe your home really is.

Install safety gates at the tops and bottoms of stairs

If you have wooden or highly polished floors, secure any rugs with sticky tape to make sure that you will not slip or trip when you are carrying your baby

Make sure there are no cords, electrical sockets or cables near your baby's cot, as they could pose a risk of strangulation or electrocution

Make sure that the mattress in your baby's cot fits snugly, so that he cannot slip between the cot frame and the mattress or get an arm or leg stuck

Check your cot for any sharp edges, rough wood that might create splinters, or loose bolts or screws

Do not hang or tie anything to the cot (mobiles and toys) as they could pose a risk of strangulation. Cut off any strings or ribbons attached to bedding or clothing

Secure all bookshelves, wardrobes and chests of drawers to the wall – they can easily topple or be pulled over

Gather up any medication and put it all away in a child-proof cupboard that will be well out of reach

Make sure that any cleaning or laundry products and toiletries are stored in cupboards fitted with child-proof catches or which are well out of reach

Get a fireguard if you have an open fireplace and secure it in place using the correct fittings

Get into the habit of keeping hot drinks, glasses and small or sharp objects well out of reach

Stock up on child-proof safety door catches and spongy protectors for furniture edges and corners

It's a good idea to get down on the floor (perhaps on your hands and knees) so that you can see things from a rolling and then crawling baby's point of view

Instead of a conventional cot you could consider a co-sleeper bedside cot. This has a removable side so that it can be attached to your bed and it allows you to put your baby to sleep in his own space. A co-sleeper can be especially useful in the early weeks and months because you can feed your baby in the night, with the minimum of disturbance to you both, and then put him back to sleep safely beside you. As he grows, you can reattach the cot's side so that it can be used as a completely separate item and relocated in his own room, if he has one.

Things you may need

Your baby will certainly need somewhere secure to sleep, but he may also benefit from a baby rocking or bouncy chair. These are softly padded seats that are low to the ground (never place one on a raised surface – keep it on the floor at all times), which allow your baby to be gently tilted so that he can watch you as you go about your life. They have a soft belt or harness, which should always be fastened to prevent your baby from rolling and tipping out. These seats should not be used for long periods of time, but are especially useful when you need to put your baby down somewhere safe while you make yourself a hot drink or take a bathroom break.

A baby bath is not strictly essential, but it can make things easier for you. You can either choose a free-standing plastic bath that you can use on the floor or place inside your full-sized bath, or the type that fits over the edges of the family bath and so requires you to do less bending. Babies can be very slippery when they are wet, so you may need to learn a few techniques for bathing him (see pages 344–5).

Baby clothes & bedclothes

It is important that your baby should be warm and comfortable in his Moses basket or cot, but it is essential that he doesn't become overheated or slip down under heavy bedclothes, as these may increase the risk of Sudden Infant Death Syndrome (SIDS) (see page 340). Babies should always be put to sleep

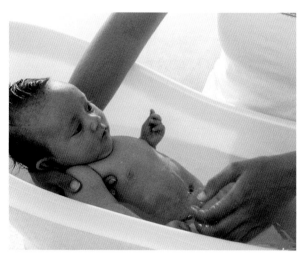

A simple baby bath is great for newborns. You can pop them into your existing bath or use them on the floor or on a stand.

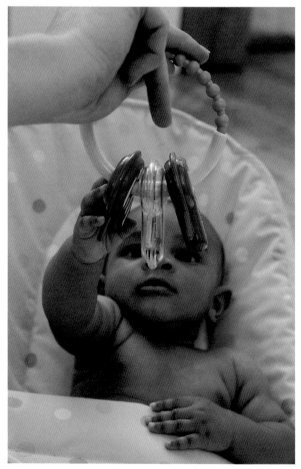

A lie-back bouncing seat is a great piece of equipment. Your baby can see what's going on and benefit from the stimulation.

NEWBORN BABY CLOTHES BASICS

6 babygros

4 sleepsuits or extra babygros

6 envelope neck or cross-over vests

4 envelope neck shirts or cross-over T-shirts

4 pairs of leggings

2 soft cotton cardigans

4 pairs socks or bootees

1 jacket for cold weather

Hats – a soft stretchy cotton one for autumn and winter and a wide-brimmed one for summer

BEDDING BASICS

1 or 2 cotton cot mattress protectors

3 cotton fitted bottom sheets

2 baby sleeping bags

2 or 3 cotton top sheets

2 or 3 cotton cellular blankets

1 woollen cellular blanket for very cold weather

on their backs in the 'feet-to-foot' position (see pages 340–1) and duvets, quilts and pillows are all unsuitable, as well as unecessary, for babies under one year of age. It is best to opt for cotton sheets and cellular blankets or baby sleeping bags. Sheets and blankets can be used in layers and allow your baby to move around in bed, but he may become uncovered. A baby sleeping bag cannot be kicked off and will keep his body at an even temperature, so he is less likely to wake up because he's feeling cold. Choose a sleeping bag that is suitable for the season – a low tog one for summer (0.5 or 1 tog) and a 2.5 tog bag for winter. If you do use a sleeping bag for your baby, you will generally only need a few bottom sheets for

the cot, but it is a good idea to have one or two cotton cellular blankets to add if the room becomes particularly cold. Some mums swear by 'swaddle'-style sleeping bags, which zip up snugly to enclose the baby's body entirely. Remember that there will be times when you will need to change your baby's bedding quickly, so make sure that you have more than one sleeping bag or set of sheets and blankets.

Baby clothes basics

Bear in mind that you may be given baby clothes as gifts, once your baby arrives, so just buy a set of basic items to start with. Don't purchase too many items in newborn size because your baby might be larger than expected and will grow out of them very soon anyway. Most baby clothes are sold in sizes determined by age (3, 6, 9, 12 months) although European clothes may be sold according to length, so for example, newborn clothes usually start at 50 cm (20 in). It may be a good idea to buy a few items one or two sizes larger than newborn, just in case, and then return smaller items if you don't use them. Remember that your baby's bones are very soft, so he must have plenty of room to grow (especially in the legs and feet of all-in-one suits). If you don't feel like pushing your newborn around the shops in the early days, top up on your basics online.

Convenience is everything

All-in-one babygros that are easy to fasten are very useful, but invest in a few separates such as soft, long-sleeved T-shirts with wide envelope necks and stretchy leggings, too, because if one item gets dirty you only need to change that, rather than find a whole new outfit. Vests can be used as an extra layer to keep your baby warm in cold weather and are ideal worn alone with a nappy at naptime when the weather is hot. Most babies (and especially newborns) dislike the process of getting dressed and undressed (see pages 346–7) so it's sensible to choose clothes that are quick and easy to put on and take off. When choosing things like sleepsuits, bear in mind that you may have to change your baby at night in dim light, so clothes need to be easy to handle. For all items of clothing opt for soft, natural fibres and run your hands over seams and labels to check that they will not cause irritation.

Too hot or too cold?

Your baby's circulatory system will be immature at first, so his hands and feet can easily get cold. Socks or soft bootees are useful indoors or out and mittens and with a warm 'snowsuit' will be needed for winter outings if it is really cold. Your baby's head will be large in proportion to the rest of his body, so a warm hat is essential for cooler months. A soft, stretchy cotton hat should be adequate for most outings, but remove it in the car so that he does not overheat. In strong sun, your baby will need really efficient protection from the UV rays so a hat with a wide brim is a must.

In general, dress your baby in layers of clothes rather than one or two thick items. That way, you can peel garments off or add more, accordingly.

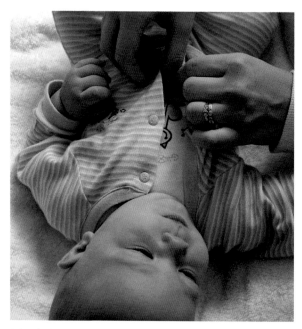

Baby clothes are cute, but they must be practical. Be sure to choose versions that are easy to get on and off.

Equipment for being out & about
Infant car seats

One of the most essential items to purchase in time for your baby's arrival is a baby car seat: you will not be allowed to leave the hospital without one. Seats for newborns are rear-facing and should be secured in the back of the car because young babies' necks are not strong enough to cope with the whiplash effect should you be unfortunate enough to be involved in a collision.

Which way should babies face?

Babies should face the rear of the car until they are at least one year old. In this position, if there is a crash, the forces exerted on impact are more evenly spread over the child's body and are less likely to result in fractures and organ damage. When buying an infant car seat, check that it conforms to the latest safety standards (see Resources) and that it will fit your car. Choose according to the weight of your baby rather than his age.

Multi-purpose seats

Many infant car seats can be taken out of the car and used as a rocking seat or slotted into a specially designed pram or buggy system. These can be convenient if your baby has fallen asleep in the car and you don't wish to wake him, but take care not to leave your baby in the seat for more than two hours in total – his breathing may become restricted because he cannot straighten his body in the sitting position. Young babies need to lie flat for a good proportion of the day (both on their backs and their stomachs – see pages 352–3).

Fitting the infant seat

Before you have to use the seat properly, practise putting it into your car and securing it with the adult seat belt, according to the manufacturer's instructions. The seat should have a three-point harness for your baby that is relatively easy to fasten and unfasten. Most baby car seats are supplied with

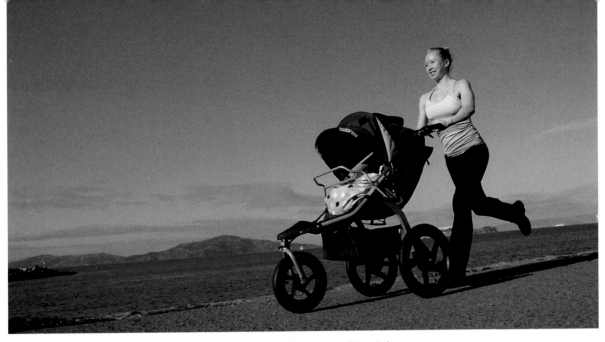

If you love to jog, why stop just because you've got a baby in tow? Acquire an all-terrain buggy and enjoy the fresh air and exercise together.

a head-hugging cushion to prevent a newborn's head from rolling about, but you may need to adjust it to fit snugly around, not under, your baby's head when you place him in the seat. Never hang or tie anything to the car seat as this poses a risk of strangulation.

Baby carriers & slings

Baby carriers can be useful both indoors and outside. However, backpack carriers with light aluminium frames are great when your baby is older, but they are not suitable for newborns. Choose a soft carrier that holds your baby on your front. It will give you greater freedom for short walks and shopping expeditions and you can also wear it around the house, keeping your baby close to you while you get on with essential tasks.

Baby carriers are sold according to your baby's weight, so check that you buy one in the right size. Most are made of cotton and have padding to support your baby's head and neck, but make sure that your baby's head doesn't fall too far forwards into your chest. A sarong-style sling can also be useful, but always make sure that it is securely tied to you and that your baby is facing upwards, with her face clear of any fabric.

Choosing prams & buggies

There is an vast range of prams and buggies to choose from, including traditional sprung suspension prams, all-terrain buggies, standard-size and double buggies and three-in-one combinations of pram, buggy and car seats. Before you buy, think about your lifestyle. Will you need to take it on public transport or in and out of shops? If this is your intention, a lightweight folding buggy may be best – but make sure that it reclines to the flat position suitable for newborns. An all-terrain model might be better for uneven terrain, but a pram may suit your life best if you are mainly around town. Check, too, that the model you choose will fit into your car. Whichever type, make sure that it is suitable to use from birth and conforms to the latest safety standards (see Resources).

WARNING

No matter how upset your baby is, never hold him on your lap in a car. If you had a crash he would be seriously injured and possibly crushed by your weight – even if you are wearing a seatbelt.

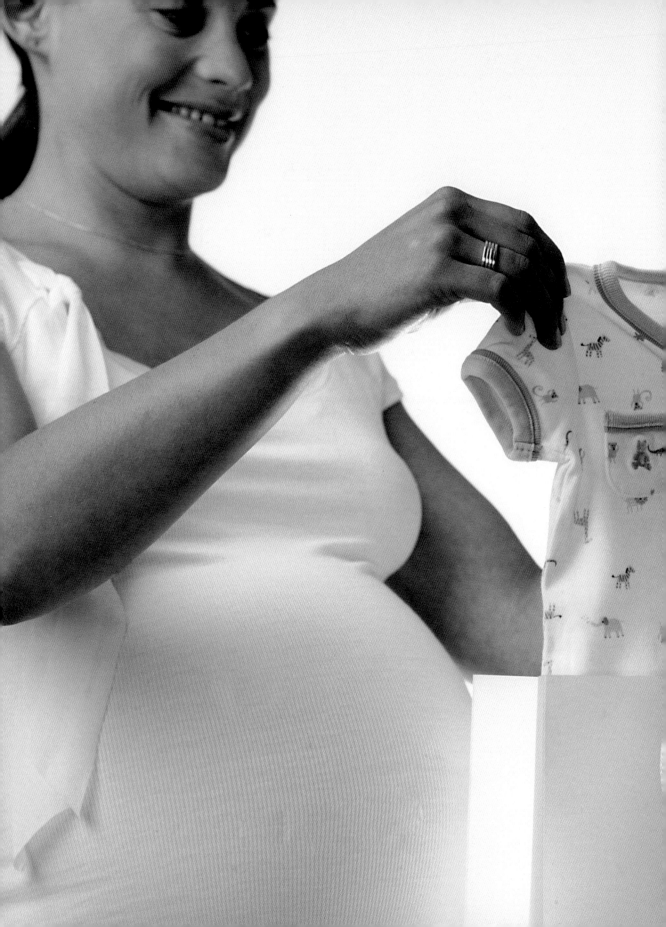

your third
TRIMESTER

Now that you have arrived at the third, and final, trimester of your pregnancy, there are a few more important things you need to know – to make sure that the rest of it runs smoothly.

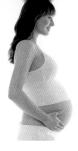

YOUR CHANGING BODY

Now that you have arrived at the last third of pregnancy, you may be feeling increasingly tired and perhaps rather large. Concentrate on building your energy resources – your baby will be here very soon.

Week 28

You may be experiencing some extremely vivid dreams, especially about birth, babies and children, which you may find disturbing. These are not omens of things to come, but your mind's way of processing the fears and anxieties that your conscious mind may be trying to push into the background (see pages 236–9). You may be waking more frequently during the night in this trimester, meaning you are more likely to remember these dreams.

Week 29

Your blood volume will probably reach a peak of about 5 litres (8¾ pt) during this trimester, though you may have a further increase between weeks 35 and 40. Most of this is fluid content or plasma and your oxygen-carrying red blood cells do not increase at the same rate, so in effect, your blood becomes more diluted. This can result in anaemia (known in late pregnancy as 'dilutional anaemia'), but while it may make you feel tired, it rarely has any serious consequences, because your blood-cell count is already much higher than normal during pregnancy. Don't worry about your baby: the lion's share of the oxygen and nutrients are going to her, so she is getting all she needs.

Week 30

You may have experienced a general backache for some weeks as your bump gets much bigger and

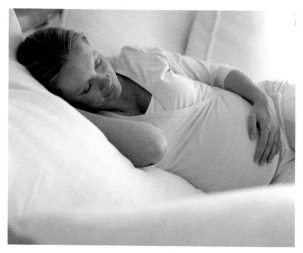

Take as many opportunities to rest as you can during these final weeks before the birth.

heavier, but now you may find that you have more specific pain, which may be due to common late-pregnancy disorders such as sciatica, coccygeal pain, sacroiliac pain or symphysis pubis dysfunction (SPD – see page 174). A chiropractor or cranial osteopath may be able to help with these conditions, but consult your doctor or midwife, too, because lower back pain should not be ignored in late pregnancy.

Week 31

Your 'nesting instinct' may have kicked in by now and you may have a strong urge to clean and organise your home from top to bottom, but take care not to do too much. You will have to resign yourself to the fact that moving around is much more of an effort now and you may feel short of breath at times. If you are normally very energetic, it can be frustrating, but while it is good to remain active, you also require periods of rest, too. Remind yourself that you need to conserve your energy for labour and birth.

Week 32

You may notice that veins just under the surface of your skin are becoming raised. This stage of pregnancy is when you are most likely to get varicose veins or haemorrhoids, which can be uncomfortable and inconvenient, but there are things that you can do to ease them (see pages 161–3).

Week 33

The top of your uterus will be at its highest point by now and may be felt about 12 cm (5 in) above your navel, but around this time, or very soon, your baby may move down into the 'head-down' position in readiness for birth. If you been experiencing shortness of breath and indigestion recently, it should now improve, but as her head presses down on your bladder you may have to urinate more frequently.

Week 34

From this week it is best to keep your knees lower than your hips as much as possible to encourage the baby into the optimal position for labour. If you do want to raise your legs, lie on your left side on a sofa and sit on an exercise ball when you are at the computer. Try some ankle rotations and flex your feet up and down when seated. Your hands may also swell and all these problems are commonly due to fluid retention. However, notify your midwife if it is severe and especially if you also have a headache – it may be a symptom of pre-eclampsia (see pages 208–9).

Week 35

You may feel an assortment of aches and pains in your pelvic area and your hip joints may feel slightly 'odd', and even painful, as your ligaments continue

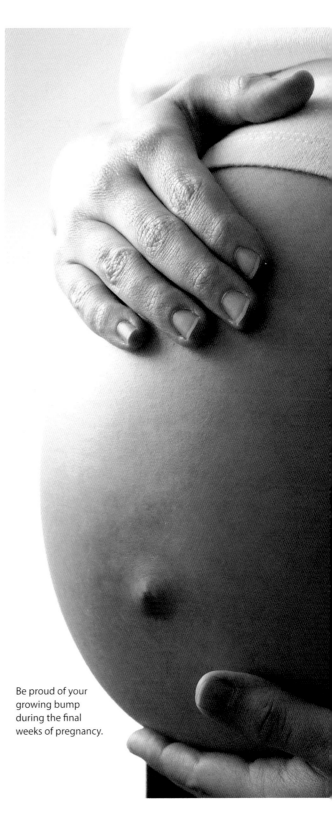

Be proud of your growing bump during the final weeks of pregnancy.

LATE PREGNANCY Q&AS

"I've noticed lumps in both my breasts that seem to be getting bigger. Should I be concerned?"

Breast lumps are common in the third trimester and form as your breasts prepare for breastfeeding. They may be quite soft, move around and be tender to the touch. Lumps should never be ignored, though, so talk to your doctor or midwife.

"When I turn over in bed or sneeze I get a pain. What is it?"

Talk to your doctor or midwife about this, but it sounds most likely to be pelvic girdle pain (PGP), also known as symphysis pubis dysfunction (SPD). It can affect one in five pregnant women and is caused by the hormonal changes that affect the way the pelvic joints work. Try keeping your legs together as you get out of bed or a car and sleep on your side, with a soft pillow between your legs to support the uppermost one. Avoid heavy pushing, pulling or lifting and make sure that you wear comfortable, flat shoes. You could also try visiting a qualified and accredited acupuncturist or osteopath.

"My baby never seems to stop doing somersaults and kicking. Is she hyperactive?"

An active baby is generally a good sign and doesn't indicate that your baby will be restless or hyperactive. However, do make sure that you are eating well and getting enough rest. Babies can respond to their mother's stress (see pages 146–7) and it may be that you need to slow down and relax more.

"Could an orgasm make me go into premature labour?"

If your pregnancy has been without complications, there should be no risk, although it may bring on a set of Braxton Hicks' practice contractions (see below). However, if you have had any bleeding or a previous premature delivery, or your waters have broken (see page 232), you should avoid having intercourse because of the risk of infection and because oxytocin, the hormone that is released during sex, also causes the muscles of the uterus to contract.

to stretch in preparation for birth (see pages 278–81). Your breasts will feel tender and much heavier and they might even leak a little milk or colostrum as they prepare for feeding your baby.

Week 36

You will be putting on weight more rapidly than ever as your body prepares for labour and giving birth. Your baby is 'filling out' now, too, and laying down vital fat stores in her body. Compared with your normal self, you may feel rather ungainly now (if you were a normal weight to start with you can expect to gain between 12 and 16 kg (25 and 35 lb) over the course of your pregnancy – see page 90), but try not to feel anxious and remember that you are doing the vital job of nourishing your baby. Pregnancy is no time for worrying about 'looking big' (it's natural) and be aware that research has shown that small babies may have significant health problems as well as a lower IQ. Don't forget that a

good proportion of the extra weight that you are now carrying is due to your baby, plus the placenta and amniotic fluid. Once your baby is born, your body will already be (and feel) much lighter and once you start looking after her – and especially if you breastfeed – more weight will drop away.

Week 37

At any time now you might experience some Braxton Hicks' (practice) contractions. The top of your fundus will harden and the sensation will travel down your abdomen, causing it to harden and then relax again. They help your uterus practise for the very strong contractions that will be needed to deliver your baby and they also help to send more blood to the placenta in the last few weeks of pregnancy. These contractions will be noticeable, but should not be particularly painful. If the pain is very strong, contact your doctor or midwife. They are most frequent around mealtimes.

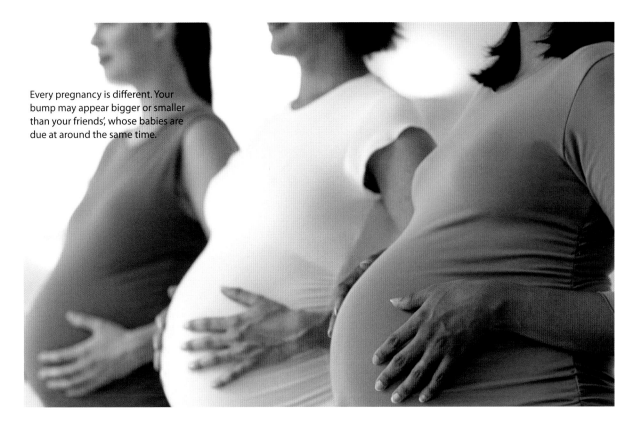

Every pregnancy is different. Your bump may appear bigger or smaller than your friends', whose babies are due at around the same time.

Week 38

You may notice an increase in vaginal secretions that may be slightly pink or brown, especially if you have sex. This is probably due to your cervix 'ripening' and softening with an increased blood supply, so it can become bruised quite easily. It is usually nothing to worry about, but if you have any bright-red blood, you will need to contact your doctor or midwife without delay.

Week 39

If this is your first pregnancy, it is likely that your baby's head will have engaged at around 36 weeks. If this is your second or third baby, her head may not have engaged until now, or it may not happen until just before labour begins. Whichever way she is lying, your baby now has very little room to manoeuvre, but you should still feel regular movements, so if there is any change in this pattern, consult your doctor or midwife.

Week 40

Although your baby may arrive this week, it is unlikely that she will be born on the exact day of her estimated delivery date (EDD) (see page 31). You will probably be experiencing quite a cocktail of feelings by now: great excitement and anticipation perhaps mixed with some fear and apprehension and then possibly a little frustration and irritation. It is difficult for you to get enough good-quality sleep at the moment, so you are bound to feel a bit irritable, but try to get as much rest as you can and practise your visualisation and relaxation techniques (see pages 144–5). At term, your placenta will measure about 20–25 cm (8–10 in) in diameter and resemble a large plate that is around 2–3 cm (1 in) thick. Towards the end of your pregnancy, the placenta is gradually using up its reserves and this is why pregnancies are rarely allowed to go on beyond 42 weeks. Your doctor or midwife will be keeping a close eye on you, though, so try not to worry.

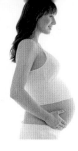

STAGE BY STAGE

Your baby is now capable of surviving (with medical assistance) if she were born at this point, but her remaining weeks in the womb are vitally important for achieving her full development.

Week 28

Although your baby now looks fully formed, many of her organs are still developing and will continue to do so even after she has been born (especially her lungs and brain). Although there is less room to move now, she may still be able to straighten up, but she is incredibly agile and can easily raise her feet above her head. So if you feel a kick at the top of your abdomen, it doesn't necessarily mean that her head is at the lower part.

Week 29

The space between the two frontal bones of the forehead has nearly closed and the bones on the right and left of the skull almost meet at the top, but there is still a gap for further growth of your baby's brain and head to take place. At last, her head looks in proportion to the rest of her body. The brain inside is taking on the characteristic wrinkled appearance as more connections are made between nerve cells (see pages 182–3).

Week 30

Your baby's skeleton is hardening now and her bone marrow has taken over the job of manufacturing red blood cells from the liver. At this stage of pregnancy it is common for many babies to move into the 'head-down' position in order to get ready for the birth, so you may experience some pressure on your pelvic floor.

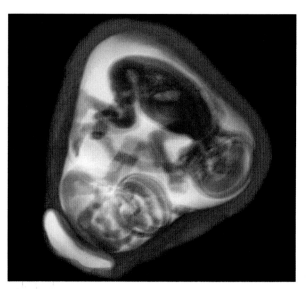

32-week-old twin foetuses.

Week 31

Your baby may be more aware of an orange glow if you stand in front of a bright light. She opens and closes her eyes frequently and her pupils dilate occasionally. Her eyes are gaining pigmentation, but true eye colour won't be established until six to nine months after birth because it needs natural light to complete the process.

Week 32

Your baby's five senses are functioning, but hearing becomes particularly important (see page 181). Although your baby will be surrounded by sound

– from the thumping of your heartbeat and the whooshing of your digestive system to the sound of blood being pumped through your blood vessels, she can hear voices from outside and can distinguish your voice above all others. Studies have shown that babies listen intently and pick up the general pattern and rhythm of their mother's native language, favouring it above others.

Week 33

There's not much room in there now and so you'll probably feel movements that are more like your baby rolling than kicking. Her head may have increased in size by 9.5 mm (½ in) because her brain has gone through another growth spurt. Try to set aside a little time each day to feel her movements. You may notice that she is less active when you are moving about, so sit quietly for a while and you may be rewarded with a kick or two. You may find that eating ice cream or sorbet produces a strong response, too! Ask your doctor or midwife how much movement you should expect to feel.

Week 34

Fat is still being laid down, which means that your baby's skin is gradually turning from red to pink. This will make her more appealing to our eyes when she is born – nature's way of helping to ensure that she will be looked after. Your baby's immune system is developing and by the time she is born it should be able to fight mild infections. She may stick her tongue out from time to time as she gets ready to suckle once she has been born.

Week 35

Although a baby of this age is still considered to be premature, 99 per cent of those born at 33 weeks' gestation survive without serious problems (see pages 194–5). The lungs are mature by now and so a premature baby delivered at this point is unlikely to suffer the breathing difficulties that can make life harder for younger babies.

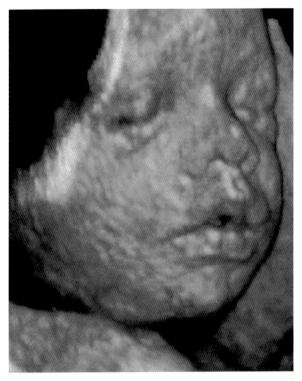

An ultrasound of a 30-week-old foetus.

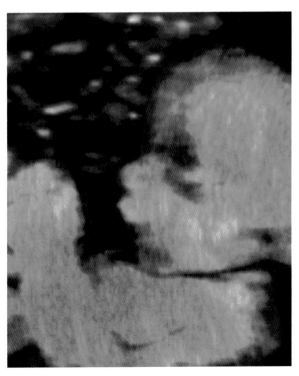

An ultrasound of a 32-week-old foetus.

Week 36

Your baby's movements will seem slower and more deliberate now. Kicks and thumps are much stronger, too, although your baby is becoming increasingly constricted. There is less amniotic fluid now, too, so you may be able to see a foot or an elbow quite clearly pushing at your abdomen.

Week 37

If your baby were to be born now she would be considered to be full term. If she is lying in the breech position (see pages 212–15) your doctor or midwife may suggest that they try to perform an 'external cephalic version' (see page 213) and manipulate your baby into the head-down position. Although they may also be able to estimate the size of your baby, it is only an estimate and you really won't know her true size until she is born.

Week 38

You could go into labour at any time now. No one knows for sure what determines the start of labour, but it is thought to be triggered by hormones produced by the baby. Her immune system is developing and you will have passed on antibodies to all the diseases to which you have gained immunity during your life. By breastfeeding your baby you can continue to boost her immune system because more antibodies and nutrients will be passed to her by your colostrum – the yellowish liquid that your breasts produce after childbirth, before your milk comes in (see pages 328–9). After sustaining your baby for so long, your placenta now begins to age and becomes less efficient. Your baby will be fine for now, but your doctor or midwife will be making regular checks on her progress.

Week 39

Your baby's neck muscles have developed so that her head can be held away from her chest, but it is also being supported by the natural buoyancy of the amniotic fluid. Once she is born, your baby will need to have her head and neck supported at all times while she is being held. The soft, fuzzy hair that covered your baby's body, known as 'lanugo' (after the Latin word for 'woolly') is partially coming away. Your baby may have actually swallowed some of it via the amniotic fluid. It will collect in her bowels and form part of the greenish-black 'meconium' the first 'solid' waste matter that she will pass after birth.

YOUR BABY'S WEIGHT

In the UK, babies weigh on average 3.3 kg (7 lb 5 oz) at birth. A third of this weight will probably have been gained by week 28, half of it by week 31 and two-thirds by week 34. The father's genetic influence on this aspect is actually quite small and the mother has the greatest influence over birth weight.

Taller, heavier women tend to have larger babies, but nutrition plays the greatest and most important part (see pages 18–19). Boy babies tend to be bigger than girls and second babies larger than first-borns. Both Afro-Caribbean and Asian babies tend to be lighter than Caucasian ones.

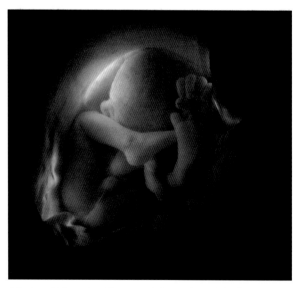

A foetus at 36 weeks – the uterus is becoming a tight fit.

COMPARING SIZE

At 32 weeks the foetus is about 29 cm (11½ in) long, or about the distance from your elbow to the base of your fingers. At 38 weeks it is about 35 cm (14 in) long, or about the distance from your elbow to the tips of your fingers.

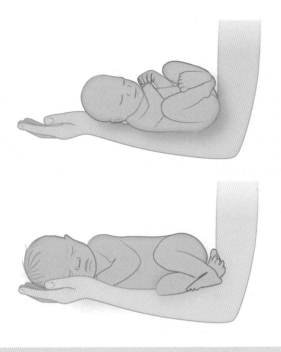

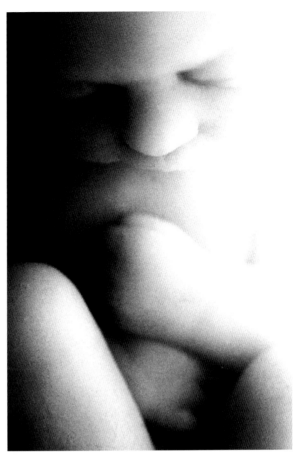

Ready to be born, this baby has reached full term.

Week 40

Your baby will be born very soon now and you will be able to see each other for the first time. All the final details of her appearance are now in place and she has eyebrows, eyelashes, and tiny toenails and fingernails. She has 300 bones in her skeleton – 94 more than you or any other adult, because the extra ones will fuse together as she grows. Her body is also made up of approximately 15 per cent fat, which will help to keep her warm and store up energy. Your baby will leave the fluid-filled uterus and take her first breath of air at any time now. When she does so, the act of breathing will trigger irreversible changes within her heart and arteries that will send the blood supply to her lungs, also helping her to expel her very first cry.

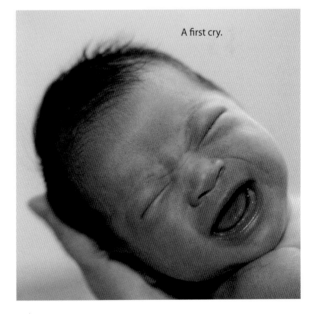

A first cry.

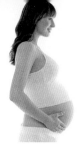

WHAT YOUR BABY SENSES

In many Eastern philosophies, at the moment that a baby is born, she is already considered to be one year old – reflecting the idea that the baby develops as a person before her birth. In the West, we are starting to realise that there is some substance to that idea.

Your baby is already using her increasingly sophisticated senses to gather and process information and from as early as 20 weeks her neural network enables her to kick and communicate with you. Gradually, her senses of hearing, touch, taste, smell and sight are being stimulated by what happens in your body – and by sensations from the outside world. What you do in terms of the food you eat, the rest you take and the way that you react to situations is all transmitted to her through hormones that are released (see pages 36–7) and what she can feel or hear from the outside world. So once your baby is born, she will certainly recognise your voice, but she may also find that the foods she receives via your breastmilk or the music that you listen to are already familiar to her, too.

Noticing changes

Your baby will pick up any changes in the pattern of your eating habits, rest and relaxation times, exercise or differences in noise level. When you are under stress and your body releases cortisol (a stress hormone) your baby responds by adjusting the amount of cortisol in her own body (see.pages 146–7). Your rest and sleep patterns also have a far-reaching effect: when researchers in Switzerland studied a group of pregnant women they were surprised to find that early-rising mothers went on to have babies who woke early, while those women who stayed up late had children who went to sleep late. By the 32nd week of pregnancy your baby will have developed four distinct types of activity pattern: active awareness, quiet awareness, active sleep and quiet sleep. Brainwave patterns have demonstrated that the active sleep phase is similar to rapid eye movement (REM) sleep. Up until 32 weeks, your baby spends a good deal of time in this active sleep phase, but after that she is more often awake and in the actively awake, or the quietly awake, periods of activity. It is thought that the smoother and more regular the rhythms of the mother's habits (eating, sleeping, exercise or relaxation), the more easily the baby will develop and settle after birth.

Touch

Touch is the first of your baby's senses to develop and begins as early as seven or eight weeks, when she also starts to move. By week 10 or 11 the palms of her hands will have become sensitive and she may feel her own face with them, though in the early stages of pregnancy it is most common for babies to turn away if their hand brushes their cheek. At first, they have little control over their movements, but in the latter stages of pregnancy, your baby is more likely to turn towards the stimulus. This may be a sign of the rooting reflex, which will be so important when she is fed (see pages 292–3). By week 14 her whole body will be responding to touch and as the

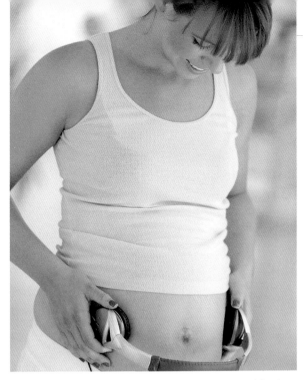

The music you play to your baby in the womb may sound familiar to her after she is born. Be sure not to play it too loudly, though.

space in the uterus becomes more confined, the umbilical cord will touch your baby more frequently – 4-D ultrasound scans have even shown babies holding on to their cords. Just as she will use her mouth to explore objects once born, your baby may suck her thumbs, fingers or toes. She may like sucking her thumb, though she doesn't yet associate the action with satisfying hunger. Shortly before birth she will be gently squeezed by Braxton Hicks' contractions (see pages 174 and 258). Besides toning your uterus in preparation for birth, it is thought that they also help stimulate your baby's senses and brain.

Hearing

This has probably been studied more than any other sense because it is the easiest one to stimulate before birth. Babies react to sound at around 24 weeks as the tiny bones in their ears harden and begin to work together. Your baby's environment in the uterus is full of sounds from your body such as your booming heartbeat and your gurgling digestive system as well as the thumping of your blood pulsing through the umbilical cord. Sounds from the world outside do

penetrate the uterus and resonate through the amniotic fluid, but in a quieter, more muffled, form. As sound waves travel towards you, a good number of them bounce off your body, while some are absorbed by your clothes and skin. Sounds that are in the high-frequency range tend to bounce back more easily, while low-frequency sounds get through, so it is likely that your baby will hear her father's voice more easily (see page 189).

Sight

From around 27 weeks your baby can open and close her eyes, but her sight will be the last sense to develop while she is in the uterus. Her environment is quite a dark one, but she may see an orange glow if you sunbathe unclothed. She can probably only perceive the tone of the glow rather than the colour because it is thought that babies' vision inside the uterus is only in black, white and grey. Colour perception is thought to develop around two months after birth and this is why so many toys for newborns are created in black and white – so that they are easier for the baby to see more clearly.

Taste & smell

From around 12 weeks your baby will be swallowing amniotic fluid and this will carry flavours and smells from the foods you eat. By around week 35 your baby's taste buds are sufficiently developed so that she can detect the flavour of the foods you have eaten in the amniotic fluid. Studies have shown that this can lead babies to develop food preferences during pregnancy, so it is a good idea to eat a wide, varied diet so that your baby has the chance to get used to many different flavours. This is called 'dietary imprinting' and if you offer a wide variety of flavours, including strong ones such as garlic, your baby may become a less fussy eater once she gets on to solids. A newborn baby's sense of smell is acute at first and it has been shown that after just three days a new baby can recognise the smell of her own mother's milk.

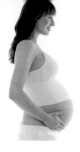

YOUR BABY'S BRAIN

Your baby will be born with around 200 billion brain cells – the most that she will ever have in her entire life. As she grows and develops, she will make vital connections between those cells. You can help her to begin the process now.

Two hundred billion brain cells, or neurons, is an extraordinary number isn't it? Neurons are the basic information-processing structures in the central nervous system and their function is to receive signals or 'information' from other neurons, to process that information and then to send an outgoing signal containing the information to other neurons. There may be as many as 10,000 specific types of neurons in the human brain, but there are three types that handle the main functions of our brain and body: motor neurons (for conveying information to make us move), sensory neurons (for transmitting information to and from our five senses so that we can hear, see, smell, taste and touch) and interneurons (which communicate signals between different types of neurons that include the cognitive information through which we are able to reason, think, plan, remember and dream).

Creating networks

Even more abundant than the neurons are 'glia', vital cells that support the neurons and which provide the structures along which the neurons can make their networks of connections. These are made via the synapses and, on average, each neuron is connected to other neurons by approximately 10,000 synapses. The number of pathways in the brain, along which the information flows, is so numerous it is greater than the number of all known stars in the universe.

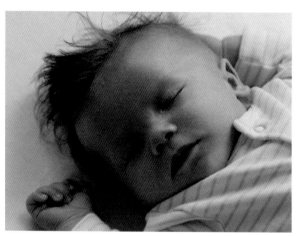

Once your baby is born, she needs plenty of sleep for good brain development.

Making connections

By the time your baby is one year old she will have lost 80 billion of those brain cells and she will continue to lose more as she grows to adulthood. This is a natural process known as 'synaptic pruning', but it is the connections between the cells that are really crucial to intellectual development. The more connections made, the greater the number of brain cells that survive: it is a case of 'use it or lose it'. If you think of your baby's brain as a computer, you can imagine a box of cells with dangling wires. The cells need to be connected to each other to work usefully, so for your baby to be able to think and solve problems, those 'wires' need to join from one

YOUR BABY'S BRAIN DEVELOPMENT BEFORE BIRTH

Weeks 3–4 The brain begins to develop from separate vesicles (tiny membrane-enclosed sacs). These join together within a few days

Week 11 The brain has formed and is already beginning to operate

Week 16 Your baby's rudimentary muscles are beginning to respond to signals from the brain

Week 20 The nerve cells that serve the senses are now forming in particular areas of the brain. The connections that will enable your baby to use her memory and to think are already beginning to form

Week 22 The 'germinal matrix' in the centre of your baby's brain is manufacturing brain cells at an astonishing rate. This extraordinary structure will no longer be needed by the end of your pregnancy and will disappear before your baby is born, but her brain will continue to expand (as connections are made) until she is five years old

Week 24 Your baby's brainwave patterns are already similar to those of a newborn

Week 27 The brain is enlarging, but it still looks smooth. There will be a growth spurt now that will not only increase the number of cells, but will develop the dendrites (the projections from each cell that receive the impulses from other neurons), which will, in turn, help your baby's brain to

make more connections. Myelin sheaths also form to protect the axons (projections that carry impulses from the cell). For the sheaths to form properly, essential fatty acids must be supplied from your diet (see page 43)

Week 29 The brain is growing so rapidly that it is pushing out the soft bones of your baby's skull

Week 30 The brain is no longer smooth, but has formed shallow grooves that make it look more like a walnut. These increase its surface area and so allow even more cells and connections to be made

Week 31 Brain cells now begin to die off. This process serves the same sort of purpose as pruning a plant does: the weaker parts are discarded so that the stronger parts will thrive. Synaptic pruning will reach a peak at around four weeks before your baby's birth. It is worth noting that most of the cells that die will do so because they have not been stimulated into action

Week 33 Rapid brain development and stronger connections between cells has resulted in the size of your baby's head increasing by around 9.5 mm (³/₈ in) in just one week

Week 36 Your baby's nervous system is now fully developed and her brain has around 200 billion cells that are ready to make more connections

cell to another, and then to another and so on. To make these connections, your baby's brain needs to be stimulated and by doing simple things such as talking and singing to your baby and stroking her through your abdomen, you can actually begin this before she has even been born (see pages 188–9).

Smooth transmission

In the third trimester of pregnancy the myelin sheath that formed around your baby's spinal cord to protect it (see pages 64 and 185) also covers the nerve fibres that enter and leave her brain. This means that the nerve impulses that carry the messages to and from the brain around the rest of the body can now be

transmitted more quickly and smoothly. This will help your baby with fine motor control (intricate or delicate movements) and to learn new skills. So every movement that she makes and each time she touches her own body or the sides of your uterus, her brain is working, receiving and sending messages.

Growth & development

Your baby's brain cells will multiply at a rate of 250,000 per minute – to help her brain to grow and develop to its full potential. Not only do you need to find ways to stimulate her (see pages 188–9), but you also need to provide her with specific nutrients, in particular, specialised fats (see pages 184–5).

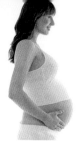

NUTRITIONAL FACTS

In this trimester your baby will be gaining weight faster than ever, but it is not the quantity of what you eat that is important – it is the quality – and there are some key nutrients that both you and your baby will need in the next few months.

Carry on eating your basic healthy diet, but pay particular attention to the following nutrients. Look at the meal suggestions in this section to get some different food-preparation ideas.

Protein

Protein is more important than ever now as your baby builds muscle and tissue. To supply the varying kinds of protein that your baby needs for a range of body functions, you should aim to eat a number of different combinations of amino acids (see page 80). You also require a good supply of protein to help you to build your reserves in readiness for labour, birth and breastfeeding.

Glycine

Glycine is an amino acid that is essential for growth and your baby receives it via the placenta and your bloodstream. In this last trimester she needs between two and 10 times more glycine than any other amino acid, so it is a good idea to increase your intake of foods that contain it (see box right).

Iron

Iron is vital for you to build up your stores in preparation for labour. It will help to give you energy and boost your immune system to enable you to fight off infection and it will also help to prevent premature labour. It is really important that you are

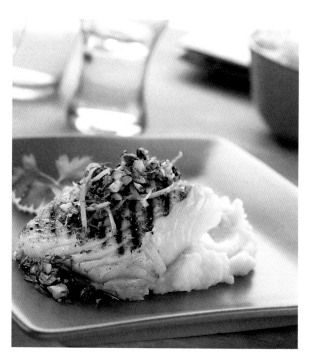

Cod is a great source of the amino acid glycine – vital for your baby's growth.

SOURCES OF GLYCINE

Baked beans	Cod	Milk
Beef	Eggs	Tuna
Black-eyed peas	Kidney beans	
Chicken	Lentils	

BOOSTING THE BRAIN WITH 'SMART' FATS

From week 28 to 40 you have a crucial window of opportunity to help your baby's brain begin to develop to its full potential:

Your baby's brain needs a distinct set of nutrients, quite different to the rest of her body's requirements. Her bones mainly need calcium and her muscles are powered by protein, but the brain needs fats and, in particular, long-chain polyunsaturated fatty acids (LCPUFAs). More than 60 per cent of her brain will be composed of fatty acids, but she cannot make essential fatty acids (EFAs) herself: they must come from you. If you do not eat food containing enough of these, her supply will be taken from your body's stores, which may result in the slightly impaired brain function that so many women complain of in pregnancy, when they find they are forgetful or clumsy. (See page 186 for sources of omega-3 and omega-6 EFAs.)

LCPs are needed for the smooth and rapid transmission of signals between nerve cells (see pages 182–3). There are basically two types that are crucial to brain function: linoleic acid (omega-6) and alpha linolenic acid (omega-3). One of the crucial forms of omega-3 is docosahexaenoic acid (DHA), which is important for cognitive brain function, vision and heart health, and may also increase your baby's birth weight. It may also help to prevent pregnancy-induced high blood pressure (hypertension) and reduce the risk of premature birth.

Choline is another 'smart' fat found in the brain that is needed for the production of cell membranes and is linked to the memory and learning centres of the brain. It is found in the myelin sheaths that protect the axons that transmit nerve signal from the cells (neurons) (see page 64). It can be found in a number of foods, but the richest source is egg yolks.

Note: It is advisable for all pregnant women to take an omega-3 supplement as it is hard to receive adequate levels needed for your baby's brain development just through your diet. Consult your doctor or midwife.

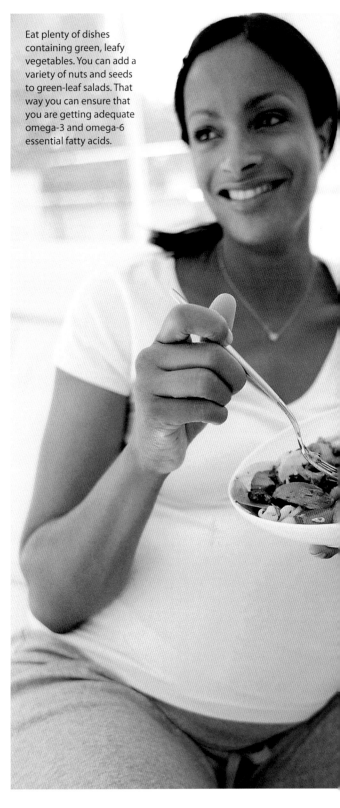

Eat plenty of dishes containing green, leafy vegetables. You can add a variety of nuts and seeds to green-leaf salads. That way you can ensure that you are getting adequate omega-3 and omega-6 essential fatty acids.

not anaemic when you go into labour as it can cause complications. You may lose up to 250 g (9 oz) of iron as a result of labour, so you don't want to start off with low iron levels.

Vitamin C

Vitamin C should be consumed alongside iron-rich foods because it helps your body to absorb the iron. You also need it to boost your immune system and to help your body heal after delivery because it aids the production of collagen, connective tissue and the repair of blood vessels. Good sources can be found in a wide range of fruits and vegetables (see page 84).

Zinc

Zinc is needed for your baby's growth (especially in this last trimester), but is vital for you, too. A pregnant woman needs around 20 mcg of zinc per day, but it can be difficult to get adequate supplies from your normal diet, so ask your doctor or midwife about taking a supplement, if necessary. A good supply of zinc may also prevent postnatal depression because research has shown that women who eat plenty of fish containing essential fatty acids and zinc during the last trimester of pregnancy were much less likely to show symptoms of depression.

Vitamin K

Vitamin K is routinely given as an injection to newborns because it plays an essential role in the clotting of blood. However you can boost your baby's supply in advance of birth by eating foods that are rich in this vitamin. Such foods include broccoli, cabbage and cauliflower. Vitamin K is produced by bacteria in the bowel, but at birth your baby doesn't yet have the colonisation necessary. When you breastfeed your baby you will be passing on some of your store of vitamin K, too.

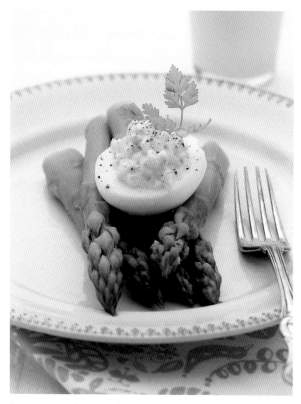
Eggs are a good source of omega-3.

SOURCES OF OMEGA-3 EFAS

Avocados	Pumpkin seeds
Brazil nuts	Shellfish (but take care during pregnancy)
Cold-water fish such as cod, herring, mackerel, salmon, sardines and tuna	
	Sesame seeds
Edible seaweed	Dark-green, leafy vegetables such as kale, mustard greens and spinach
Eggs	
Flaxseed/flaxseed oil	Walnuts
Hempseeds/hempseed oil	

SOURCES OF OMEGA-6 EFAS

Flaxseed/flaxseed oil	Olive oil
Hempseeds/hempseed oil	Pine nuts
Grapeseed oil	Pumpkin seeds
Olives	Sunflower seeds

MEAL IDEAS FOR THE THIRD TRIMESTER

Choose from the following (organic options if possible):

Breakfast

Cereal such as branflakes with semi-skimmed milk, topped with sliced banana and sunflower seeds

Home-made muesli made from oats, fortified wheatgerm, sliced or grated Brazil nuts, dried apricots and raisins, and seeds with semi-skimmed milk

Wholemeal multigrain toast with butter and scrambled eggs, and grilled tomatoes

Natural yogurt with mashed strawberries, raspberries and/or blueberries, topped with sliced almonds

Sardines and grilled tomatoes on wholemeal toast and a glass of juice (orange or grapefruit)

Lunch

Wholemeal bread or pitta sandwich filled with tuna, hummus or avocado and kidney beans, salad and sunflower seeds

Baked potato with cottage cheese and a watercress, spinach and tomato salad topped with sunflower seeds and/or pine nuts

Lentil and tomato soup and wholemeal multigrain bread spread with butter or polyunsaturated margarine

Baked cheese and mushroom omelette with tomato and pine nut salad

Smoked mackerel with baby new potatoes baked in their skins, and an orange, watercress and rocket salad sprinkled with sunflower seeds or pine nuts

Supper

Baked or grilled salmon or cod with parsley sauce, steamed new potatoes, asparagus, broccoli, or cauliflower and peas

Stir-fried chicken with fresh ginger, cashew nuts and baby corn served with brown rice and steamed broccoli

Quorn Bolognese made with sofrito of celery, carrot, onion, garlic and mushroom with wholewheat spaghetti, grated cheese and a green salad

Curry made with lentils, split peas, kidney beans and chickpeas, onion, garlic, tomato and spinach, served with brown rice and natural yogurt

Grilled tomatoes and lean beef or lamb steak with steamed or mashed potatoes, kale, peas and runner beans

Desserts

Baked apples filled with dried apricots, raisins and sultanas

Vanilla panna cotta made with skimmed milk and served with fresh blackcurrant coulis

Fresh fruit salad of apples, pears, bananas and grapes, macerated in orange juice and sprinkled with sliced almonds and Brazil nuts

Snacks

Fresh berry and yogurt smoothie

Raw vegetable sticks including celery, carrot, peppers and cucumber and hummus

A selection of nuts and seeds, olives, grapes or prunes

Celery sticks with cottage cheese, walnuts and apple

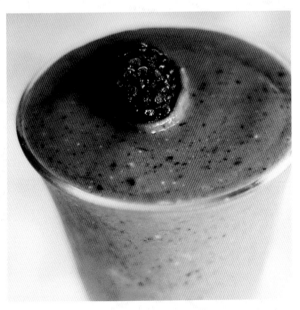

A smoothie makes a delicious, refreshing and nutritious snack.

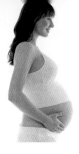

bonding and stimulating

MIND-BODY-BABY

This is the time to really focus on your baby and build your
relationship with her. She will be here very soon and if you stroke
her, talk and sing to her now she will already know your voice and
recognise your soothing touch when she is born.

Now that so much more is known about
babies, both in the uterus and at birth, we
can see that the relationship you forge
with your baby when she arrives can really be a
continuation of the connections that you began
when you were first pregnant (see pages 110–11
and 144–5). In this last trimester, your baby is both
physically and mentally mature enough to send and
receive signals from you and those closest to you. At
the start of this trimester, in your 28th week, your
baby will be at least 26 weeks old, and if she were
born prematurely, she would undoubtedly be
communicating with you. So apart from the obstacle
of your abdomen, why shouldn't she respond to
stimulation from you while still in your uterus?

Using touch & sound

You can use touch and sound to send messages to
her and you can respond to her movements, too.
By interacting with your baby you also strengthen
the bond between you. If a sudden, loud noise
startles her and she kicks, you can soothe her with
your voice and caress your abdomen. By gently
stimulating your body you will not only reinforce
your emotional bond, but you may also help her
intellectual development, too. It is thought that by
communicating with your baby in the uterus, you
may boost her intelligence and lessen the risk of her
developing attention deficit disorder (ADHD).

Playing music (particularly classical) to your unborn
baby is also thought to promote intellectual
development – perhaps by stimulating more
connections to be made between the neurons (see
pages 182–3). And music that babies hear repeatedly
when they are waiting to be born and which are
associated with their mother's periods of relaxation
has been shown to be familiar to them once they
have arrived, and importantly, to soothe them if they
are distressed.

Chemical messages

It is also clear that while positive experiences such
as listening to music, or reading aloud will calm your
mind and slow both your heartbeat and your baby's,
if you are under stress yourself, or fearful, the
opposite will happen and your baby's heart will race
even faster than yours. Do not be surprised if you feel
some frantic kicking when you become angry or
anxious. Your baby is reacting to 'chemical' messages
from you – your stress hormones.

Brief upsets that are swiftly resolved will not
actually harm your baby, but long-term distress
may affect her own ability to cope with emotional
difficulties (see pages 146–7) and this could have
long-term implications. Research has shown that
women undergoing prolonged emotional stress
during pregnancy tend to have smaller babies who
are more likely to cry and more difficult to comfort.

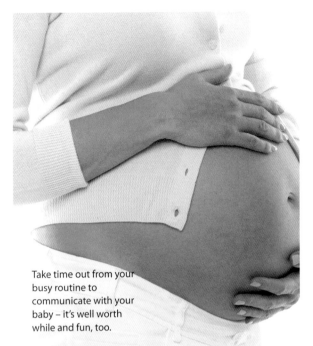

Take time out from your busy routine to communicate with your baby – it's well worth while and fun, too.

Giving attention to your baby

It is important that you make time to be 'with' your baby and give her your undivided attention. In this trimester you are working towards her birth and you need to gather strength and slow down. One of the best things you can do for your baby now is curtail your activities, if you can, and if you work, perhaps start maternity leave well in advance of the birth. It's understandable to want to spend as much time as possible with your baby after she is born and before your maternity leave is up, but your relationship with her needs investment from you now, too.

You need to be emotionally and physically prepared for the labour and birth. Getting ready for your baby is about more than buying equipment. What your baby needs most is you, so use this trimester to prepare for your 'babymoon' (see page 221) and then forget the chores for a while. Now's the time to nurture yourself and your baby.

WAYS TO COMMUNICATE WITH & STIMULATE YOUR BABY

Talk to your baby You can read to her or give her a running commentary on what you are doing as you carry out tasks such cooking or preparing her nursery

Play music to your baby If there's a soothing piece that you particularly like, play it often when you are relaxing. The combination of the gentle sound and the 'happy hormones' that you release as you enjoy it will calm her in your uterus – and may continue to do so after she has been born

Sing to your baby Singing relieves stress and increases lung capacity, which will help to make you stronger going into labour. It will also make you feel good and encourage your body to release all-important 'happy hormones'. Your baby will love to listen and will feel the vibrations from your voice. She may even 'remember' the tune after her birth

Play gentle touching games with your baby When she gives a kick, respond by stroking the opposite end of your abdomen, where her head may be. Or give a gentle pat or press where her foot has just struck. Then do it again if she repeats the kick

Dance and sway as you listen to music The movements that you make will improve your circulation and the amount of oxygen in the blood that will be sent to your baby. Dancing will also encourage your body to release feel-good hormones that will, in turn, encourage your baby to produce 'happy hormones' of her own. She will also hear the sound and feel the rhythm

Encourage your partner to talk and sing to the baby, too The low-frequency sounds of the male voice are more easily heard than female ones, but don't forget that your baby will hear and feel your voice through the vibrations that travel through your body, too, so she will know yours best of all

Each day, make time to use your visualisation techniques to focus your mind on your baby (see pages 110–11 and 145). Lie down comfortably, place your hands on your abdomen and stroke your bump. Imagine what it will be like to hold your baby in your arms and visualise a warmth from your heart travelling down to your baby. Talk to her and tell her how much you love her and want her

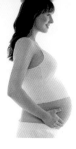

EXERCISE FOR STAMINA

In this last trimester you will be focusing more and more on the approaching labour and birth of your baby. So you need to change the emphasis of the exercise you take. Building stamina is the key to your routine now.

If your pregnancy is going smoothly, without complications, there is no reason why you should not continue with gentle exercise up until the day that you give birth. However, the key thing to remember is that the exercise really should be gentle, so you need to opt for less-strenuous types of exercise or reduce the intensity of what you do. Yoga can be particularly helpful to your preparations for labour and birth because it will teach you how to focus on your breathing (see page 147). Swimming, too, is especially useful because it exercises almost every part of your body and the natural buoyancy of the water makes you feel almost weightless, so there is far less pressure on your back, legs or any aching areas. When sitting, try to avoid lying back and instead sit on your haunches with your chest supported on an exercise ball. This helps encourage your baby to adopt a 'back to front' (her back to your front) position that can make labour easier than a back-to-back position (see pages 212–15).

Building stamina

If you have remained reasonably fit throughout your pregnancy you should have already built up some stamina, but now increasing endurance levels is key. If you are aiming to have an active labour you need to build strength and stamina in your lower body. Squats are one of the best ways of doing this and should form an integral part of your exercise routine.

Squats

Make sure that you always do a brief warm-up before carrying out any exercise and if you are doing squats, try standing with your hands against a wall so that you can raise your heels off the ground without toppling over. By doing this, you will warm up and contract the muscles in your calf before you stretch them in a squat.

This exercise is particularly useful for opening out the pelvis and encouraging your baby to engage (see page 214) and it will also improve the flexibility of your pelvic joints. But take care to do any pelvic exercise gently because your ligaments will be stretched and softened by your pregnancy hormones (see pages 36–7). To do some squats:

- Using a chair for support, stand facing it with your feet apart, in line with your hips.
- Turn your feet out slightly, then slowly bend your knees, gently lowering your body into a squatting position. Hold on to the chair for support and keep your knees in line with your feet.
- Hold for a few seconds only, then gently raise yourself up before repeating once or twice.

Good stretches

At this stage in your pregnancy you are likely to be experiencing some backache, but spine mobility exercises can help to relieve discomfort. Get into an

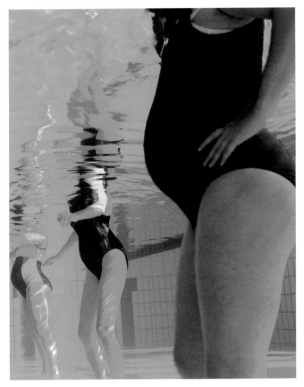

Aquarobics have been shown to help women get into good pscyho-physical condition and deal with pain in labour better.

STAYING SAFE DURING EXERCISE

Make sure that you are always well hydrated. Keep sipping water as you exercise

Make sure that you are well nourished so that your blood sugar is properly balanced (see page 147)

Don't exercise to the point where it is difficult to keep up a conversation

Avoid exercise if you have any kind of infection (including an ordinary cold) because it means that your body is already having to work hard to fight off illness

Stop exercising immediately if you experience any pain, bleeding or contractions and call your doctor or midwife

Keep a check on how your baby reacts when you exercise. You should feel a number of kicks within the first twenty minutes after exercising. A lack of movement indicates that your baby could be distressed, because she is conserving her energy. If this happens you will need to rethink your approach to exercise and perhaps try to find another type of activity. Consult your doctor or midwife

all-fours position on the floor and 'draw' large circles with your hips in a clockwise, anti-clockwise direction, then combine the two movements to make a figure of eight.

Aquarobics

Research has shown that a course of organised water aerobics can reduce the amount of painkilling medication that women request during labour.

A team of researchers led by Rosa Pereira from the University of Campinas, in Brazil, investigated the effects of aquarobics classes on a group of 71 expectant mothers. Half of the women were randomly selected to attend three 50-minute sessions a week over the course of their pregnancy – the others did not take part. The results showed that only 27 per cent of women in the aquarobics group requested analgesia in childbirth, compared to 65 per cent in the control group.

There has been concern that exercise during pregnancy may interfere with the demands of the placenta and the growing baby, and so increase the risk of abnormalities or cause poor development or growth. However, the researchers in Brazil found that there was no harmful effect on the cardiovascular health of the women who did water aerobics.

It was found that the regular practice of moderate water aerobics during pregnancy did not affect the health of the mother or the child. In fact, women in labour made fewer requests for analgesia, which suggests that it can help women get into better psycho-physical condition.

Whatever form of exercise you choose, whether it is a full-body routine, yoga, aquarobics or just a walk around the block, make sure that you do your pelvic floor exercises (see page 141) every day and pay special attention to your posture (see page 140). You'll be glad you made the effort.

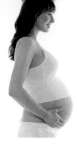

SMALL/LARGE FOR DATES

Occasionally a baby will be found to be growing either too slowly, so that she is too small, or too quickly, so that she is overly large. Both these conditions can present issues that you should know about.

Small for dates

This is is sometimes also called 'foetal growth retardation', but is most commonly written on medical notes as 'intra-uterine growth restriction' (IUGR). The condition may result in a baby weighing less than 2.5 kg (5½ lb) at term and is usually the result of a foetal abnormality or the under-nourishment of the baby, which may be caused by a problem with the placenta such as pre-eclampsia (see pages 208–9), an infection such as rubella (see page 71) or by smoking or alcohol intake, drug abuse (see page 103) or the mother's poor nutrition. The dating scan in the first trimester provides the baseline measurement from which all subsequent checks can be measured, so routine antenatal care is designed to spot IUGR early.

Any reduction in the healthy functioning of the placenta or the flow of blood to your baby will result in IUGR because your baby's supply of nutrients and oxygen will be compromised. Smoking is a common cause and the mother's poor nutrition is frequently the reason for small babies in developing countries, but it is also seen in the UK. Women with an underlying medical problem (see pages 72–3) are also more at risk of having a baby with IUGR because their placenta may develop inadequately, so this is one of the reasons why such women may have more antenatal appointments than those with lower-risk pregnancies. IUGR is also more common in women who have had many pregnancies and it seems to run in families. It also develops in around 20 per cent of all twin and multiple pregnancies and is more likely with identical twins because they share a placenta, so there is always the risk that one baby will receive more blood supply than the other (see page 197).

Around five per cent of IUGR babies will have a chromosomal abnormality such as Down's syndrome (see page 154) or a congenital abnormality such as a problem with the heart, skeleton or kidneys. If there is a possibility of infection being the cause it may be due to rubella, cytomegalovirus (herpes), syphilis or toxoplasmosis. Both syphilis and toxoplasmosis can be treated with antibiotics during pregnancy. Rubella and cytomegalovirus present more difficulties, but cases are rare.

What can be done to help?

If IUGR is suspected, you will be given more ultrasound scans, not only to measure your baby, but to check the amount of amniotic fluid around her and to monitor how fast the blood is pulsing through the umbilical cord. A problem with either of these things can indicate that the placenta is functioning inadequately. A small baby is also likely to be less active and practise her breathing less often. A heart trace is likely to be used in conjunction with these checks and the results of all these examinations should yield a diagnosis.

If you have had a number of consecutive ultrasound scans that show poor, or even nonexistent, growth or that the amount of amniotic fluid in your uterus has decreased (see below) it may be necessary to deliver your baby earlier than your EDD (see page 31). This can only be possible, though, if your baby is more than 24 weeks (when it is judged to be 'viable' outside the womb) and will only be considered if the doctors think that your baby will do better in a special care baby unit (SCBU – see pages 298–301). If this is the case, then the baby may need to be delivered by Caesarean section and you will probably be given an injection of steroids to help her lungs to mature (see page 195).

Large for dates

Heavier and taller women tend to have larger, heavier babies, but big babies are not always the result of inherited traits. The most common cause of overly large babies is diabetes (see page 72). This can cause babies to be born with polycythemia (an excess of red blood cells), poorly developed and immature lungs, jaundice, poor temperature control and hypoglycaemia (too-low blood-sugar levels). The babies of some diabetic mothers may also be smaller than normal (IUGR) and if the mother's diabetes is poorly controlled there is also an increased risk of still birth or intrauterine death.

What can be done to help?

If diabetes is diagnosed during pregnancy it may be treated and controlled with dietary measures and insulin. If your baby seems to be especially large, you may be offered early delivery either by induction or Caesarean section. Depending on whether there are any other complicating factors, you may need to deliver your baby at a hospital that has a SBCU (see pages 298–301) in case she requires extra help. If you are diabetic, you will probably also need insulin intravenously during labour and birth.

AMNIOTIC FLUID – TOO MUCH & TOO LITTLE

Polyhydramnios means that there is too much amniotic fluid in the uterus. Your symptoms may include a taut and tense abdomen, which is difficult to feel the baby through, abdominal discomfort and indigestion, heartburn and breathlessness. Most cases are mild and simply the result of a build-up of fluid towards the end of pregnancy. About 50 per cent of those diagnosed will find that the problem decreases after a time and they will go on to deliver healthy babies. It is more common with twins because of the increased surface of the placenta, or placentas, but it may also be due to the development of gestational diabetes (see page 72) or a foetal abnormality that prevents the baby from absorbing amniotic fluid.

Polyhydramnios is most commonly diagnosed using ultrasound and if the condition is considered severe you may be offered amniocentesis (see page 155) to drain excess fluid away. If the condition is allowed to continue and your waters break (see page 232) prior to labour, there is an increased risk of cord prolapse.

Oligohydramnios is when there is too little amniotic fluid. It is usually due to IUGR (see facing page) or ruptured membranes, but it can also happen in the latter part of a normal pregnancy. The amount of amniotic fluid in the uterus is a good indicator of the health of your unborn baby, so if a scan shows it to be significantly reduced close to your baby's EDD (see page 31) the decision may be taken to deliver her early. It is more rarely seen in early pregnancy (at the 20-week scan) and is likely to indicate an abnormality of the foetal urinary or digestive system.

The main risk at this point is that the baby's lungs fail to develop properly (pulmonary hypoplasia) as it is the swallowing and 'breathing in' of the amniotic fluid that helps lungs develop. There is the risk of club foot developing, too, because the baby will not have enough space for normal growth. Most women with oligohydramnios have normal pregnancies, however, and the condition may be helped by bed rest and an increased fluid intake, intravenously (IV) and by drinking more water.

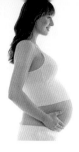

born a little early

PREMATURE LABOUR

Not every baby is born between 37 and 40 weeks. In the UK about 10 per cent of births are defined as being premature, but thanks to the huge advances in neonatal medicine and care, many of these babies who have not had any serious complications in the uterus will catch up and grow up to be perfectly healthy.

Antenatal care is designed to try to identify women at risk of having a premature baby, and every effort is made to try to help you carry your baby for as long as possible (unless she has problems indicating she might be better looked after in the outside world). In general, the longer a normal, healthy baby can stay inside the womb and the heavier she is, the better are her health prospects after her birth and the less time she is likely to need to stay in a special care baby unit (SCBU). For a baby born very early – at 23 weeks for example – the risk of handicap is very high, at 99 per cent, but by 26 weeks that risk will have dropped to 25 per cent and by week 30 the risk is greatly reduced. However, only 1.5 per cent of premature births occur before 32 weeks, so the risk of long-term health problems and handicap to most premature babies is very small.

Why premature births happen

The reasons for premature birth are still unclear. But there are several possible causes.

In some women the cervix shortens during pregnancy and this process seems to be implicated in more than half of the cases of premature labour.

Smoking increases the risk of premature birth by 25 per cent and alcohol or drug abuse also pose a serious threat (see page 103).

Health conditions, such as diabetes (see page 72), can also raise the risk.

Women with gum disease are six times more likely to go into premature labour. This is thought to be because harmful bacteria appear to target the placenta and amniotic fluid. Smoking lowers resistance to bacteria in the mouth.

Placental problems (particularly if nutrition the baby is receiving from it is inadequate) may cause the baby to release hormones that trigger labour.

If the baby is stressed it sends a signal to accelerate birth because conditions in the uterus are worsening. If a woman is stressed her adrenal glands may also release hormones, which may prompt an increased production of oestrogen, which can trigger labour. Or stress may be due to levels of a protein found in the vagina and cervix when a woman is about to go into labour.

Infection of the urinary tract or the vagina is another common factor, with around 20–40 per cent of premature labours being attributed to this.

If you have had a previous premature birth, then statistically, you are more likely to have another.

Your doctor may have to intervene if you have pre-eclampsia, high blood pressure, diabetes or placental insufficiency, placental abruption or placenta praevia.

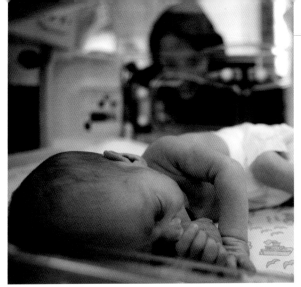

A little extra help at the start of life can usually ensure healthy growth and development thereafter.

Issues for premature babies

Immature lungs One of the main problems for premature babies is the fact that their lungs have not had time to develop fully and they will not be sufficiently elastic to enable the baby to breathe unaided. Surfactant (a detergent-like substance needed to coat the alveoli and keep them open as they inflate with each breath) is not produced in the baby's lungs until week 26. Without it, the walls of the alveoli are liable to collapse. Doctors may spray artificial surfactant into the lungs and although after 35 weeks there is usually a sufficient amount naturally occurring, she may still require the insertion of tiny tubes in her nose to ensure that she is getting enough oxygen.

If your baby has to be delivered before 35 weeks you will probably be given an injection of steroids to help her to produce surfactant more rapidly. These steroids also encourage fat to be laid down under the skin to help keep the baby warm, but they take around 24–48 hours to work, so the staff will always try to delay delivery at least until they have had time to take effect.

Difficulty feeding Premature babies also commonly have difficulty taking their feeds. The sucking reflex is not fully developed before 35 weeks and the digestive system is unable to cope with large quantities of liquid. This means that these babies are usually fed with small quantities of milk via a tiny tube and at frequent intervals.

WARNING SIGNS

If you experience abdominal pain, bleeding, contractions or your waters breaking contact your doctor or midwife without delay. If there is any sign of infection, you may be given syntocinon intravenously to speed up and increase contractions (see page 233). If your baby shows signs of distress or is in the wrong position for birth, she may be delivered by Caesarean section (see pages 286–9).

If your waters have not broken, but you have contractions, or have had a 'show' (see pages 232–3) then you may be asked to go to hospital, where you may be given drugs that relax the uterus and help stop contractions. You will need complete bed rest and careful monitoring. If your membranes are still intact and contractions mild, you may be able to halt the onset of labour, but without the use of drugs. Once the contractions have stopped you should be able to go home, but bed rest is still best and you should abstain from sex.

If your contractions are stronger and become established, however, there is little that can be done to delay labour much beyond another 48 hours. This time is still crucial, though, because it gives a chance for you to receive steroid injections to help mature your baby's lungs and it will also allow the staff looking after you to transfer you to a hospital that has a SCBU and is better able to look after you.

Vaginal delivery may be more rapid than it would have been at full term because your baby will be smaller. However it is also likely that she will not yet be in the head-down position, so a Caesarean section delivery is far more common in these circumstances. If your baby is in distress a Caesarean section will be performed mostly for speed of delivery, but it may also be done to protect her head. This is because premature babies' skull bones are much softer than full-term babies' bones.

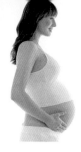

ANTENATAL CARE

Towards the end of this trimester, your doctor or midwife will monitor your progress carefully. You may want to discuss your options for birth in greater detail now, so take advantage of specialist knowledge to help you make your plans.

At each of your antenatal appointments you will have all your usual routine checks. These will include:

- Urine tests to check for the presence of proteins or sugar, which might indicate risk of pre-eclampsia (see pages 208–9) or diabetes (see page 72).
- You may be weighed.
- You will have your blood pressure taken.
- The height of your fundus (the top of your enlarged uterus) will be measured. If the height of this is either higher or lower than your EDD (see page 31) would suggest, you may be offered an ultrasound scan to check the size of your baby and the levels of amniotic fluid present.

- You will have your abdomen palpated to determine which way your baby is lying in the womb (see pages 212–15).
- You may also have a blood test at 28 or 32 weeks to check for anaemia and for any sign of unusual red blood cell antibodies that could cause problems with bleeding during delivery.
- If you are rhesus negative (see page 33) your blood will be checked to make sure that you have not produced any rhesus antibodies and you will also be given an anti-D injection.
- If any other complications are suspected at this stage you may be offered further ultrasound scans.

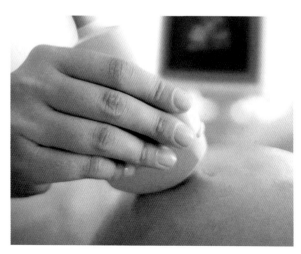

An ultrasound scan being given in the third trimester.

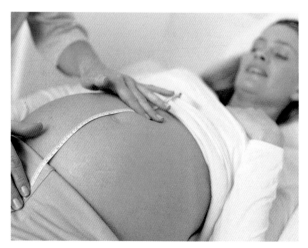

Measuring the height of the fundus.

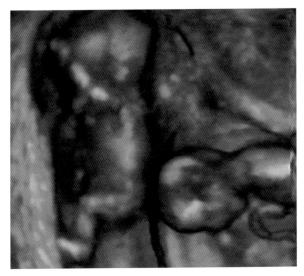

An ultrasound scan of non-identical twin foetuses at 16 weeks.

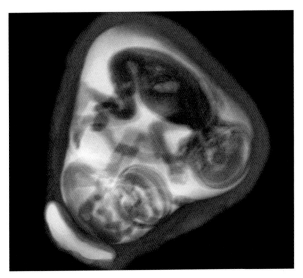

A coloured magnetic resonance imaging (MRI) scan of 32-week-old twin male foetuses.

Antenatal care for twins

Carrying twins, or more, increases the risk of complications, especially: premature birth (see pages 194–5); IUGR (see page 192); pre-eclampsia (see pages 208–9); anaemia and placenta praevia (see page 209). So if you are expecting twins, your pregnancy will be more closely monitored than for a single baby. Around 50 per cent of twins are born early, either spontaneously, or, more frequently, by planned induction (see pages 226–9) or Caesarean section, and so twins are more likely to need special care. They tend to be smaller than single babies, but no matter what their birth weight, newborns also often need help with breathing and feeding because these reflexes are less well developed.

Common complications with twins

Antenatal care in the last trimester will be carefully managed. High blood pressure is more common in multiple pregnancies, at about three in every 10 women compared with one in 10 among single pregnancies. Cervical weakness can also be a problem because of the added weight of two babies (and perhaps two placentas) on your cervix. Your 20-week scan will let your carers see whether your cervix is

beginning to shorten and dilate – you may be given a surgical cerclage (see page 121) to keep it closed until labour is due. If you are having identical twins sharing one amniotic sac, there is a risk of the umbilical cords entangling. This is potentially dangerous because their blood supplies can become restricted or even cut off, so you will be closely monitored and your babies will most likely be delivered by Caesarean to avoid delivery problems.

Polyhydramnios (see page 193) is more common for identical twins and in most cases the cause is unknown, but it may be due to twin-to-twin transfusion syndrome (TTTS) when connections form between arteries and veins in the placenta that identical twins share, so that blood goes from one baby to another, one twin 'donating' blood to the other. Consequently one twin may be much smaller and weaker than the other, so early delivery may be necessary to give the smaller baby a better chance.

In general, one twin will be born larger and heavier than the other, but unless there is a marked difference, this will not be a cause for concern. Even in the uterus, one twin is often more active and quicker to react to stimulus than the other and will have a faster heartbeat and a stronger kick.

Where do you want to give birth?

This is an important question because it will set the tone for the kind of labour and delivery that you aim for. The key thing is that it is an aim, because it is impossible to predict how things will progress and it is essential that you remain flexible in attitude and are prepared to change your plans. 'D-Day' (Delivery Day) is not really what these nine months have led up to – it is having a healthy baby that is important, not the way that she arrives. That said, if you are prepared for labour and birth it can make it a much more rewarding experience, so it is important to know exactly what all your options are so that you can make the decision that is right for you.

Reviewing your plans

You may have expressed a preference about your baby's place of birth earlier in your pregnancy, but you can review your choices in this last trimester and change your mind. Where you give birth may be dictated by whether yours is a high-risk pregnancy (see pages 32–3), any complications that you may have developed or whether there is a pre-existing condition (see pages 72–3).

If you are having twins or triplets, for example, you will be scheduled for a hospital delivery, and as this will have been clear from early on in your pregnancy, you may be content with it. If, however, your pregnancy started without any difficulties and you were hoping for a home birth, but subsequent events have made that impossible, it is natural to feel a little disappointed. However, try to use this time to adjust. You may at least be able to exercise choice over the hospital that you give birth in.

If your pregnancy has been straightforward, you may have grown in confidence over these past months and be keen on giving birth at home or at a midwife-run birthing centre. However, 97 per cent of babies in the UK are born in hospital and you may prefer yours to be among that number. If you know a little more about what each environment offers you will be able to make the right choice.

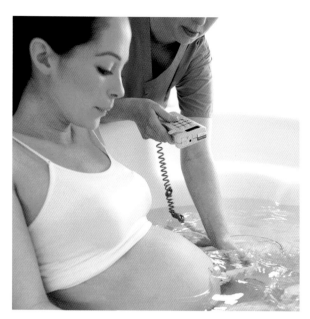

Many hospitals now have birthing pools available. If you want one for your home birth, you will need to hire one well in advance.

Hospital care

If your pregnancy has been uncomplicated then you have probably been looked after by your doctor and midwife, with perhaps only visits to hospital for routine scans and tests. You may be able to choose this or another hospital for your baby's birth, so it is worth asking your doctor or midwife for advice. Bear in mind the practicalities of getting there. If you have had some antenatal care carried out at a hospital under an obstetrician or midwife, you may be more inclined towards continuing with it there.

Find out who will be responsible for looking after you at your preferred hospital. Then find out about the maternity unit. Most UK hospitals have birthing rooms where you can go through labour, delivery and some recovery time, before you go on to the ward, but a few let you stay in the same room with your baby until you go home.

A hospital birth may mean a certain loss of privacy, but it does give you access to specialist expertise and life-saving equipment, if necessary. You can use many forms of natural pain relief in hospital, such as hypnobirthing (see page 144) and massage,

QUESTIONS TO ASK AT THE HOSPITAL

What is the policy on induction?

Is there a time limit on 2nd-stage labour?

What are the Caesarean rates and how do these compare with the national average?

Can I move around during labour and can I choose the position that I give birth in?

Are epidurals available 24 hours a day?

Is continuous foetal monitoring used routinely?

Does the hospital have a special care baby unit (SCBU) or do sick babies have to be transferred to another hospital?

Am I limited in the number of people who can be in the birthing room with me?

Do you have a birthing pool, or pools, and how many midwives are experienced in water births?

Are there likely to be medical students or student midwives present?

Can I bring in birth aids such as a birthing ball, homeopathic remedies, aromatherapy oils or music?

Can I eat and drink during early labour?

What are the visiting hours? Can my partner visit me and our baby outside these times?

How are newborns identified and what security systems are in place?

---

just as you would with a home birth, but you should also be able to have partial or full pain relief (see pages 244–51) and if a Caesarean is necessary it can be performed without delay (see pages 286–9).

Birthing centres

You may be able to choose to give birth at an NHS or private birthing centre, where you will have the care of community or private midwives, some of whom you may know from your antenatal care. Birthing centres are midwife-run and although a few are attached to hospitals, most are independent from them, and so they do not have doctors or specialists on site. This is a low-tech option, but intervention rates tend to be lower than in hospitals and may suit women who want a more natural approach but not a home birth.

Pain-relief options such as birthing pools, TENS and gas and air (entonox) may be available (see page 244), but other forms of pain relief such as epidurals (see pages 246–7) will not, because they must be administered by an anaesthetist. Keep in mind, too, that if problems do arise you may need to be transferred to hospital, so perhaps check where this is and how long it might take to get there.

Home birth

You may prefer to give birth at home, perhaps with family members there. If you have small children, think hard about having them present and ask someone they know to care for them (see page 217).

You are legally entitled to a home birth, but it is not always possible because of midwife shortage. Your midwife will be responsible for organising your care, but if you cannot get the support you want, you may be able to seek help from your local head of midwifery services or the supervisor of midwives. Or try contacting the consultant midwife at the hospital, who is there to promote normal childbirth and may be able to help you. Most women opt for a home birth to avoid medical intervention so bear in mind that certain pain relief, such as epidurals (see pages 246–7), will not be available.

For many women, fear can intensify pain (see page 238), so for some women being at home allows more control, leading to less fearfulness. At home you can use natural pain relief (see pages 252–7) and your midwife may bring entonox with her. You may also be able to hire a birthing pool. Remember that situations can change and your midwife may want to transfer you to hospital if there are problems.

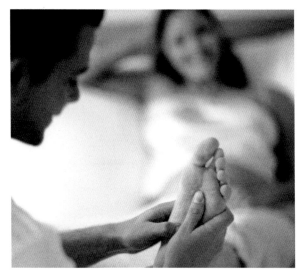

The right birth partner is important. Your baby's father may be the one – if not, select someone who can support you fully.

Birth partners

Who you choose to be with you at the birth is an important personal decision. Most fathers attend their baby's birth and there is no doubt that it is a momentous, life-changing experience that strengthens the bond between father and baby. Although your partner may be keen to be there to support you, some fathers find it difficult. Watching the person you love go through pain can be hard and some men just feel they can't face it. If this is the case for your partner, it may be better to find someone else who can fully support you, but consider your choice carefully – once you have extended this invitation it may be difficult to retract it.

A position of responsibility

Being present at a birth is an honour, but it also carries responsibilities. If you plan to ask more than one person to attend, check with your midwife or hospital first to make sure that they are able to accommodate more than one partner. Even if you are having a home birth, it is best to speak to your midwife (out of courtesy, if nothing else) and whoever is present must be prepared to leave the room if asked to do so by the midwife.

STEM CELL HARVESTING

Stem cells have the ability to develop into different types of cells, which are the building blocks of blood, organ tissue and the immune system. Studies have shown that they may be used to treat up to 70 diseases and conditions (especially those that involve the malfunction or destruction of cells such as leukaemia), so some parents have them collected and stored as a kind of health insurance for their baby's future. Stem cells are found in the blood of the baby's umbilical cord, but shortly after birth they travel to her bone marrow and transform into blood-manufacturing cells.

This is partly why stem-cell harvesting is controversial. If the cells are to be collected, the baby's cord must be clamped as soon as possible and the blood withdrawn, but this means that the third stage of labour is interrupted and the baby may not get as much of this kind of blood as she would if the clamping didn't happen quite so swiftly. If you do wish to collect these cells, you will need to ask your hospital at least eight weeks in advance whether they have the facilities to do so. You will also need to make private arrangements to pay for the blood to be collected, frozen and stored.

CIRCUMCISION

It is estimated that around 30,000 boys are circumcised in the UK every year, mostly for religious reasons. It is not routinely available on the NHS because there are no medical reasons for having a newborn boy circumcised.

If you are considering circumcision for your baby boy, you need to know that it is not risk free. It is painful and so requires local anaesthesia, the administration of which is not pain free. General anaesthesia of newborn babies is risky and so generally to be avoided. There is also a small risk of infection, excessive bleeding or scarring, so it is an issue that you need to discuss properly with your family and your care providers before making a decision.

YOUR BIRTH PREFERENCES

You might like to fill out this chart to take to the hospital with you. Show it to your midwife and discuss it with her. Let your birth partner have a copy, too. Be prepared to be flexible and change your decisions, should the course of your labour make it necessary.

My birth partner

My partner

Mother or other relative

Friend/other children

Doula (or other support)

Induction

I would prefer not to be induced

I would consider being induced for medical reasons

I would consider having my membranes swept, but would prefer not to have chemical induction

I would prefer to be induced

Monitoring

I would prefer not to have continuous foetal monitoring unless there are signs that my baby is distressed

Labour

I want to be able to walk and move around, if possible

I would like to be able to eat and drink in early labour

I'd like to be able to use a birthing pool for at least some of my labour

Pain relief

I wish to give birth without pain-relief medication

I would like an epidural as early as possible

I would like an epidural later

I would like to have medication available, but only given to me if I ask for it

Managed delivery

I would prefer ventouse (vacuum version) to be used rather than forceps, if assisted delivery becomes necessary

I would prefer not to have an episiotomy unless it is necessary

I would rather have an episiotomy than risk tearing

Caesarean

If I need to have an emergency Caesarean I would like my partner to be present at all times

If I need to have an emergency Caesarean I would like to see my baby as soon as possible afterwards

I would prefer to have an epidural or spinal block, if possible

I would prefer to have a full anaesthetic, but I would like my baby to be handed to (name of person) after the birth

After the birth

I would like to hold my baby immediately after delivery

I would like to wait until my baby's cord has stopped pulsing before it is cut

I would like my partner to cut the cord

I would like to have syntocinon to speed up delivery in the third stage

I would prefer not to have syntocinon to speed up delivery in the third stage

---

If you are unsure about asking a member of your family or a friend, consider employing a 'doula', who is an experienced woman offering emotional and practical support before, during and after childbirth. Doulas usually have good knowledge of female physiology and can provide physical support (for example, massage), but they are not medical care-givers. You need to inform your midwife in advance. Make sure that even if your partner will not be your birth partner, he knows what your birth preferences are (see above) and is familiar with the practical details of getting you to hospital. Whoever is at the birth with you will need to know what you want, what to expect and what they can do to help. By attending antenatal classes together, you may have formulated a list of birth preferences, but it is useful to draw up a list of things your birth partner can do to help (see pages 260–1).

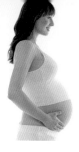

WHEN TO STOP WORK

If you intend returning to work after your baby has been born you will need to have a clear idea of your rights and responsibilities. You also need to think carefully about when is the right time for you to stop work and concentrate on your baby.

Many women continue working for as long as possible before their baby is born so that they can use the majority of their maternity leave after the birth. This is fine, but you should be alert to signs that your body might be under strain. You need plenty of rest in the first trimester, when your baby's organs and body systems are first forming (see pages 62–5) and in the second trimester you will probably have had a burst of energy, with luck feeling in 'blooming' good health. In the third trimester it can be tempting to assume that your baby is fully formed and is just growing bigger. But important developments are taking place such as the 'wiring' of your baby's brain (see pages 182–3). However, you are getting ready for labour and birth, so you need to take good care of yourself, too. Plenty of rest and relaxation, some exercise to boost circulation and re-oxygenate your blood are important (see pages 190–1), as is a well-balanced, nutritious diet (see pages 78–85).

When to give up work

The time for stopping work is your decision, but consult your doctor or midwife. If you have had any complications, you need to review your plans, but even if your pregnancy has been trouble free, consider slowing down. Once your baby is born, you will be on call to feed, change and comfort her, so your mind and body need to be in tip-top condition.

Maternity leave

You are entitled to take up to one year off work and still have the right to return. You cannot be sacked on maternity leave and if you are made redundant you are protected. Your employer is also not allowed to demote you on your return to work. However, some employers assume that pregnant employees will be less committed to their jobs, both now and in future, so if you think you could be sidelined, be clear about your plans. You are entitled to change your mind about your period and timing of maternity leave.

Procedures & practices

There may be a well-established procedure for taking maternity leave and arranging cover at your workplace, but if not, take care not to undersell yourself, for example, by suggesting that someone might be able to do your job part-time.

You may be asked to go to KIT (Keeping in Touch) days, which means doing up to 10 days' work while you are still on maternity leave. These are arranged by mutual consent and enable you to maintain working relationships and keep abreast of developments. You should be paid for these days, but the rate is at your employer's discretion. If you are self-employed be clear about how much leave you will take and when.

Rights and benefits frequently change and the maternity pay that you receive from your employer will depend on your contract, how much you earn

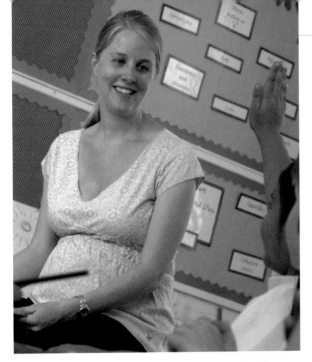
Familiarise yourself with your rights well in advance of taking maternity leave.

and how long you have been working. Your year's entitlement is broken up into blocks of time: the first is known as Ordinary Maternity Leave (OML) and lasts for the first 26 weeks of your leave; Additional Maternity Leave (AML) may be up to a further 26 weeks, bringing the total to 52 weeks. There are two types of materity pay: Statutory Maternity Pay (SMP) and Maternity Allowance (MA). How much you earn and how often and how long you have worked for will determine which you qualify for. If you find that you do not qualify for either, you may be able to claim other benefits instead.

The earliest you can begin maternity leave and claim maternity pay is 11 weeks before the due date, but if you have to stop work before your maternity leave date, your employer may insist that you take the time as maternity leave and not as sick leave. You are legally obliged to take at least two weeks off work after the birth and you will need to give your employer at least four weeks' notice of starting and finishing your leave. If you return to work from OML you are entitled to go back to the same job, and if that job no longer exists, your employer must offer you a similar one with equal pay and conditions.

Paternity leave

Fathers-to-be may be entitled to Ordinary Paternity Leave (OPL) and may also qualify for Ordinary Statutory Paternity Pay (OSPP), but many employers have their own paternity-leave arrangements that are more generous than the statutory entitlement. These are usually included in the individual's employment contract, but if the Statutory (Ordinary and Additional) Paternity Leave arrangement is better and you qualify for it, you may choose that instead. If you qualify, you can take one or two weeks' Ordinary Paternity Leave, but you cannot take odd days off and if you take two weeks they must be taken together. If you are a new father and your partner is returning, or has returned to, work you could also have the right to up to 26 weeks' Additional Paternity Leave, but certain conditions apply, so you would need to be sure that you qualify.

Fathers or same-sex partners do not have a legal right to time off to accompany their partner to antenatal appointments, but many companies will allow employees take holiday or time off in lieu.

When you schedule your paternity leave is up to you. You may want to have time off as soon as the baby is born, but if you already have arranged for someone to help out in the first few days, you may consider postponing parental leave slightly. It will help if you can plan a 'babymoon' (see page 221) so that you can get to know your newborn.

EXTRA RIGHTS & BENEFITS

During your pregnancy and up to a year afterwards, you will be entitled to free prescriptions, free eye treatment and NHS dental care. Ask your midwife for an application form. Once your baby is born you may be entitled to Child Benefit. It is important to apply as soon as possible because claims are only backdated for up to three months. If you give birth in hospital, you may be given an application form there, or you can or ask for one at your local post office or apply online (see Resources).

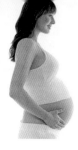

COMMON COMPLAINTS

The third trimester is likely to find you uncomfortable anyway, but a selection of minor ailments might be adding to your discomfort just now. However, there are several things you can do to make life easier.

Oedema, carpal tunnel syndrome & leg cramps

Oedema is the swelling of the ankles or hands and is common towards the end of pregnancy. Carpal tunnel syndrome happens when the hands become so swollen that it restricts the nerves in the wrist, which may result in numb or tingling fingers (especially at night). Leg cramps are often experienced at night and are also be known as 'restless legs'. The symptoms are usually cramping or an unpleasant prickling feeling in the legs and the condition is often a sign of mineral deficiency.

Nutrition

To relieve the swelling of oedema:
• Try eating more garlic and onion, which improve the circulation, and opt for foods that are natural diuretics such as artichokes. asparagus, black-currants, celery, grapes and parsley. Vitamin C may also help, so eat more citrus fruits, strawberries, dark-green, leafy vegetables, tomatoes and peppers.

For carpal tunnel syndrome

• Increase your intake of B vitamins, which are essential for healthy nerve function. Foods that are rich in these include bananas, chickpeas, egg yolks, wholemeal bread, sesame seeds and yeast extract.

For leg cramps

• These can indicate a deficiency of calcium and magnesium, so increase your intake of milk and milk products, small bony fish such as sardines and

SELF-HELP TIPS FOR OEDEMA, CARPAL TUNNEL SYNDROME & LEG CRAMPS

Do not be tempted to drink less fluid. Your body needs plenty of liquids (especially water) to flush out toxins and supply your baby with enough nutrient-rich blood	To alleviate swelling, put pillows or cushions under your hands and arms when resting
Opt for sea or rock salt rather than refined versions	Wear comfortable shoes – perhaps ones that are larger than your usual size – or do without them completely sometimes
Make sure that you rest with your legs elevated for at least 20 minutes, four times a day and rotate your ankles constantly	Avoid socks or stockings that have tight bands around the ankles, thighs or calves
To relieve cramp, flex your legs and stand with your feet on the ground while curling your toes	Take a little gentle exercise such as a daily walk or swim
Avoid crossing your legs or ankles while sitting	Crouch on the floor and gently press your hands flat on the floor to stretch your carpal tunnels

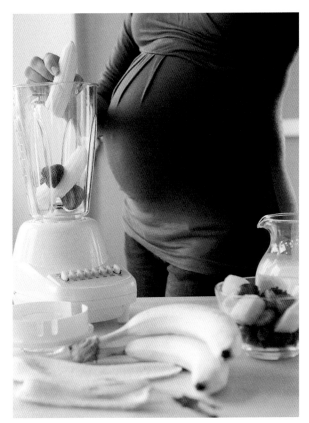

Bananas, rich in B vitamins, make a great quick, healthy snack. Increase your intake of these to help carpal tunnel syndrome.

green, leafy vegetables (for calcium) and eat more dried apricots, nuts, wholegrains, soya products and green, leafy vegetables such as spinach and kale (for extra magnesium).

Complementary therapies

Consult your midwife or doctor before you try any complementary therapies and make sure that your practitioners are fully qualified and accredited.

Acupuncture Acupuncturists take the view that carpal tunnel swelling is the result of an imbalance in the spleen and kidney meridians and so will insert needles in your wrist and your 'stomach' point, which is just below your knee. This cannot 'cure' the problem, but it can give welcome pain relief for around 24 hours.

Aromatherapy Avoid using aromatherapy essential oils for massage, but try combining a few drops of lavender or cypress oil with some carrier oil (such as sweet almond or grapeseed oil) and adding it to a bowl of tepid water to soak your feet in. If in doubt, check which oils are safe to use (see page 41).

Homeopathy Take care to follow the manufacturer's dosage instructions, but remedies are best prescribed by a professional homeopath to match your precise symptoms. Contact a registered homeopath.
- For oedema: natrum muriaticum 30c
- For carpal tunnel with a tingling sensation and numb fingers: arsen alb 30c
- For cramp that is worse at night: calc carb 30c

Massage Use 10 ml (1 tsp) natural plant oil such as grapeseed, wheatgerm or soya oil and stroke one hand after another from your ankle up to your knee or use both hands at the same time. Stroke towards your body (not away from it) and apply pressure to stimulate the flow of blood through your veins.

Osteopathy To ease swollen hands and carpal tunnel syndrome, an osteopath may gently manipulate your wrists to stimulate and improve lymphatic drainage.

Western herbalism Try applying a 'poultice' of green or white cabbage leaves on the swollen area to draw out excess fluid. Chill them in the refrigerator first. They should also help relieve discomfort. Try drinking dandelion or nettle tea (both have a diuretic effect). They will stimulate your kidneys to produce more fluid and therefore your body can expel it as urine. Dandelion is also a good source of vitamins A, C and E as well as calcium and potassium.

WARNING

If you have carpal tunnel syndrome, you should take extra care when you are carrying hot liquids because of the risk of spilling. If your swelling seems severe and is accompanied by a headache, speak to your doctor or midwife because this could be an indication of pre-eclampsia (see pages 208–9).

SELF-HELP TIPS FOR SLEEPLESSNESS

Take time to unwind before going to bed. Try to get to bed early so that you have plenty of time to relax and gradually drift off to sleep

Try to get some fresh air and exercise each day (such as walking or swimming). It will help you to feel physically tired and reduce your stress levels, too

Avoid having caffeine and stimulants

Make sure that your bedroom is well aired and a pleasant temperature

Make sure that your bed is cosy, but not too hot. Your body temperature will be higher than normal, so you may want to opt for a cotton sheet and layers of soft, light blankets that you can throw off, or add, as necessary

Try putting soft pillows or cushions under your bump and between your legs (to support your hips), and wear a soft sleep bra to make sure that your breasts are supported

Increase your intake of tryptophan-rich foods such as tuna, eggs and dairy products (see nutrition, below)

If heartburn or indigestion is a problem, try eating smaller meals more frequently, but avoid eating too late in the evening and try sleeping propped up a little, against some soft pillows

Ask your partner to give you a gentle massage (but don't lie on your bump or flat on your back)

Try sleeping on your left side because it will relieve pressure on your major blood vessels

Take a warm (but not hot) bath containing a few drops of lavender oil mixed with a little carrier oil (see page 40)

Try not to panic and try out some relaxation and visualisation techniques (see pages 110 and 144)

If all else fails, catch up on your missing sleep with some relaxing naps during the day

Sleeplessness

Difficulty sleeping may occur during all three trimesters, but by the third it is often due to the sheer size and weight of your bump. It may also be because you have so much to think about. However, there are quite a few simple remedies that may help.

Symptoms

You may experience difficulty falling asleep or when you are asleep be restless, experiencing vivid, even disturbing, dreams. You may also feel worried and be more tired and irritable than usual.

Nutrition

• Insomnia can be caused by a vitamin-B deficiency. Eat more bananas, chickpeas, egg yolks, nuts, pulses, sesame seeds, wholegrains and yeast extract.
• Calcium also calms the nerves, so increase your intake of almonds, yogurt, soya products, dried apricots and milk (which also contains tryptophan – an amino acid that helps you to sleep).

Complementary therapies

Consult your doctor or midwife before you try out any complementary therapies and make sure that all practitioners you choose to be treated by are fully qualified and accredited.

Acupuncture An acupuncturist will need details of your sleep patterns and will treat the appropriate meridian. Research has shown that acupuncture can stimulate the production of seratonin, which can be deficient in people who suffer from insomnia.

Aromatherapy Try combining a few drops of lavender oil with some carrier oil (such as sweet almond or grapeseed oil) and adding it to a warm bath. You could also try burning sweet mandarin oil (which is reputed to have calming qualities) in a vaporiser. If you are in any doubt, check which oils are safe to use (see pages 40–1).

Homeopathy Take care to follow the manufacturer's dosage instructions, but remedies are best prescribed by a professional homeopath to match your precise symptoms. Contact a registered homeopath.

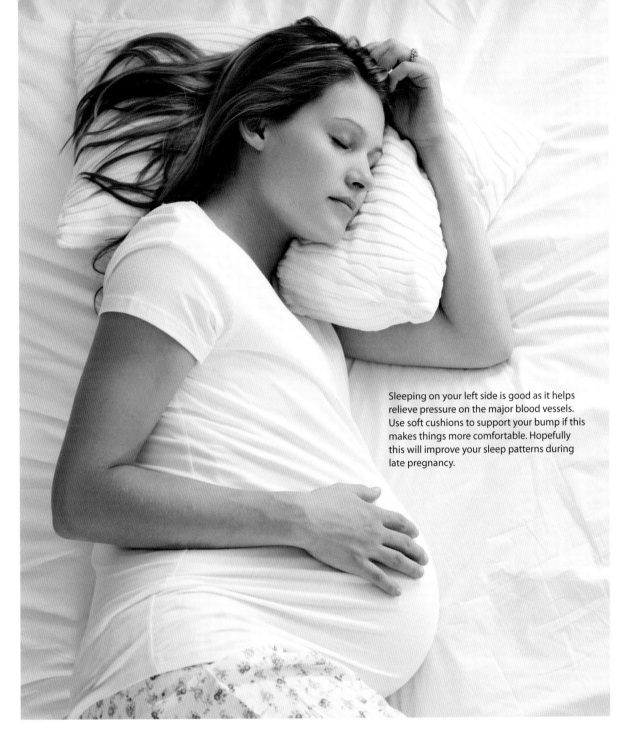

Sleeping on your left side is good as it helps relieve pressure on the major blood vessels. Use soft cushions to support your bump if this makes things more comfortable. Hopefully this will improve your sleep patterns during late pregnancy.

- For an overactive mind that refuses to shut off: coffea crudum 30c
- For vivid dreams and anxiety: aconite 30c

Flower remedies Try putting two drops into a cup of cold water and having it twice a day – and again before you go to bed:

- White chestnut for worries
- Red chestnut for negative, frightening thoughts
- Rock rose for terrifying thoughts

Western herbalism Try drinking a cup of chamomile or lemon balm tea before you retire for the night.

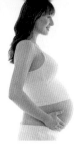

taking care in

LATE PREGNANCY

Most pregnancies will be trouble free, but there are a few conditions in late pregnancy that will need careful management. If any of these complications affect you, then it may be helpful to understand the nature of the problem and how it may be treated.

Pre-eclampsia

Also known as 'pregnancy-induced hypertension' (PIH) or toxaemia, pre-eclampsia affects around 8 per cent of pregnancies in the UK and is usually a mild condition that can be treated fairly easily. It happens most often in the latter half of first pregnancies and the only proper cure is the delivery of the baby.

However, if your case is mild, you may simply be prescribed bed rest at home, with close monitoring of your blood pressure from your doctor or midwife. If your blood pressure is fairly high, you may be admitted to hospital, but unless you are very close to your due date, your carers will do all they can to prolong your pregnancy and avoid delivering your baby prematurely (see pages 194–5).

If the blood flow to the placenta is affected, however, your baby may at risk of developing IUGR (see page 192) or having a reduced supply of oxygen, which can have serious consequences. If you are 26 weeks' pregnant, or more, then induction is very likely to be advised.

Severe pre-eclampsia can be life-threatening to both you and your baby because it can lead to eclampsia, which can cause convulsions and coma. It is now rare in the developed world, but if it does occur it requires emergency treatment with anti-convulsive drugs and immediate delivery of the baby by Caesarean section.

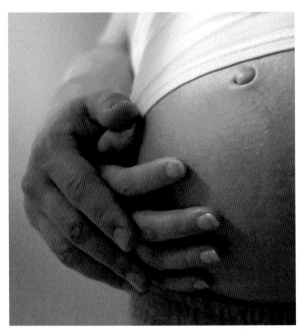

Late pregnancy is the time to take things as easily as you can. That way you can avoid, or alleviate, many potential problems.

The cause of pre-eclampsia is not clear, but it does seem to run in families and is more prevalent among both younger and older mothers. You will also be at greater risk if you are overweight, have diabetes or kidney disease or already have high blood pressure. Hypertension (high blood pressure) is one of the main symptoms, but severe swelling of the hands, feet and legs, as well as the presence of protein in the urine are all possible indicators. Headache accompanied by vomiting, blurred vision or flashing lights in front of the eyes or a pain in the upper abdomen are all symptoms. Fortunately, antenatal care and the routine checks that your doctor or midwife make are designed to detect such problems as early as possible.

Placenta praevia

Around one in 200 pregnancies may be affected by placenta praevia. In cases of partial covering, vaginal birth may still be possible, but with complete obstruction, a Caesarean is the only way. It seems more likely if you have had several pregnancies, if you have had a previous Caesarean resulting in scarring, if you have had fibroids or if you have a multiple pregnancy. You may have no symptoms at all, but there might be painless vaginal bleeding. The condition is usually spotted at the 20-week scan and is monitored with further scans. Bed rest may be recommended if you have light bleeding, but there is an increased risk of haemorrhaging after the birth, so a Caesarean may be advised.

Placental abruption

Normally, the placenta does not come away from the wall of the uterus until the baby has been born (see pages 296–7), but sometimes part of it (or, more rarely, all) will separate before the baby has been delivered. If there is vaginal bleeding it may be detected quite easily ('revealed' abruption), but in some cases, the blood collects between the placenta and the uterine wall ('concealed' abruption) and it is betrayed by sometimes severe abdominal pain and tenderness. It is more common among women who smoke, take cocaine or crack cocaine or who have high blood pressure or poor nutrition. This is a potentially life-threatening condition for the baby and you will need to be seen by a doctor immediately. If the bleeding is not severe, then bed rest may be sufficient to manage the condition, but a large abruption would make it necessary to deliver the baby by induction or Caesarean.

Obstetric cholestasis

This is a rare liver disorder caused by bile salts being deposited under the skin – the main symptom is an intense itching of the palms and soles. Itching is common in pregnancy because of the increased blood flow, but if it is severe and not accompanied by a rash, then it might be due to this condition. The reduction in the amount of bile in the liver can lead to a deficiency of vitamin K, which is responsible for helping the blood to clot. It increases the risk of bleeding in mother and baby and although it can be treated with ursodeoxycholic acid, it is most likely that induction will follow at 37 or 38 weeks.

Premature rupture of the membranes

Usually, just before labour starts or when it has begun membranes that enclose and protect the amniotic sac break. But in around one in 14 women they rupture before then. Smoking certainly seems to increase the risk, but it is unclear what the cause may be, although it is thought that there may be a link with vaginal infection. If the membranes do rupture, then the amniotic fluid will leak either in a trickle or a sudden gush. The baby will then be at increased risk of infection and cord prolapse. If it happens at 37 weeks or more, then labour is likely to follow, but if not, labour may be induced. If it happens before 37 weeks, then you may be admitted to hospital for monitoring for signs of infection or foetal distress.

MONITORING FOETAL MOVEMENTS

Towards the end of your pregnancy, especially, you need to keep a check on the number of movements that you feel your baby make. Space will get tighter for your baby, but you should still be conscious of at least 10 definite movements per day. If you are very active, you may find it difficult to keep track of them, so stop what you are doing for an hour and concentrate on what your baby is doing. If you notice that the number or pattern of movements has changed call your doctor or midwife straight away so that they can check that all is well.

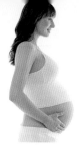

preparation time

COUNTDOWN TO LABOUR

Getting ready for labour draws on mental, physical and emotional reserves. It can be hard to think beyond the birth, which undoubtedly requires huge amounts of energy, but you also need to be prepared for afterwards. You'll need time to heal and cope emotionally with the impact of this life-changing event.

With most major events you can work towards a precise date, but with labour you only have a 'guesstimate'. Try to make time to do some thorough preparation.

What to do at 34 weeks

• If you work up until your due date it will be difficult to find time to prepare mentally and emotionally for labour and your baby's arrival. Now is a good time to plan for the coming weeks.

• List the things you have to do and review your work–life balance. If you are planning to work until a few weeks before the birth, but you are getting tired, think about stopping earlier.

• Get some early nights. Use relaxation techniques learned at antenatal classes or yoga or hypnobirthing techniques (see page 144) to relax.

• Seek help for minor ailments.

• Book in for a breastfeeding class. You will feel more prepared when the time comes to feed your baby.

• Start doing perineal massage. Research suggests that daily massage in the last six weeks of pregnancy may help to prevent perineum tears. Begin by emptying your bladder and soaking in a warm bath to soften the tissues. Use a mirror to become familiar with the area. Place some simple plant oil (such as soya or grapeseed) on your thumbs or index fingers and put it into the vagina for at least 5 cm (2 in), pressing down towards the rectum. Gently stretch the area in a U-shaped motion, holding firmly, so you experience tingling, then release and carry on massaging. Do this every day for 5–10 minutes.

• Keep exercising – aquarobics are especially helpful for toning the muscles.

• Use mind–body techniques such as visualisation (see pages 110 and 144) to communicate with, and stimulate, your baby and try to 'tune in' to what she is sensing (see pages 180–1).

• Stock up on iron-rich foods to prevent anaemia.

• Start taking raspberry leaf (either tea or in tablet form). Raspberry leaf extract is rich in vitamin C and can help tone the uterus and ripen the cervix.

What to do at 35 weeks

• Do pelvic floor exercises every day (see page 141).

• Continue to get a little gentle exercise every day: swimming, walking, yoga or gentle stretching.

What to do at 36 weeks

• If you are starting to think 'I hope I won't go into labour today' you are doing too much. Slow down!

• It is normal to feel fed up with being pregnant by now and understandable, especially if you are tired,

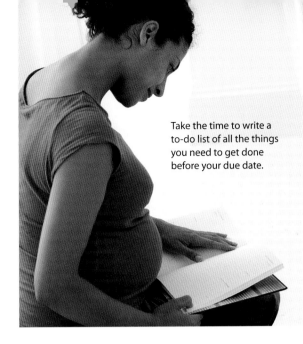

Take the time to write a to-do list of all the things you need to get done before your due date.

uncomfortable and sleeping badly. Try a massage and pamper yourself a little.

- From 36 weeks consider having weekly acupuncture to help you prepare for labour. Research has shown that it can reduce the chances of going overdue and may increase the chance of a shorter, easier labour.
- Now is the time to do any last-minute baby shopping, but consider doing it online.
- If you have not stopped work, consider doing so.
- Give yourself time to emotionally and psychologically prepare not only for birth but for motherhood, which will last a lifetime.
- Try to do something you enjoy every day – relish these last few weeks.

What to do at 37 weeks

- You could go into labour any day now and you may be feeling anxious about the birth. Keep practising your relaxation and hypnobirthing techniques.
- Keep up with your weekly acupuncture sessions.
- Proper rest is more important than ever. Try to have a few hours with your feet up in the afternoon and make sure you get to bed early.
- Continue with your daily gentle exercise.
- Make sure you are getting a good supply of vitamin C and zinc through your diet and perhaps top up

with good pregnancy supplements. Both are essential for hormone production before delivery.
- Pack your hospital bag (see pages 219–20).

What to do at 38 weeks

- Start to increase your intake of complex carbohydrates (see page 79).
- Attend your weekly acupuncture session.
- Order a TENS machine (see pages 252–3).
- In the ten days before your delivery date, you could take the homeopathic remedy caulophylum 30c or arnica (for seven days – before bedtime). This dose is recommended, but it is always best to consult a registered homeopath. Increase your intake of red raspberry-leaf tea to four cups a day.
- Eat lots of magnesium- and calcium-rich foods (see page 85).

What to do at 39 weeks

- Increase your intake of foods that contain co-enzyme Q10 because it improves the cells' ability to use oxygen. Good sources include broccoli, cauliflower, oranges, strawberries, beef and fish such as herring and salmon. (Or take a supplement, but check with your doctor or midwife first).
- Keep your weekly acupuncture appointment.
- Make time do enjoyable things with your partner.
- Eat plenty of foods that are naturally rich in vitamin K (see page 186), which is vital for blood-clotting and is needed by the baby, who cannot manufacture it for herself until several weeks after birth.
- Take arnica 6c to prevent post-birth bruising.

What to do at 40 weeks

- Have your regular weekly acupuncture session and talk to your acupuncturist about how to get your labour started.
- Practise using your TENS machine, so that you will know how to use it in labour.
- Stay positive. Labour and birth can be an incredible, positive, life-enhancing experience. Believe in your own power and ability to labour and give birth.

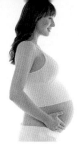

OPTIMAL POSITIONS

Your pelvis is designed for childbirth. However, the way your baby is positioned at the end of your pregnancy will have an impact on the sort of labour you have. Therefore, it is a good idea to try to encourage your baby into a good one.

These days, so many women work right up until a few weeks before they have their babies, but think about it: if you are sitting at a computer all day, driving in a car and then slumping on the sofa, exhausted, these positions won't help to get your baby into the right one. The back of your baby's body is heavier than the front, so her back will tend to roll towards the direction you're leaning in. If you're leaning back, therefore, her back may roll towards yours and she will be in a posterior position (see pages 214–15). So if you lean forward, her back may roll toward your front – an anterior position. Also, if you can sit with your knees below your hips, it will create more space for the baby's head to lie in the front of your pelvis.

An active birth

If you are planning an active birth (one where you move around), thinking about how your anatomy works can really help. Active birth allows you to maximise the space in the pelvis anatomically by at least 30 per cent – and don't forget that the hormone relaxin softens the ligaments of the pelvis so that it can expand as birth takes place. A little extra space is also added by the coccyx (the 'tail' bone at the base of your spine), so when you are upright during labour you ensure that you are giving your baby the maximum amount of space in your pelvic cavity. When your body is upright, gravity can help, too,

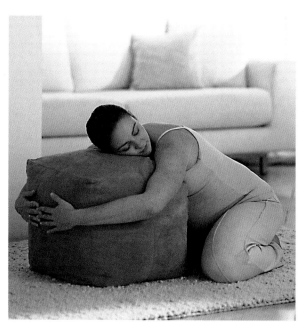
Leaning forwards on a large cushion or beanbag relieves pressure.

so that your baby will naturally descend through your pelvis. This also means that if your baby's head is well applied to the cervix, it will help with dilatation of the cervix, which in turn means that you will have better, more effective, contractions.

How you may be able to help

If you are having a single baby who is head down, then this advice may be useful to encourage your baby to adopt an optimal position such as lying with

OPTIMUM POSITIONING FOR BIRTH

There are a number of natural, straightforward things you can try to get your baby into an optimum position:

Regularly use upright and forward-leaning postures when sitting or moving around. This allows more available space in the pelvis for your baby to turn

Sit with your knees lower than your hips, keeping your back as straight as possible. Use pillows or cushions in the small of the back and under your bottom, to tilt yourself forwards

Use an upright dining chair when you are reading and rest your elbows on the table, keeping your knees apart while you lean forwards

You can also use the dining chair to sit facing the chair back. Lean towards its back and rest your arms on it

When watching television, try to kneel on the floor and lean forwards over a large beanbag or floor cushion

When driving, put a wedge cushion under your bottom to tilt your pelvis slightly forwards (rather than back, as many car seats tend to be designed to do)

Swim using breaststroke or crawl rather than backstroke

When resting or sleeping, lie on your side, preferably on your left side, with a pillow between your legs and your uppermost knee resting on the bed

When you get Braxton Hicks' contractions, try to adopt postures where you are leaning forwards. This will increase their effectiveness and help your baby to manoeuvre herself into the best position

her back to your left side or front (LOA – see pages 214–15). However, it may not be suitable for all pregnancies, so you should check with your midwife or doctor first.

Breech babies

Between weeks 32 and 36, most babies settle into a head-down position – the best position for birth, but around three or four in every 100 pregnancies are breech presentations, meaning that the baby's bottom is closest to the cervix and delivered before the head.

In most cases there is no obvious cause for this, it may simply be that this position is more comfortable for the baby, but there are some factors that may contribute and these include: premature or growth-restricted babies; twins; excess amniotic fluid that allows the baby to move around more freely than other babies at this stage of pregnancy; placenta praevia, where the placenta is low and prevents the baby's head from engaging, or very rare causes of congenital abnormality of the baby's limbs or spine, (although this will normally have already been detected by ultrasound scan).

External cephalic version (ECV)

Many babies will naturally turn in the last four weeks of pregnancy, but if this does not happen you may be offered an ultrasound scan. If your baby is still breech you will be referred to a consultant obstetrician, who (if there are no other complications) may perform an External Cephalic Version (ECV). This is usually done at or after 36 weeks, when the risk of prematurity has passed and is successful in around 50 per cent of cases.

The procedure involves gentle manipulation and massage of your abdomen. First, you may be offered an injection of salbutamol to relax your uterus, then an ultrasound Doppler scan is used to assess the exact position of the baby and to check the placenta. Electronic monitoring of the baby's heart beat (CTG) will be carried out before and after the procedure to check the baby's well-being and there should be immediate access to emergency delivery facilities (such as theatre for Caesarean section) if complications arise.

The ECV should only be performed by an experienced practitioner, so make sure that your consultant has carried out the procedure successfully a number of times before. The baby's position will then be checked at your next antenatal appointment. If your baby is still in the breech position, an elective Caesarean section will be scheduled for week 39 of your pregnancy.

Presentation, position & lie

In the last month or so of your pregnancy it becomes more important for your midwife or doctor to assess the presentation, position and lie of your baby. The 'presentation' simply means which part of her is closest to your cervix and will therefore present itself to the outside world first.

The 'lie' is literally the way that she is lying: longitudinal means a vertical position and may be written in your notes as (L/long), transverse (T/Tr) which means she is lying horizontally across your abdomen or oblique (Obl), which means she is in a diagonal position. The 'position' records where your baby's spine and the back of her head (known as the occiput) are in relation to the inner (front) wall of your uterus.

Best position

The best position for your baby to be in for birth is head down (known as cephalic – C/Ceph), with her back against your abdomen and facing your back. In this position, she can fit through your pelvis as easily as possible. She can 'flex' her head and neck and tuck her chin into her chest, so that the narrowest part of her head (the back) is pressing on your cervix, helping it to dilate. The flexible bones in your baby's skull also allow her head to change shape and negotiate the birth canal during birth.

This position is also known as know as 'occipito-anterior' (OA), meaning that the back of the baby's head, or 'occiput', is at the front (usually written in your notes as 'anterior'). Most babies lie in this position, which may be written in your notes as LOA ('left occipito-anterior') if the baby is lying to your left or, less commonly, ROA ('right occipito-anterior') if she is lying to your right.

Some babies lie with their back against their mother's spine, which is known as an 'occipito-posterior' (OP) position. In this position, labour tends to take longer because the baby can't tuck in her chin properly and so getting through the pelvis is more difficult.

COMPLEMENTARY THERAPIES

Note: Check with your doctor or midwife first before you use complementary therapies. Only use them if you are NOT carrying twins and if you have never had a Caesarean section delivery.

Moxibustion

Use a qualifed and experienced practitioner for this technique. It has been practised in Traditional Chinese Medicine (TCM – see pages 38–9) for centuries, but it should not be used for women with high blood pressure or those who have had any bleeding during pregnancy.

The smouldering end of a stick of the herb moxa will be held close to, but not touching, the relevant acupoints. This is to send gentle heat up along the bladder meridian, which in TCM is thought to be linked to the uterus. This is best done between 32 and 36 weeks and must be practised for 15 minutes once or twice a day. If your baby turns during treatment, you should stop at once and have the position checked by your midwife.

Homeopathy

Pulsatilla 30c may be recommended to help turn a breech baby and it is usually prescribed three times a day over four days, but remedies are best prescribed by a professional homeopath to match your precise circumstances. Contact a registered homeopath.

Engagement

Your baby's head may engage (drop into your pelvis) as early as 36 weeks or as late as the start of labour. Engagement has occurred when more than half the baby's head has passed below the top of your pelvic brim (bone). Your doctor or midwife may gently palpate your abdomen and record it in your notes as:

(High/Fr) If all of your baby's head can be felt in the abdomen it is called 'high' or 'free'.

(NE/Neng) If more than half your baby's head can be felt above the pubic bone it is not fully engaged.

(E/Eng) If less than half the baby's head is felt above the pubic bone, it means it is engaged.

COMMON BIRTH POSITIONS

These are some common ways in which your baby can present before birth. Remember that the position can change just before labour – or even during it.

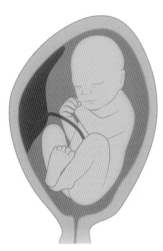

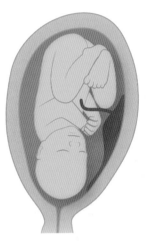

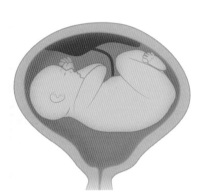

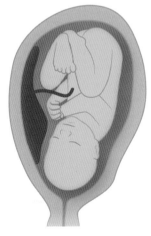

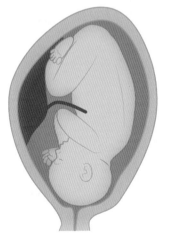

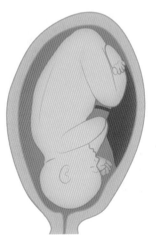

Transverse The baby lies across the mother's abdomen. If the position does not change, the birth will be made possible by a Caesarian section.

Breech The baby's bottom is lying next to the cervix rather than the head, which is positioned at the top of the uterus.

Right posterior (ROP) The baby faces the mother's front, slightly to the right, with her spine along the mother's spine. Labour may not start naturally.

Left posterior (LOP) The baby is slightly to the left. The labour may last a little longer and be somewhat more painful in the mother's lower back.

Left anterior (LOA) The baby faces the mother's back and her spine is along the mother's abdomen.

Right anterior (ROA) The position is slightly to the right and her head can flex. The smallest part of it lies next to the cervix.

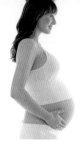

LATE PREGNANCY

As you get closer to the birth of your baby, there may be a number of issues that you may not have considered up until now. Here are some commonly asked questions.

If this is your first baby, are you wondering how this event will affect your other relationships – with friends, colleagues and family? Will people treat you differently or think of you differently?

Perhaps you have other children to consider and wonder how they will cope with your absence from home. Or perhaps you are a single parent wondering how things will be in hospital without a partner.

LATE PREGNANCY Q&AS

"I'm expecting identical twin girls (if the scan is right) and I'm worried about how my partner and I – and other people – will tell them apart."

When your babies are delivered the staff will put little name bands on their ankles or wrists, so try to decide on names in advance. You can change your mind later if necessary. Even identical twins are not identical in every way, because one is often slightly larger than the other (see page 197). When leaving the hospital, parents have been known to mark one baby's toenails with nail polish or even to put a marker pen dot on the foot of one baby to ensure they know who's who.

You and your partner will soon get to know your twins and their personalities and you may notice quite quickly that one is more dominant than the other. You may want to think about how you will present them to the world, though. If they are identical, it is easy for other people to forget that they are individuals with different personalities, likes and dislikes. If you want people to treat them as individuals, then think about the outward signs of their 'twinness'. If you dress them alike, it will be harder for people to tell them apart. As they get older you may find that they both like a particular colour, so try to find clothes or toys in that colour, but perhaps in a different shade or design.

"I'm really excited about the birth of my first baby, but my best friends from work (none of whom have children) have hardly been in touch with me since I went on maternity leave and I'm beginning to feel a bit left out and hurt."

This is a very common situation. It is inevitable that things will change when you have a baby and you are the first in a group of child-free women. The others may feel that you need a little time to yourself, though they are bound to come visiting once you have actually had the baby. However it is likely that you will have less in common with them (at least for a while).

Try to concentrate on the new networks of friends that you can make through your pregnancy or baby groups. Join an aquarobics class for pregnant women or an antenatal group (if you haven't already) (see pages 158–9). These will help you to build a support network because you will all be going through the same thing at roughly the same time and it is surprising how that can forge very strong bonds (among the women and among their partners). Your baby will also have the advantage of a ready-made group of baby friends who will always be at just the right stage for her to play with as she grows up.

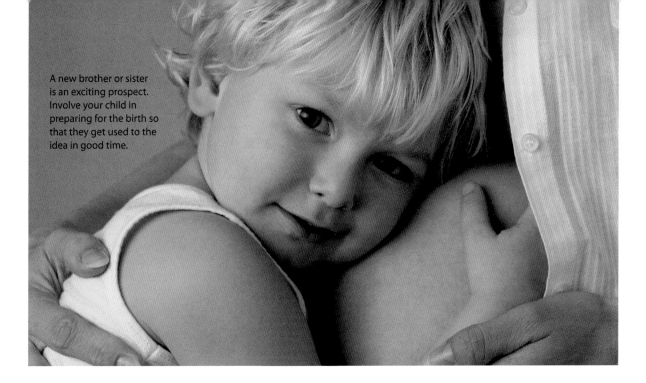

A new brother or sister is an exciting prospect. Involve your child in preparing for the birth so that they get used to the idea in good time.

"I already have two children and they are excited about having a new brother or sister, but I am worried about how they will feel as they watch me go off to hospital for the birth. What can I do to make things better?"

Try to make plans so that they don't have to watch you go. Make sure that they know and understand what is happening and prepare them in advance. Try to arrange a few 'trial runs' with a good friend or relative whom they know well and who is prepared to look after them when the time comes. Perhaps you can arrange for them to have a treat while you are away, so that they are occupied with an enjoyable activity rather than worrying about you.

"I'm going to be a single parent and I'm dreading having my baby in hospital and being the only one without a partner. My best friend says she will be with me at the birth if I want her to, but I'm not sure what to do. "

The birth of your child will be an incredible experience, but also tiring and possibly painful. If your friend is someone you trust, you can only gain by having her there – not only to support you – but to share in your joy, too. You will always have that shared memory and your baby may one day be

glad to hear about his or her birth from another perspective as well. Don't worry about what other people may think. You will not be the only woman giving birth without a partner and hospital staff are trained to respect everyone equally.

"I want to tell my mother about the names we are considering for our baby, but my partner says we should wait. Do we have to?"

Deciding on your baby's name can be fun, but it is for you two to do. The problem with discussing it in advance is that everyone has an opinion. Your relatives may have a name that is 'traditional' in the family, and that they want passed on, and friends may like a particular name for their own children (if and when they have them) that they may not want you to use. If people give you a negative reaction you may find it upsetting and if they list alternatives, you may feel awkward rejecting them. If you wait and announce it once the baby is born it is unlikely that anyone will challenge your choice. It may be a good idea for you and your partner to separately note your favourites and then consider each other's list. You could include a family name as a middle name. Reserve a few alternative first names, though. When you finally meet your newborn, you may feel your chosen name just doesn't suit.

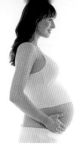

what you will need

PLAN FOR THE BIRTH

When you first realised that you were pregnant, it probably felt as if your labour and birth were a long time away, but it is amazing how quickly nine months can go by, so the sooner you get organised the easier things will be when your baby is here.

Preparing for a home birth

If you are having a home birth, most things that you will need are likely to be found in your home anyway, but the main extra is probably some plastic sheeting to protect floors, sofas and beds. You may want to have your own pain-relief strategies such as a TENS machine (see pages 252–3) or some natural pain relief such as homeopathic remedies. Ask your midwife for a list of things you might need, but here are some suggestions:

• Plastic sheeting and old sheets and towels.
• Light food and drink for labour (see pages 240–1).
• Food and drink for your birth partner, midwives and your other children.
• Hot-water bottles.
• Hand mirror for watching the crowning.
• If you plan to have a water birth, you'll need as many old towels to hand as possible.
• Disposable bed mats (to protect your mattress and to wrap the baby in if she is cold.
• Refuse sacks – one for dirty towels and sheets and one for waste.
• A container for the placenta (although NHS midwives usually carry bags for the placenta if they are taking it away for disposal).
• A bucket in case of vomiting.
• Maternity sanitary pads.
• Disposable or large cotton knickers.
• An old T-shirt, a short, front-opening nightdress, dressing gown or a man's shirt (you need to be able to put your baby on to your skin as soon as possible after the birth).

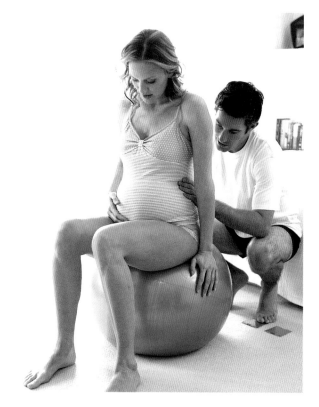

Your partner will be invaluable for helping you to relax during the early stages of labour at home.

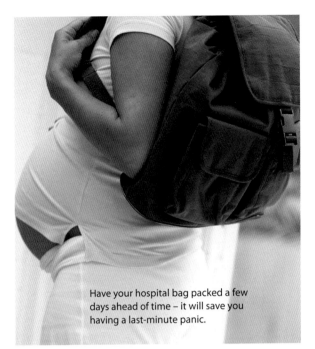

Have your hospital bag packed a few days ahead of time – it will save you having a last-minute panic.

FOOD & DRINK IN LABOUR

The National Institute for Clinical Excellence (NICE) recommends drinking water in labour. Light snacks are fine, too, as long as you haven't had opioid-based pain relief (see pages 244–50). It is important to keep up your energy levels because a lack of it can make contractions less efficient. If your body cannot get enough carbohydrates to fuel it, and your blood-sugar (glucose and glycogen) levels are too low, then you will produce ketones, which interfere with the body's capacity to circulate oxygen around itself. Fluid is vital, too, because if you become dehydrated you will require intravenous fluids, which will then restrict your movements. An energy drink designed to give sustained energy release is ideal (isotonic sports drinks are not recommended), so look for those containing a maltodextrin and fructose, or at least drink watered-down fruit juice or cordial.

Your hospital bag

It is a good idea to pack your hospital bag about four weeks ahead of your due date – even if you are expecting to have a home birth – because events may force a change of plan. Take enough with you for a few days' stay (just in case you need to stay a little longer) and don't forget to pack things for your labour and recovery time afterwards. Perhaps make a list and show it to your partner, so that he knows what you have packed and why.

For labour

- Phone numbers for your midwife, partner, relatives or doula.
- Copies of your birth plan (at least one for the hospital staff and one for your partner, so that he can make sure that your wishes are being considered if you are unable to do so).
- Pain relief such as a TENS machine.
- Any natural remedies (such as homeopathic ones) that you wish to use.
- A list of people and contact numbers for those you'd like to be contacted after the birth.

- Relaxation aids such as music and books.
- Your own pillows and towels may make you feel more comfortable.
- A watch with a second hand so that you can time your contractions.
- Oils or lotion for massage.
- A cool bag to keep water and snacks cold.
- Bottles of water.
- Nutritious snacks (for you and your partner).
- An old T-shirt, short, front-opening nightdress or man's shirt that opens down the front (you need to be able to put your baby on to your skin as soon as possible).
- Large, comfortable, dark-coloured cotton knickers.
- Socks to keep your feet warm.
- Mobile phone.
- Camera or video camera.
- Money (in case you have to stay in hospital for longer than expected).
- Toiletries, including your toothbrush and toothpaste, a flannel, soap, shampoo and moisturiser.
- Hand mirror for watching the crowning.

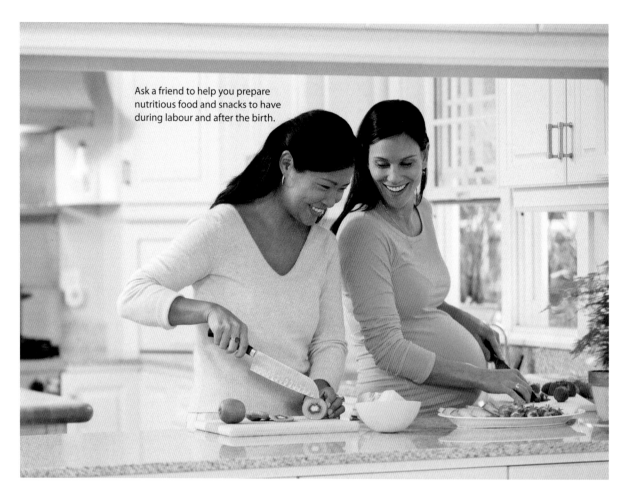

Ask a friend to help you prepare nutritious food and snacks to have during labour and after the birth.

For after the birth

- Spare pair of pyjamas or nightdress and dressing gown.
- Slippers for walking around the ward/to and from the bathroom.
- Maternity sanitary pads.
- Nursing bra (and possibly nipple cream).

For your baby

- Nappies, wipes, nappy sacks, travel changing mat.
- Baby clothes (soft, cotton babygros in more than one size), a cotton hat, vest and cardigans.
- A few muslin cloths.
- A hooded towel and flannel.
- A soft blanket.
- A car seat.

Planning for post-birth nutrition

Snacks to eat throughout labour will ensure that you have enough energy for the birth. They should be small, and quick and easy to prepare, easy to eat and safe to store without a fridge if you are in hospital.

- Plan which foods you need and buy or prepare in advance for both labour (see pages 240–1) and post-birth nutrition (see pages 314 and 320).
- Make a list of snacks to take and instruct your partner how to make them.
- Buy a picnic coolbag and some cool/icepacks.
- Buy plastic storage boxes with tight-fitting lids, plastic food bags and foil for packing everything.
- Pack flexible straws so that your partner can hold drinks for you while you are in labour.

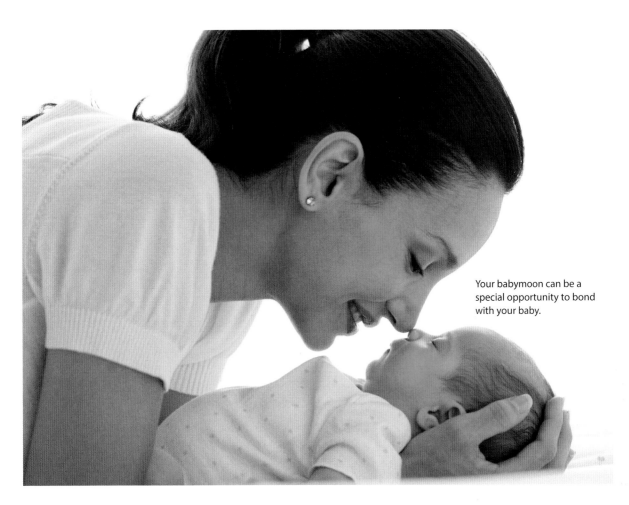

Your babymoon can be a special opportunity to bond with your baby.

Planning a 'babymoon'

Rather like your honeymoon, a 'babymoon' is a few days reserved for time alone at home as a family with your new baby. It's a good idea to discourage too many excited visitors – they can prove very exhausting. You will undoubtedly be tired yourself and your newborn will probably sleep a surprising amount in the first few days at least (labour and birth are tiring for your baby, too), so these early days may be the ideal time for you to gently get to know one another without too many distractions. The time may also give your partner a chance to nurture you both and if you make the necessary preparations (see right), you can dispense with many everyday chores, so that you can both concentrate on the wonder of being with your new baby.

THINGS TO DO

Keep a notebook for all your lists. As you think of things, jot them down and cross them off as you achieve them

Make sure your baby's car seat fits in your car and that you know how it works

Do some batch-cooking of your favourite meals and freeze them so that you can have home-cooked food without the bother of having to make it on the day

Order your groceries (plus nappies and toiletries) online. Create and save some shopping lists, then you can just activate them as and when you need to

Let people know that you will be having a babymoon and schedule visits for a convenient time afterwards

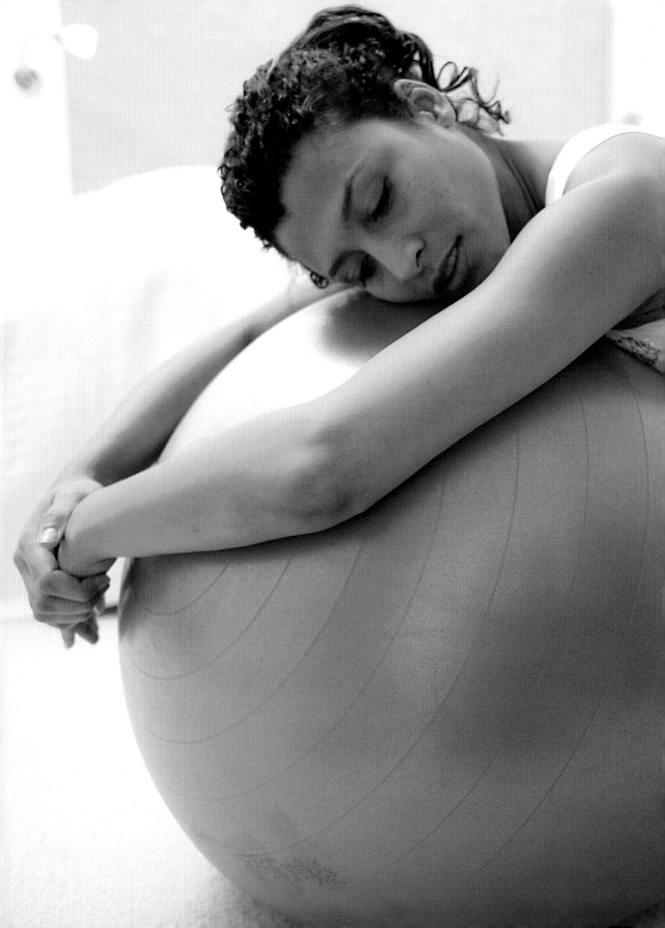

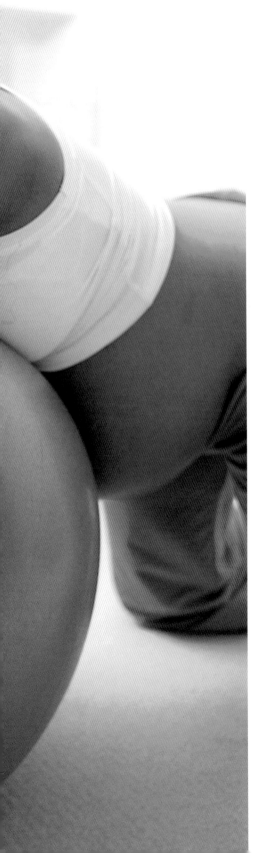

chapter 6

labour &
BIRTH

Getting ready for labour and the birth of your new son or daughter is an exciting time. There is a lot to take on board, but with a little careful planning and preparation you will be ready for the big day – and all the days to follow.

BEING OVERDUE

If you have reached the magic 40 weeks of pregnancy and there is no sign of labour starting, you will be described as being 'overdue', but although few babies do arrive on time and anything between 37 and 42 weeks may actually be considered normal, your doctor or midwife will want to keep a close eye on you.

The precise trigger for labour is unknown, so it is not clear why it should start late, although this is more likely to happen if it is your first baby. Around 45 per cent of pregnancies do go on into the fortieth week, but after that most women give birth, so that only about 15 per cent will continue beyond 41 weeks. After this time, there is a risk (though relatively small) that your placenta will function less efficiently and so your baby's health could be compromised. This is why your medical professionals will want to carry out regular assessments to check that all is still well.

Dates & assessments

The accuracy of your expected delivery date (EDD) will be checked first using a combination of your last menstrual period (LMP) and your early dating scan. Depending on whether you have had any complications during your pregnancy, you may be advised to wait a little longer, but at 41 weeks you are likely to be assessed again at a clinic or hospital.

You will probably have an internal examination and if your baby's head is engaged and your cervix is soft and dilated, your doctor or midwife may suggest that they 'sweep' your membranes (see page 227) at the top of your cervix, to release prostaglandins (chemicals that may help to trigger contractions –

see page 233). If this is not an option, you may be offered a chemical induction of labour (see page 228). If you do not want to be chemically induced, there are some natural alternatives that you may try in order to kickstart your labour (see page 229).

Research shows that induction is more likely to lead to a longer labour and further intervention (such as forceps or ventouse delivery – see pages 284–5), but there is no firm evidence that it results in a higher rate of Caesarean sections (see pages 286–9). However, letting a pregnancy go beyond 42 weeks increases the risk of the baby becoming distressed or being still born.

It is unusual for late babies to need to be delivered immediately, but if this is the case, a Caesarean section would be recommended.

Post-maturity assessment

Your doctor or midwife will probably check the size of your baby and carry out an ultrasound scan to check the amount of amniotic fluid surrounding him. This will give them a good idea of the well-being of your baby and the efficiency of your placenta, but you may also have a Doppler ultrasound scan to check the blood flow in your placenta.

If the placenta is still working well, then the blood should flow easily, with a peak in pressure at the start

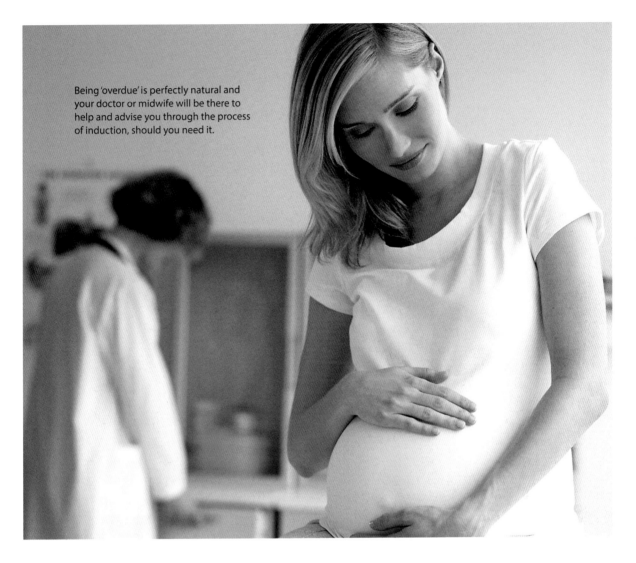

Being 'overdue' is perfectly natural and your doctor or midwife will be there to help and advise you through the process of induction, should you need it.

of a cardiac cycle (one cardiac cycle is completed when the heart fills with blood and the blood is then pumped out of the heart into the arteries, to be transported around the body with each heartbeat), and there should be some reduction in pressure at the end, but the flow should be continuous.

If there is a problem with the placenta, it will be resistant to blood flow and the pressure may drop to such an extent that there is little or no flow at the end of the cardiac cycle. This may mean that your baby is receiving an insufficient amount of oxygen, so the prompt delivery of your baby would certainly be recommended.

Biophysical profile

You may also have a biophysical profile performed on your baby, but this is usually only if there are major concerns about growth. The profile is done rarely and is not the norm. It uses tests to estimate the baby's health and well-being. A scoring system is used to record his movements, muscular tone and posture, breathing movements, the amounts of amniotic fluid and the results of a CTG (cardiotocograph). Low levels of amniotic fluid and a poor CTG showing a pattern of heart activity with little variation would indicate that the baby's health was compromised with prompt delivery would be advised.

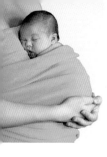

all the options explained

INDUCTION

Most women would, of course, prefer to go into labour naturally and spontaneously. However the safety of you and your baby is the most important consideration and in some circumstances it may be safer to speed up the process of labour and birth than to leave the pregnancy to continue.

When induction may be offered

You may be offered induction if:
- Your health or your baby's health is compromised for some reason and an early birth is advisable.
- Your baby is 'overdue' because you have reached 41 weeks of pregnancy, or more.

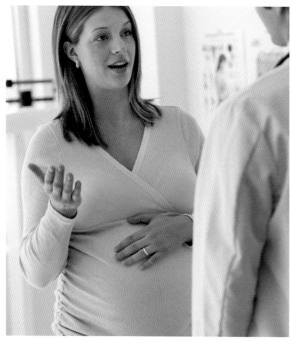

Take every opportunity to inform yourself about your possible induction – the health professionals are there to advise you.

- Your membranes have ruptured, but labour has not yet started.
- If you are an 'older' mother.
- If your obstetric history makes induction necessary.

The reasons for induction

If you have been offered induction, you need to understand why. It may be suggested because you have high blood pressure (see page 73) or have an existing condition such as diabetes (see page 72). However, a common reason for induction in otherwise normal pregnancies is that the baby is 'overdue' (see pages 224–5). Some doctors will let a low-risk pregnancy carry on for up to twelve days after the expected date of delivery (EDD), but few will allow it to continue far beyond that date. If you are more than 37 weeks' pregnant and your membranes have broken (i.e. the waters have broken), but you have not gone into labour within one to four days, induction will be strongly advised because of the possible risk of infection (especially from the group B streptococcus bacteria).

Planning an induction

Induction is planned in advance, so you should have the opportunity to discuss the advantages and disadvantages with your doctor or midwife, but it is your choice whether to proceed or not. Rather than one single action being performed to bring on labour, induction is a process and one intervention may lead on to another. Therefore induction is only suggested if there are good reasons for it.

A membrane sweep.

This is the first stage of induction and can be performed either by your community midwife or at the hospital prior to medical induction, if you wish – it may be uncomfortable though not painful. A sweep enables the midwife to try and separate the membranes from the cervix, however it is only possible if the cervix has already opened. It is more likely to be successful if it is done after 41 weeks, or even at 10 days overdue.

Your midwife uses her finger to 'sweep' the neck of your uterus and the process may be performed twice. The aim is to encourage your body to release prostaglandin, the hormone that softens and stretches the cervix.

Once this happens, labour should start within the next 48 hours, but there is also a risk that your waters could be broken, too. If this does happen, further intervention is necessary to induce labour because of the risk of infection. You may have a bloody 'show' (see page 232) afterwards. If the membrane sweep does not get labour started within a few days, then the following procedures will be offered:

Cervical 'ripening' A prostaglandin pessary will be inserted into your vagina and sometimes gel is applied to the cervix, too. This is always done in hospital and it may be enough to start your labour, but it can take a while.

The baby is monitored before and after the insertion of the prostaglandin. Occasionally the pessaries can cause strong, painful contractions that can be difficult to cope with and cause your baby stress. If so, you may need continuous foetal monitoring (see pages 276–7), making it harder to have an active labour (see pages 270–1) and you may

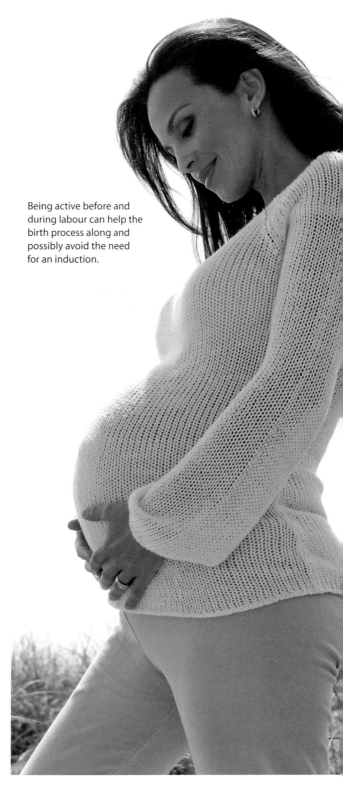

Being active before and during labour can help the birth process along and possibly avoid the need for an induction.

INDUCTION Q&AS

"Do I have the right to refuse induction?"

You have the right to refuse intervention and if induction is considered you should have the opportunity to discuss your options. It is best to take the advice offered – going overdue can be a risk and records of the baby's movements in late pregnancy may not be made. If you still want to delay induction you may be asked to attend your hospital at 41 weeks – so that you and your baby can be monitored (see pages 276–7). If results are satisfactory, you may continue to wait, but you will probably be assessed at two-day intervals until you reach 42 weeks. By then, you will probably be advised that induction is the safest option (see pages 226–7).

"If I am induced, can I still have a home birth?"

Apart from having a membrane sweep, all other procedures have to be carried out in hospital, so if you had those, you would have to remain there for labour and delivery.

"Is there an alternative to induction?"

If you have been offered an induction after 42 weeks and you are otherwise healthy, you should also be offered cardiotocograph (CTG) monitoring of your baby's heartbeat, a scan to check the amount of amniotic fluid surrounding your baby and a biophysical profile of the baby's health (see page 225). You may also want to try out natural alternatives (see opposite).

If you are advised to have your labour induced it is likely that you will have a few days' notice, so you may be able to try a few alternative methods such as intercourse, acupuncture, reflexology, homeopathy or cranial osteopathy. Only try alternative or complementary therapies if you have reached your EDD, your pregnancy has been without complications and you have no existing health problems. Make sure, too, that you see a qualified and accredited practitioner.

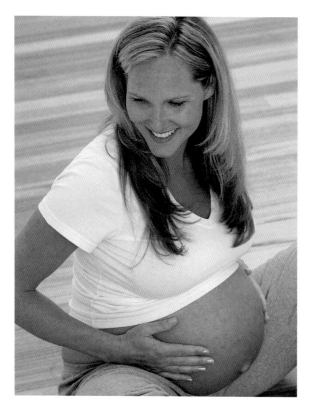

need to review your methods of pain relief (see pages 244–57).

Artificial rupture of membranes (ARM) This can only be done if your cervix is dilating (see page 232). The midwife uses a plastic hook to break the membranes and it can be very uncomfortable. Contractions may be stronger and more painful, so you need to review pain relief (see pages 244–57).

Synthetic oxytocin (syntocinon) This is an artificial form of oxytocin, which causes your uterus to contract. It is administered intravenously, only when the membranes have been ruptured first. It increases the frequency and strength of contractions so the baby will be monitored continuously throughout labour and you may need to review your pain-relief options. This, in turn, means that your labour may need further intervention (such as forceps or ventouse delivery, or a Caesarean section).

Carry on with your life as normal – you may find that you do not need to be induced after all.

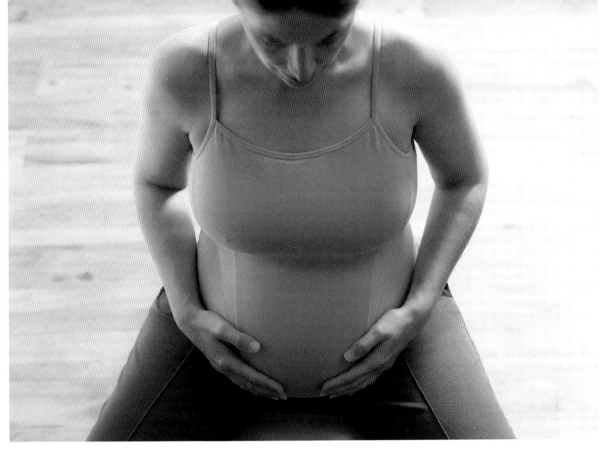

Mild exercise may do the trick if you want to avoid having an induced birth.

Avoiding induction

If you want to avoid having to have an induced birth, you could try out the following:

- Have sex – semen is rich in prostaglandins (the hormones that stimulate contractions), but you must be sure to avoid intercourse if your waters have already broken. This is because of the increased risk of infection. Otherwise, kissing, stimulation of your nipples and orgasm can all increase your natural oxytocin levels.
- Try eating spicy foods – sometimes a bowel movement as a result of eating hot food might bring on contractions.
- A good walk – or mild exercise such as yoga or squatting on a low stool may encourage your baby's head to press further on your cervix and stimulate contractions. Swimming is not recommended after 37 weeks because the risk of infection is high and you may not be aware of ruptured membranes.

- Acupuncture – an acupuncturist may insert needles in your lower back and in your hands and legs, but you will need to have more than one treatment for there to be any significant effect. Ensure you consult a qualified therapist experienced in this procedure.
- Reflexology – a reflexologist would be likely to treat the pituitary and uterine reflexes. Ideally, though, this works best as part of a treatment programme to aid labour that is begun in the 12th week of pregnancy.
- Cranial osteopathy – a qualified cranial osteopath might stimulate the pituitary gland to encourage it to produce the hormones necessary to start labour.
- Herbalism – raspberry-leaf tea four times a day.
- Homeopathy – you might take secale 30c or caulphyllum 30c until your contractions start. However it is important that you should consult a qualified homeopath, so that any treatment you have can be tailored to suit your individual circumstances and needs.

YOUR LABOUR

The prospect of going into labour and meeting your baby for the first time is exciting, but also daunting and you may be feeling apprehensive. Understanding what happens to your body and why, during labour and birth, will help you prepare and feel in control.

Although the process is the same for every woman, each labour has its own rhythm – it's probably best to ignore the clock and follow the pace that your body is setting. Experienced midwives can tell a great deal about the pattern of behaviour a woman displays at the different stages of her labour, and will use these cues to guide her through each stage.

Early labour

In early (latent) labour your body is simply preparing the cervix and uterus for the real work ahead and you may experience niggly period-type pains in your lower back. You may also feel some cramping and contractions that send shooting pains. These may be coming regularly, but they don't last for very long.

It is easy to get excited about the start of labour and convince yourself that this is really 'it'. Many women then pour a great deal of energy into this initial phase, only to end up disappointed and exhausted by the time they get into established labour. For this reason you will probably be encouraged to stay at home for as long as possible during this stage unless there is some other reason why you should go into hospital.

Many women don't expect the early part of labour to go on as long as it can do – especially if it is a first child. For some women, more effective contractions

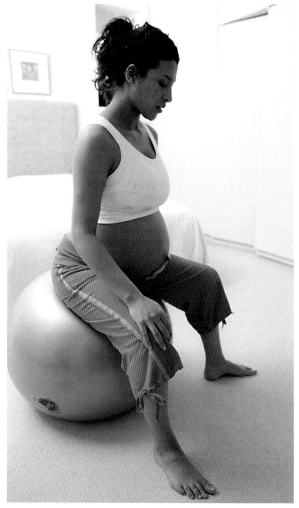

A 'birthing ball' helps you make a natural rotating hip motion, encouraging the descent of your baby through the birth canal.

DILATATION

The baby's head starts to move into the birth canal during this first phase of labour, which can last many hours.

The cervix gradually becomes softer and thinner, dilating all the time and allowing the baby's head through.

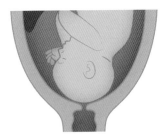

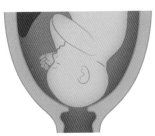

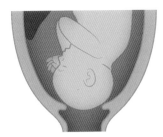

The early stage is accompanied by sporadic contractions.

The baby's head drops down as the cervix dilates to 6 cm (2 in).

The cervix is fully dilated to 10 cm (4 in) at the end of the first stage.

may come on fairly fast with little build-up and labour progresses quickly. However, for others this phase may seem to go on 'for ever' and may last for several hours, or even days. Having a long early phase doesn't necessarily mean that you will have a long first stage, though. Once your cervix has become fully dilated your labour may progress quickly.

The stages of labour

Labour is divided into three stages. It usually lasts between 12 and 18 hours altogether if it is a first pregnancy and tends to be shorter (six to 14 hours), in subsequent ones, but these are only average times and your labour may be either longer or shorter.

The first stage This is usually the longest stage and is when your cervix gradually opens up (dilates), to eventually allow the baby through. When you reach 4 cm (1½ in) dilatation you are considered to be in 'established labour'. Your contractions will usually intensify once you have dilated to 6 cm (2 in). Transition may start at around 7 cm (2¾ in), normally the time just before the second stage. At 10 cm (4 in) you have reached the second stage and may feel the urge to bear down.

The second stage This begins once you are fully dilated and will involve some intense pushing and

CERVICAL EFFACEMENT

As late pregnancy progresses prostaglandins work on making the cervix softer and Braxton Hicks' contractions thin out the cervix, making it shorter in length. Gradually the uterus draws it upwards and eventually the cervix becomes fully dilated, allowing the baby to pass through it.

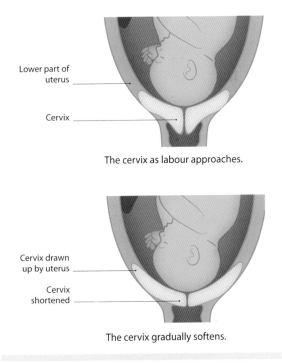

Lower part of uterus

Cervix

The cervix as labour approaches.

Cervix drawn up by uterus

Cervix shortened

The cervix gradually softens.

bearing down until your baby moves down through the birth canal and is born into the outside world (see page 281).

The third stage Your baby will have been born and you may well be preoccupied with cuddling him. Your placenta will now come away from the wall of your uterus and be delivered, along with any remaining membranes. You may be so absorbed with your baby that you are unaware of this happening. You will also be cleaned up and your perineum inspected after the delivery of the placenta. Any tears will be sutured (see pages 282–3) if need be.

Waters breaking (membrane rupture)

Most women experience their waters breaking during labour, but it can also happen before it starts, though it will trigger the release of prostaglandins, the hormones that will stimulate contractions, so labour is likely to start within 24 hours of rupture.

The waters are the amniotic fluid that your baby has been cushioned in and when it is time for your baby to be born, the amniotic sac breaks and the fluid drains out through your vagina. This may happen as a slow trickle or a sudden gush, so be prepared by keeping a sanitary pad (not a tampon) to hand if you are going out, and you might want to put a plastic sheet on your bed. Amniotic fluid should be clear and a pale straw colour, although it may be slightly blood-stained to begin with. If you are losing blood or the liquid is smelly or coloured yellow, green or brown it means that the fluid contains meconium (your baby's first bowel movement), which should be passed after he has been born. If this has happened before delivery it could be a sign that he is in distress and so you will need to contact your midwife and get to hospital as soon as it is feasible.

If your waters break before your labour begins, contact your midwife, doctor or the hospital for advice. Without amniotic fluid, your baby is no longer protected from infection, so avoid intercourse. Once your waters have broken your contractions are likely to intensify as your baby's head will be pressing more firmly on your cervix.

CERVICAL DILATATION & THE 'SHOW'

During pregnancy your cervix will have remained closed and it should have remained firm throughout, to support the weight of your uterus and the growing baby. It is also sealed against infection by a mucus 'plug'.

During the first stage of labour your cervix has to open to create enough space for your baby to be born. This happens gradually (around 0.5–1 cm per hour) so that by the end of this stage your cervix will be fully dilated, or open to about 10 cm (4 in) in diameter (see page 231). To get to this stage, the cervix must first soften and shorten (efface, see page 231). To get a clearer idea of how your cervix has to change, touch the tip of your nose. It will probably feel firm and resistant. Now if you touch your lips, they feel much softer and yield easily to the pressure of your finger. Your cervix will change from being firm, like your nose, to being soft and stretchy, like your lips.

Your cervix may have begun to soften in the latter stages of your pregnancy and you will probably have been unaware of it, but you may now notice a change if you have a 'show'. This is when the mucus plug comes away from the cervix and is expelled through the vagina. It looks jelly-like and may be pinkish brown and stained with blood. There should only be a little blood, so if there is a lot, contact your midwife or doctor for advice.

The plug may come away in one, or several, thready, mucousy parts and some women don't even notice it – in fact not every woman has a show (there is no need to worry if you don't). Labour may start after this or it may be delayed for a few days. If you have had a show it is best not to have intercourse.

CONTRACTIONS

At the start of labour, contractions are often infrequent, mild and felt in the lower abdomen. Many women compare this discomfort to period pain. Depending on the position of your baby, the pain may be felt in your lower back as well.

Babies who lie against their mother's spine are called 'posterior' babies and this usually causes a considerable amount of back pain as the pressure is felt in all the nerves, which are so rich around the sacrum. Trying to get your baby into an anterior position beforehand is therefore very beneficial (see pages 212–15).

As labour progresses the contractions become closer together and are much stronger. In the beginning they may last only 30 seconds, but as they become more efficient they will last up to 60 seconds. As the large muscle of the uterus contracts, so it helps to move your baby down deeper into your pelvis.

If the waters have already broken, the baby's head will be in direct contact with the cervix and this may speed up dilatation. It often takes longer to get to 5 cm (2 in) when women have their first baby, than it does to get from 5–10 cm (2–4 in).

Remember that as labour progresses and contractions become more painful, you will have more of your own pain-relieving hormones in your body, helping you to cope better. Labour is hard work, hence its name, but the pain of contractions can be manageable.

Towards the second stage of labour contractions should be coming every two minutes and lasting for 60 seconds. It is normal for the woman to experience 5 contractions in 10 minutes. However, just before the second stage begins, contractions often tail off, giving the woman time to prepare to birth her baby. This is sometimes described as the 'rest and be thankful' stage.

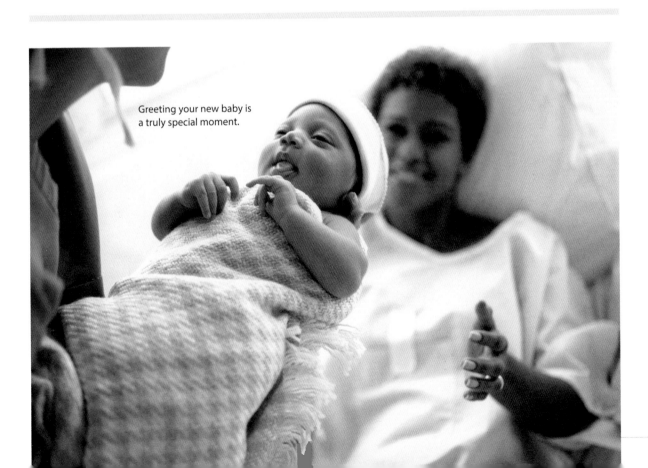

Greeting your new baby is a truly special moment.

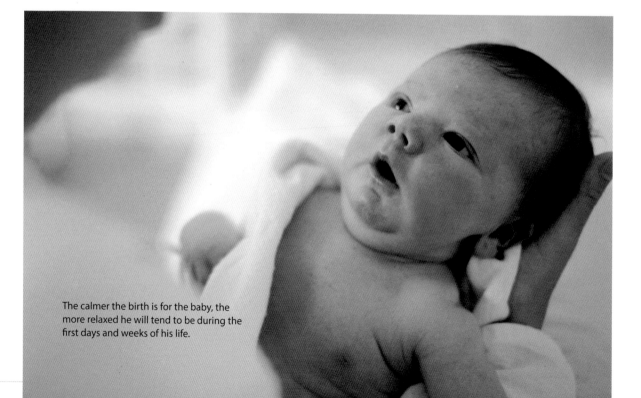

what your baby experiences

LABOUR & BABY'S BIRTH

Your baby in labour is going on a journey – from your uterus into the outside world – and it is important that it should be as quick and easy as it can be, so that his start in life can be as relaxed as possible.

In 1974 a French obstetrician published a book about childbirth with a truly revolutionary question at its heart: What does the baby experience during birth? Frederick Leboyer wrote *Birth Without Violence* because he believed that obstetricians, midwives and parents were ignoring the individual at the centre of the story – the baby.

Nearly 40 years on, many of Leboyer's ideas have become standard procedures, so that delivery rooms are now quieter, more softly lit and calmer places. Unless your baby needs urgent medical assistance, he will no longer be taken away from you immediately, but will be placed on your chest or tummy, permitting the all-important skin-to-skin contact.

Birth Without Violence looked at the process of labour and birth from the baby's perspective and now, because we know so much more about what the baby experiences, we can try to make his journey into the outside world much more gentle.

Your baby's birth may be quick or slow, easy or difficult, but however it proceeds, it will be full of new and strange sensations for him. Fortunately, he is

The calmer the birth is for the baby, the more relaxed he will tend to be during the first days and weeks of his life.

intense. During each contraction the blood flow is reduced to the uterus, but the effect will be partly counteracted by the placenta, which will store oxygenated blood in between each one.

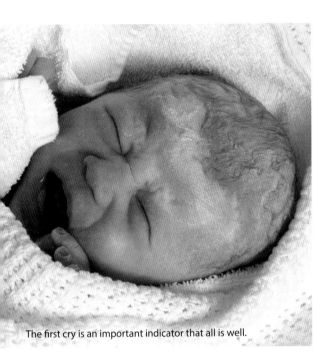

The first cry is an important indicator that all is well.

Helpful pressure

The pressure your baby feels with each tightening is actually helpful in preparing his body to function in the outside world. The pressure exerted on his head triggers the release of hormones from his thyroid and adrenal glands that will help him regulate his body temperature after delivery. As your baby's head passes through the cervix he has to rotate by 90 degrees (or 180 degrees if he is in the occipito-posterior position – see pages 214–15) to fit the contours of your pelvis. And as he moves into the birth canal the pressure also compresses his chest, expelling fluid from his lungs and preventing him from breathing and therefore inhaling blood and fluid. On his way through the birth canal his umbilical cord becomes compressed so he may be somewhat compromised, but once delivered, the pressure on his chest and head ceases triggering an instinctive response: his lungs expand as he inhales.

well equipped to cope. Even when your cervix is fully dilated at 10 cm (4 in) it would seem a very tiny space for a baby to get through, but the plates of his skull are not yet fixed in place and are soft, so they can mould to the right shape to get along the birth canal. This is why some newborn heads can seem an odd shape (don't worry, though, they return to normal within 24 to 48 hours).

Awareness of contractions

It is thought, too, that the neural connections that would cause babies to interpret the pressure that is exerted on them during birth as pain are not yet in place, or 'wired-up', during labour. At the start of labour (unless your membranes have already ruptured), your baby's head will be cushioned by the amniotic fluid as it presses on your cervix, but once your membranes, or 'waters', have broken, the pressure will increase (see page 232). Your baby will be aware of the contractions and although he will have been used to some tightening and relaxing of the uterus when you had Braxton Hicks' contractions, these 'real labour' ones will feel more

The umbilical cord

Your baby's umbilical cord will continue to pulse after birth, so that he has a 'double lifeline' of oxygen. Once it is clamped and cut, dramatic changes take place in your baby's heart and lungs. While he was inside you, his heart had to pump blood around his body and along the umbilical cord, so little of it went to his lungs. Now, though, he has to supply his own oxygen by breathing, so when he takes his first breath, the tiny air sacs (alveoli) in his lungs expand and the oxygen in the air that fills them causes the blood vessels in his lungs to relax, which allows more blood to flow through them. Shortly after birth, the openings in his heart that enabled the blood to be previously diverted from his lungs will close and so when his cord is clamped and cut, the blood supply to it will have shut down.

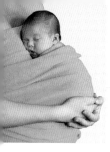

preparing for labour

MIND-BODY-SOUL

How you feel as you approach labour and birth can have a huge impact on the way it progresses – and a relaxed, positive frame of mind can help you get through it with greater ease, even perhaps alleviating some of the pain.

Confidence and positive thoughts help things along during labour, but fear can actually slow things down. If this is your first baby, or you have had a previous birth that was difficult, you may be feeling anxious. It may be that you are worried about how you will cope with the pain, you might be frightened of tearing or defecating accidentally, or it may be that you are fearful for your baby's health. If you do have such anxieties, it is important that you try to face them, discuss them and deal with them in advance (see below). When you do go into labour you should only be concerned with what is actually happening now, not what you fear might happen. It is important, too, that you are flexible in your approach. Labour rarely goes exactly to plan, so try not to get preoccupied by what you would like to happen. Think of it as a momentous act of letting go on every level – mentally, physically and emotionally. With that in mind, try to be prepared for most eventualities, review your birth preferences (see pages 198–201) and use them as a basis for an action plan. Make a list of all the complementary therapies that you would like to use (see pages 254–7) and then work out strategies with your birth partner, so that you know what you want to use, and when and what to use if events force a change of plan.

Practise using your TENS machine (see page 252) and work out which positions you would like to use

DEALING WITH FEARS

List your fears in question form, for example:

What if I can't cope with the pain?

I want a natural birth, but will I let myself down and regret it later if I have to take pain-relief drugs?

What if I shout or scream during labour?

What if I accidentally open my bowels during labour?

What if I bleed or tear?

What if my partner faints?

Will my body go back to normal again after the birth?

What if something goes wrong?

Try to analyse what you are frightened of and why and then talk to your midwife. She (or he) will be used to answering such questions and you will find that she will have sound, reassuring answers for you – all based on experience. Just by voicing your fears and anxieties you may find that they are lessened and you can deal with them more calmly.

Then write a list of responses to your fears and a list of what makes you feel good and safe. Show it to your birthing partner.

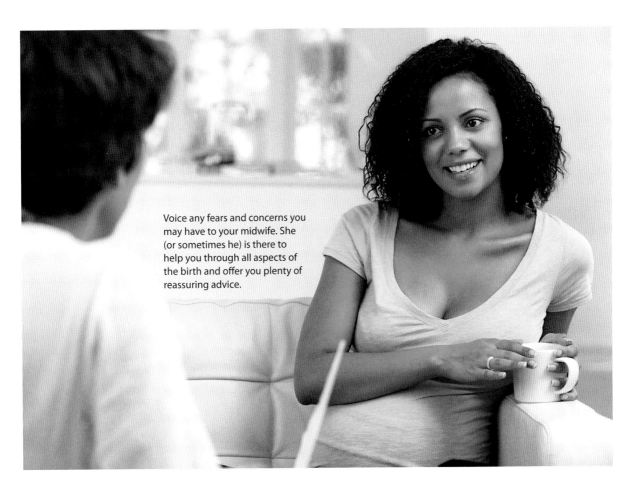

Voice any fears and concerns you may have to your midwife. She (or sometimes he) is there to help you through all aspects of the birth and offer you plenty of reassuring advice.

at each stage of labour (see pages 270–1 and 279). If your male partner is to be with you during labour and delivery, make sure that you are both happy with that arrangement. If you feel that you could do with some extra support, don't be afraid to say so, and if your male partner is reluctant to attend the birth at all, consider whether it might be better to invite a close female friend instead. Whoever accompanies you during your labour, the vital thing is that you should be able to trust them completely.

Riding the storm

Labour is often likened to the sea. It can be unpredictable, with periods of calm and then waves of activity (such as strong, painful contractions) that threaten to overwhelm you. You need to try to ride these waves and swim through both the stormy periods and the calm. But this kind of relaxed state, where you focus inwards and take your cues from your own body rather than from outside events, takes practice. Keep doing your visualisation (see pages 144–5 and 241) and hypnobirthing (see page 144) exercises and pay attention to your breathing (see page 147).

The brain in labour

Our brain has evolved by building layer upon layer, from a 'reptilian' brain to a 'mammalian' one and finally to a 'rational' brain – which is the 'higher' brain (also known as the 'frontal lobes' or 'neo-cortex'). This is the part of our brain that differentiates us from animals and it has two hemispheres, or halves: the left and right. Generally speaking, we function in 'left-brain' mode for most

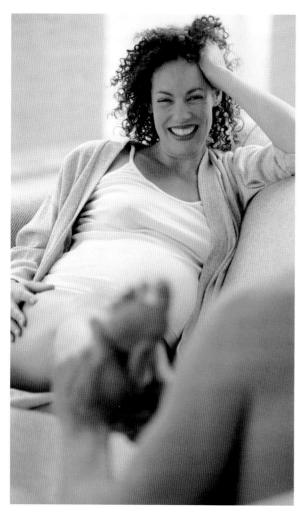

Your partner can help you relax with a gentle foot massage.

your 'right-brain' function during labour:

- Ask to visit the labour ward in advance and try to see a delivery room so you know what to expect.
- Prepare your partner, so that if you are having a hospital delivery he can act as a sort of 'buffer' for you and help to answer questions when you are being booked in. Dealing with questions will mean that you have to switch back to 'left-brain' mode, but if you are both prepared for this, you can then get back into the right 'zone' once you are warm and comfortable.
- Stay at home for as long as you can during the early part of labour and create a comfy 'nest' in bed or on the sofa, where you can rest from time to time.
- Dim the lights (bring an eye mask to hospital).
- Keep the noise level low, with soothing music (bring earplugs with you to hospital in case you are disturbed by noises there).
- Scent the air with relaxing aromatherapy oils (see pages 40–1).
- Bring familiar blankets and pillows to hospital with you. When you are in strange surroundings you can feel very exposed and it is surprisingly common for labour to actually slow down and contractions to stop on the way from home to hospital. Therefore make your environment in hospital as comfortable (and comforting) as you can.

The fear factor

Most women are fearful about labour and childbirth on some level, but nature has tools that you can use to help you cope. Endorphins are your body's natural painkillers, which can build up and increase as labour intensifies, but fear can prevent this build-up and instead cause your body to release adrenalin (the hormone that is activated by the fight-or-flight instinct). If your body is flooded with adrenalin, it will block the release of the endorphins. To try to prevent that kind of panic reaction, you need to practise your hypnobirthing, meditation or visualisation techniques for 20 to 30 minutes each day (see pages 144, 110 and 241).

of the time. The left hemisphere is responsible for logical, analytical thinking and is where we make decisions. During labour, women need to switch into 'right-brain' mode, which is more closely associated with our intuitive side and which, when we feel calm, releases endorphins – the hormones that make us feel good. It is this part of the brain that you can activate by practising visualisations and meditation.

Preparing for labour

When you are in labour you need to feel safe, warm and calm so try to prepare for as little disruption as possible. Try these tips for activating and maintaining

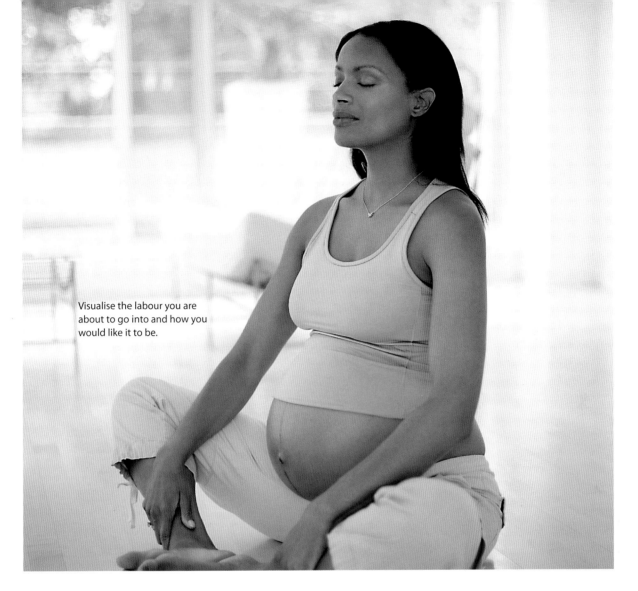

Visualise the labour you are about to go into and how you would like it to be.

Harmonising mind & body

Try out this simple exercise to help you to harmonise your mind and body and induce a calming state of deep relaxation in preparation for labour and birth. In this way you can go into labour in a positive frame of mind and so be better equipped to cope with all the outcomes:

- Make yourself as comfortable as you can.
- Sit alone quietly and try to clear your mind of all the things that need to be done. Instead, focus on the present moment.
- Close your eyes and focus on your breathing.
- Inhale and exhale naturally. Simply observe how you are breathing and don't try to change the pace.
- Carry on for a few minutes and as you exhale, imagine what kind of labour you would like.
- Visualise yourself taking up positions that will help your baby to descend the birth canal.
- Think about what it will be like having your birth partner there with you and consider how he or she will be able to help you.
- Think about each contraction coming like a wave. Ride on top of it – don't let it push you under. Consider how you will calmly breathe through it and how it will help your cervix to open.
- Visualise your baby descending through the birth canal and being born.

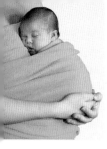

FUEL FOR LABOUR

Preparing your mind and emotions for birth is crucial, but of equal importance is your physical well-being and, just like an athlete preparing for a marathon, you need to build your energy reserves.

You have probably been eating a well-balanced diet (preferably organic) during pregnancy, to nourish both you and your baby (see pages 78–85, 136–7 and 184–7). Now you need to build on those months of healthy eating and stock up on complex carbohydrates (see page 79), so that your muscles and liver can store the glycogen that will deliver energy to your uterine muscles. Complex carbohydrates will also help to keep blood-sugar levels stable and your energy in steady supply. To help your body convert glucose into energy you will need to eat foods that contain plenty of vitamins and minerals (see right).

Energy production

When your body's cells require energy they take it from the glucose in your blood. If there are insufficient amounts from the food in your last meal, your body will draw on its long-term store known as glycogen. Simple carbohydrates are broken down by the digestive system and absorbed into the bloodstream quickly, but that means they are used up quickly, too, so you need to eat complex carbohydrates, which are broken down slowly and so release their energy gradually. To make sure that your glycogen reserves are well stocked eat plenty of vegetables, wholegrain foods and pulses (preferably organic). To convert the food into energy you also need to produce certain enzymes and for this you need the specific vitamins and minerals listed here:

B vitamins: B_1, B_2, B_3, B_4, B_6, B_{12} These convert food into energy and are found in milk, poultry, meat, eggs, vegetables, watercress, nuts, pulses and wholegrains. In addition, folate is found in broccoli, spinach, nuts, seeds and wheatgerm (see page 84).

Vitamin C aids the absorption of iron and the repair of tissue. It is found in citrus fruit, blackcurrants, tomatoes, broccoli and peppers (see page 84).

Vitamin K aids blood-clotting and is found in avocado, broccoli, beans, cabbage, lettuce, cauliflower, spinach and watercress (see page 186).

Iron maintains muscles and produces haemoglobin for red blood cells. It is found in red meat, prunes, apricots, nuts and pumpkin seeds (see page 85).

Calcium and magnesium maximises the efficiency of contractions and are found in milk, cheese, parsley, beans, nuts, raisins and seeds (see page 85).

Choline helps smooth transmission of signals between nerves and muscles. It is found in fish, eggs, nuts, pulses, soya beans, wholegrains (see page 185).

Chromium maintains properly balanced blood sugar and is found in eggs, chicken, wholemeal bread, peppers and potatoes.

Co-enzyme Q_{10} increases the efficient use of oxygen by the muscles. It is found in fish, meat, eggs, soya beans, broccoli and spinach.

Zinc helps to boost your hormone production and aid your body's ability to heal after delivery. It is found in beef, nuts, bananas, wholegrain foods and sweetcorn (see page 85).

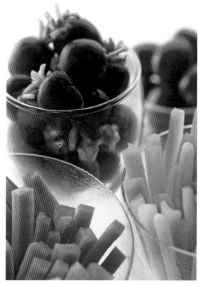

Carrot and celery sticks, strawberries and tomatoes make ideal snacks in labour.

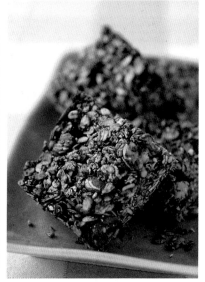

Homemade nut and seed flapjacks are delicious and sustaining in labour.

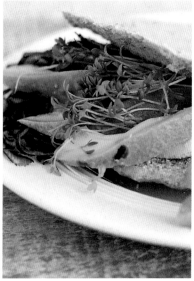

Sandwiches filled with cheese, cress and avocado will boost your energy levels.

FOOD & DRINK

In labour you will need to keep properly hydrated and you should also pack small, light snacks (preferably made from organic foods) to eat. Choose from the suggestions below. Make a list ahead of time for your birth partner to follow (see pages 262–3) – that way you don't need to be involved and it's one thing less to think about.

Mini wholemeal pitta pockets containing cheese, hummus, yeast extract or honey (but don't put in too many chopped-up ingredients – they may fall out and be messy to eat)

Tiny sandwiches with their crusts removed. Use thin-sliced bread and butter. Try using thinly sliced cucumber with a little salt and fresh black pepper or cooked chicken slices

Falafels and hummus

Crudités – sometimes the crisp, clean taste of raw vegetables is very refreshing. You could soak some kitchen towel in very cold water, squeeze it out and lay it in the bottom of a plastic storage box. Put in carrot, celery, cucumber, baby tomatoes and peppers and a mini tub of hummus

Cubes of cheese and seedless grapes

Fresh fruit– a pot of washed and prepared strawberries, blueberries and mango will keep fresher than hard fruits. Watermelon is also very refreshing and thirst-quenching. Pack a couple of small bananas and easy-to-peel clementines

Small tubs of yogurt

Mixed seeds are tasty and easy to nibble on

Make flapjacks with honey instead of syrup and add some sunflower, sesame and pumpkin seeds. Add chopped, dried bananas or apricots. Dried fruit – Medjool dates (but make sure that they are stone-free) are particularly energising, as well as little boxes of raisins, mango slices, dried bananas and apricots

Oatcakes – plain or flavoured

To drink

Fruit smoothies

Diluted fruit juice

Pure fruit cordials

Water

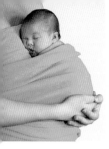

TOP TIPS FOR LABOUR

If you feel a little overwhelmed by all the information about your forthcoming labour, perhaps just read through the most important points listed below.

- **Stay upright and mobile** 'Upright' might not mean standing – it might be a supported squat, or kneeling upright with your arms around your supporter. It's important to remember that gravity helps and your pelvis can open more easily if you are not sitting or lying down, and that your baby can find his way down through the birth canal more easily when you are in an upright position.

- **Go with your body** It will probably give you strong messages as to which position works best for you. This may mean swaying your hips, walking up and down stairs or sitting astride a chair. If your labour gives you a lot of backache, you may want to be on all-fours, or kneeling and leaning over a beanbag or a big pile of pillows – to take the weight of the baby off your back.

- **Make a noise** Labour may be more painful than you were expecting, but you don't have to grin and bear it. Groaning, moaning, rhythmically chanting, swearing and singing have all been found to help women in labour. Making a noise is a fantastic way to relieve tension and connect with the more instinctive parts of your brain – those that direct your body in labour.

- **Choose a good birth partner** A good supporter can have an profound influence on your labour. Studies have shown that having a really supportive companion can reduce the need for painkillers and even result in fewer medical interventions. While most women choose their partner and/or a doula, some feel that their mother, sister or a friend will be the best person to give the love and encouragement that they need. It is important that your chosen companion feels confident and relaxed in the role of labour supporter, so bring them along to antenatal classes with you. They need to prepare for the birth, too (see pages 260–5).

- **Use visualisation** It can help if you try to see, in your mind's eye, what is happening to your body and your baby as labour progresses (see pages 234–5 and 239). Visualise the cervix opening a little more with each contraction and your baby moving further down the birth canal. Because labour is directed by both your hormones and your mind, what is going on in your mind can influence what is happening to your body as you give birth.

- **Be informed** Prepare yourself for the birth with antenatal classes, books and videos. Find out what classes are available in your area (for example hypnobirthing, active birth and National Childbirth Trust) and then decide which will be best for you – or go to them all. When you understand what is happening in labour, the intense and unusual sensations are not so frightening. You'll recognise each stage as it comes and feel more confident about trying different ways of coping.

- **Try water and massage to help relieve pain** There are several ways of helping to relieve pain without using drugs. Most women find a bath or a shower helpful. If you are using a bath, keep the water at

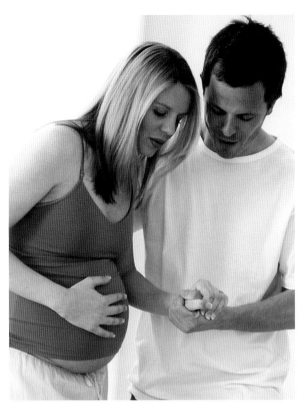

Remaining mobile in labour will help things move along more quickly. Ask your birth partner to support you while you walk.

about body temperature and try other positions besides sitting or lying – kneeling forwards might feel good. Massage, too, can help relieve pain – firm massage with the heel of the hand can help with pain in the lower back. Sometimes you may need to be held or gently stroked.

• **Communicate with your carers** Most women find it reassuring to get to know their midwife or main carer before the birth. You can talk through your anxieties and express your hopes and fears about labour – perhaps concerning medical intervention. Everyone takes a slightly different approach, so your medical professionals will not know what you want unless you tell them. Writing a realistic birth plan will make your ideas even clearer to them and perhaps clearer to you as well. A written birth plan can be particularly valuable if a new midwife takes over your care mid-labour.

• **Remain at home for as long as you feel comfortable** This depends somewhat on the length of journey you have to reach the hospital. If you have a 40-mile journey, you may not want to delay setting out. Although you do hear stories of babies being born on the way to hospital, there are far more women who say that they wished they had spent more of their early labour in the comfort and privacy of their own home. At home you feel more relaxed, there is more to distract you, more space to move around in and you can have nourishing snacks and drinks, which you may find some hospitals still frown upon.

• **Think positive** Think of the progress you have made, rather than all the work you still have to do. Concentrate only on the next contraction – not on the possible 100 still to go. Tell yourself how well you are doing. If you have coped with the last contraction, you can probably cope with the one to come. Explain to your partner beforehand that some well-timed praise will help you cope with pain better. Keep an image of your baby in the forefront of your mind and remember that a contraction never lasts longer than a minute.

• **Relax** This might be the most important thing that you can do for yourself in labour – and it may only be possible if you have all the other things in place. Relaxation does not mean relaxed muscles – it also means having a calm mind and feeling confident that birth is a natural process and that your body is strong enough to cope with it. Then you can afford to let go, let the 'old', or primitive, part of the brain take over and go with the rhythm of your contractions. Concentrating on slow, rhythmic breathing will help. Every birth, particularly the first, is a journey into the unknown. You cannot know for certain whether it will be a quick labour or a long, drawn-out one, whether the pain will just be uncomfortable or more difficult to bear. A straightforward birth cannot be guaranteed, but with the right love and support, even a complicated birth can be a happy and enriching experience.

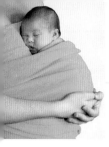

PAIN RELIEF IN LABOUR

You cannot predict how you will react to discomfort and pain in labour and so it's important to remember that your pain-relief requirements may change during the different stages of labour and birth. Keep an open mind and remain flexible in your approach – and remember that there's no need to suffer unnecessarily.

We all have different pain thresholds and experience labour in different ways. This means that it's hard to know exactly how you'll react to pain and what you will require when the time comes – especially if this is your first baby. However, it's important to be aware of all the options. There is a range of analgesics on offer, depending on your needs, how your labour is going and whether you are having a home birth or going into hospital. Discuss your choices with your midwife, so that you are fully informed. Never feel a 'failure' if you wanted to have an analgesic-free birth, but this ends up being impossible.

TYPES OF MEDICALISED PAIN RELIEF

There are three main groups:

1 Analgesic drugs relieve pain, or the perception of pain, by dulling the receptors in the brain that receive pain messages sent to them by the nervous system:
Inhaled analgesic – entonox (gas and air/oxygen)
Systemic analgesics – pethidine, diamorphine

2 Regional anaesthetics that block pain:
epidurals, spinal blocks, pudendal blocks, cervical blocks

3 General anaesthetics, which cause a loss of consciousness resulting in no pain being experienced

Analgesic drugs
Inhaled analgesic

Entonox (gas and air/oxygen) is the only inhaled analgesic. It is composed of 50 per cent nitrous oxide and 50 per cent air/oxygen, numbing the pain receptors in the brain. Entonox briefly dulls your perception of pain and may give you a sense of well-being at its peak. It does not make you unconscious, but it does make you feel light-headed and briefly detached from reality. It works quickly, but its pain-relieving effects wear off almost instantly.

Entonox is stored in a cylinder and administered to you via a pipe, using either a facemask or a mouthpiece. It is used widely during labour, its popularity partly due to the fact that it works quickly and partly because it is held by you – so that you are in complete control of it (the perfect pain-relief choice for a birthing-pool labour). Although the gas does cross the placenta, it is eliminated quickly and has no adverse effects on your baby. It is available in all hospitals and birthing centres and midwives attending home births can bring it with them.

Systemic analgesics

Pethidine affects the whole body and is a synthetic version of morphine and diamorphine. It is the most widely used type of analgesic, but as a narcotic

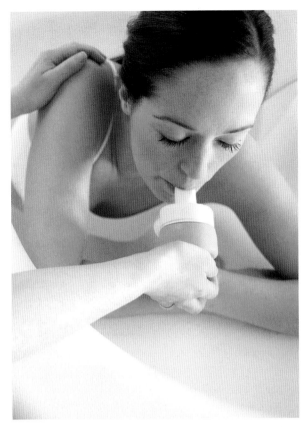

Entonox (also known as 'gas and air'/oxygen) is easy to use and control, and the effects soon wear off.

HOW TO USE ENTONOX

Most maternity units favour mouthpieces over facemasks as the rubber in them has been reported to make some women feel nauseous. The mouthpiece also has the advantage of giving you something to bite on as contractions increase in intensity. Entonox takes about 15 to 20 seconds to work, so to use it most effectively you need to wait until the beginning of a contraction, then inhale deeply and slowly (through your nose with a facemask or through your mouth with a mouthpiece).

Once you have done this for five or six breaths the entonox reaches a certain level in your brain and you will experience some pain relief. At the height of its effectiveness, it may also make you feel floaty and possibly quite dizzy – though this passes quickly and may only be experienced initially.

Keep breathing in and out with the mouthpiece or facemask in place until the contraction has subsided. Do not be tempted to use the gas in between contractions because it will have no pain-relieving effect and may make you feel nauseous and disorientated.

opioid drug it reduces pain and also makes you drowsy. Pethidine targets particular receptors in your spinal cord and brain so that pain messages are dulled, but unlike entonox, it doesn't give you a sense of well-being and some women report that it makes them experience a loss of control, but without adequate pain relief.

Pethidine is the only form of medical pain relief that midwives are authorised to administer without a doctor being present. This means that it can be given by them both in hospital and when they are attending home births. It is injected (usually in the upper thigh or bottom) and it takes effect within 15 to 20 minutes, before wearing off completely after about three or four hours.

This form of pain relief is used in as many as 40 per cent of all deliveries. It can cause nausea and vomiting, so an anti-nausea injection may also be given to you at the same time. The drug should not be given in the last two or three hours before the birth, but if it is, your baby can be given an injection of naxolone to help counteract the effects. Pethidine has been found to make affected babies a little slower to take to breastfeeding, but overall its effects are not long-lasting.

Diamorphine is a semi-synthetic derivative of morphine and it is increasingly used in maternity units these days because it seems to be more effective than pethidine in terms of pain relief. However, it does have some similar side-effects to pethidine, since it causes a certain amount of drowsiness and respiratory depression in both the mother and the baby. This means that the administration of it needs to be very carefully timed.

Regional anaesthetics

Epidurals

An epidural is a local anaesthetic that numbs the nerves in your abdomen. For around 90 per cent of women who have one, an epidural gives complete pain relief and can be particularly helpful if yours is a long or painful labour. The anaesthetist is the only person who can administer the epidural, so perhaps it is wise to check that your hospital has 24-hour anaesthetic cover. If you think you may want an epidural, talk to your midwife when you arrive at hospital, so that the anaesthetists can be alerted.

Medical complications Epidurals may not be suitable if you suffer from inherited or acquired bleeding disorders or if you are taking anti-coagulant drugs following thrombosis. The main risk with an epidural is that your blood pressure may fall, but that is why an IV drip with vital fluids is inserted before the procedure begins and why your blood pressure is carefully monitored afterwards. There is also a very small risk of infection, but this is more likely with an existing infectious condition and so in such cases an epidural is unlikely to be recommended. Around one in 100 women develop a headache after an epidural, which may be due to the membrane around the spinal cord being punctured by the needle and fluid leaking out. If this happens, your headache can normally be treated with ordinary painkillers and the tiny hole heals by itself. If it does not heal easily, then you may be given a 'blood patch' to seal it over. This is done in the operating theatre.

There are other minor side-effects associated with epidurals. Some women experience itching – a reaction to the opioid element. In this case, a greater proportion of anaesthetic will be used with a lesser proportion of the opioid. Your back might also feel a little sore for a couple of days, but an epidural will not cause long-term backache.

As well as these side-effects, an epidural can be less effective than it should because the anaesthetic has failed to spread evenly in the epidural space – so pain relief is only experienced on one side. The anaesthetist will try to reposition the tube and administer another dose. If this fails, then the epidural will be begun again. The epidural procedure may sound rather complex and worrying, but it is important to know that it is virtually impossible for it to damage your spinal cord or cause paralysis.

TYPES OF EPIDURAL

High-dose epidural A conventional, high-dose epidural may also block the nerves that control your bladder and it might be problematic for you to pass urine, meaning you will need a urinary catheter. Your legs will feel heavy and numb, so it will probably be difficult for you to remain in an upright position. It may also make it harder for you to push your baby out. Your midwife may place her hand on your abdomen and be able to tell you when to push, but if your pelvic floor muscles feel heavy and numb, you may need assistance with the delivery (see pages 284–5).

Lower-dose, or 'mobile', epidural Many hospitals now offer lower-dose epidurals, which use a combination of local anaesthetic and an opioid painkiller (if the contractions are still too painful, the amount of painkiller can be increased). A lower-dose epidural blocks the pain fibres of the nerves, but allows the motor fibres to work, so you can better control your leg movement. It also allows some movement (to an extent) and you can adopt different positions, taking advantage of the effects of gravity in labour. You will not feel the need to empty your bladder, so you will need to be catheterised. The anaesthetic effect of a low-dose epidural does not last as long as a high-dose one and it may need to be topped up every hour or so. This can mean that it is better tailored to the exact stage of your labour and with a slightly lower dose, just before your baby moves into the birth canal, you can push more effectively.

HOW EPIDURALS ARE GIVEN

You will be asked to lie on your left side, curled over, or to sit upright, leaning forwards. It is important that you keep absolutely still (the anaesthetist will pause the procedure each time you have a contraction). Before the epidural procedure starts the anaesthetist or midwife will firstly put an intravenous drip into the back of your hand or lower arm. Fluids given via this drip will counteract, if necessary, any fall in blood pressure once the epidural is sited. You will then have your lower back cleaned with antiseptic and sterile covers are placed over it.

Local anaesthetic will be injected at the site of the epidural to numb your skin, then a fine, hollow needle will be carefully inserted between two of the vertebrae in your lower back and into the epidural space, which lies between your bones and your spinal cord (protected by a thick membrane called the 'dura'). The procedure should not be painful, but you will feel a pushing sensation as the anaesthetist finds the epidural space.

Once the anaesthetist has checked that the needle is in the correct place, a test dose is given via the thin, hollow epidural catheter. Once this is safely in place the needle can be removed. The tube is then secured with sticky tape and the remainder is run over your shoulder, where it is taped to your skin. The tube will remain in place until your baby is delivered, but it is pliable and safe to lie on. Once everything is in place, you will be given the first full dose of anaesthetic, which will feel cool as it passes down the fine catheter in your back. It will take about 20 minutes for the epidural to become fully effective and the effects should last for one or two hours. The epidural can then be topped up with anaesthetic, when necessary, by your midwife.

After the epidural has been fitted, your blood pressure will be checked every five minutes for approximately 30 minutes. Your baby's heartbeat will also be monitored using a CTG (see pages 276–7). In most maternity units an epidural is accompanied by continuous foetal monitoring, which means that your contractions and your baby's heart will be tracked by a machine. This is done by placing a 'belt' around your abdomen. If it is not possible to get a good recording of the baby's heartbeat for any reason via the abdominal transducer, a small clip may need to be attached to the baby's head.

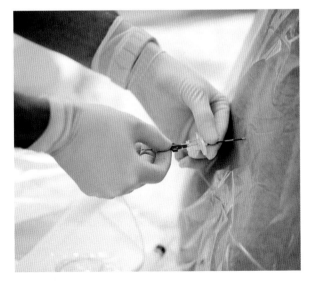

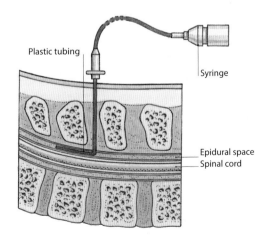

When an epidural is administered the needle is inserted between two of your vertebrae.

Plastic tubing

Syringe

Epidural space
Spinal cord

Spinal block

The spinal block procedure is very similar to an epidural, but the pain relief is achieved by passing a thin, hollow needle between your vertebrae and actually piercing the membrane ('dura') that covers the spinal cord. The anaesthetic is then injected into the fluid surrounding the spinal cord and the needle is removed. No tube is left in place. The needle used for spinal blocks is finer than that used for an epidural, so although the dura is pierced, there is less risk of a leakage of spinal fluid. A lower dose of anaesthetic is needed and it takes effect almost immediately, rather than after the 15 to 20 minutes that an epidural takes to become fully effective. For this reason, spinal blocks are a method of pain relief often favoured for emergency Caesarean sections (see pages 286–9) and obstetric procedures. However the disadvantage is that the anaesthetic can only be administered once in this way. Many hospitals now use a combined spinal block and epidural (CSE) so that the block delivers instant pain relief, but the epidural allows for more pain relief once the operation is over.

Pudendal block

This is local anaesthesia for the vagina and perineum and is achieved via injections in the vaginal tissues that surround the left and right pudendal nerves. It reduces pain in the pelvis when an instrumental birth is necessary and if you do not have adequate pain relief on board. It has no effect on the sensation of the contractions, only blocking those nerve receptors deep in the pelvis. The needle used is large, so normally the area is sprayed with local anaesthetic before the injections are given. Once injected, the anaesthetic takes effect quickly and so it is often used just before a forceps or ventouse delivery (see pages 284–5) in less-complicated births. The pudendal block can also be administered by a doctor rather than an anaesthetist, so it is more commonly used in birthing centres (see page 199), where anaesthetists, epidurals and spinal blocks aren't available.

ANAESTHETIC Q&AS

"What if my epidural doesn't work?"

Occasionally, the anaesthetic does not spread through the epidural cavity evenly. The anaesthetist will adjust the position of the tube and ask you to lean in a certain direction – to help the mixture to cover your nerve endings evenly. If this does not work, the epidural may be resited.

"I'm due to have an elective Caesarean, but I'm scared of being awake and in pain with an epidural or spinal block. Should I ask for a general anaesthetic?"

The team will reassure you and with an epidural or spinal block you should have complete pain relief. You will feel a pushing or pulling sensation as your baby is delivered, but you will not see the procedure because of a screen. It will be better for your baby if you can have an epidural or spinal block, because unlike a general anaesthetic, the medication does not cross the placenta (see pages 76–7). If you have regional anaesthesia you will see your baby straight away.

General anaesthetics

Most Caesareans are carried out using regional anaesthesia such as epidurals, spinal blocks or CSE, but in some cases general anaesthesia is necessary. Possible reasons for this include: your own request because of a phobia or being extremely worried; or it is advised because of problems with your spine (making an epidural too difficult); pre-eclampsia (see pages 208–9); coagulation problems making excess bleeding a possible risk; an existing heart condition; or an obstetric emergency such as placental abruption or cord prolapse. A general anaesthetic may also be suggested if you have anterior placenta praevia (see page 209).

How general anaesthesia is administered

If you have a general anaesthetic all the preparations will be carried out in the operating theatre while you are still awake. You may be given a drink of sodium citrate to reduce the amount of acid in your stomach.

Then just before you become unconscious your partner will be asked to leave the operating theatre. You will be given a urinary catheter to keep your bladder empty and antiseptic will be applied to your abdomen. A wedge will be used to help you lie on your left side and breathe deeply through an oxygen mask to increase your oxygen levels. Only when everything is absolutely ready will you be given the drugs that will put you to sleep. This is to minimise the time that your baby is exposed to anaesthetic.

As you go to sleep

The oxygen mask will be held over your mouth and nose and you may feel pressure on your throat. This is to minimise the risk of food and acid coming up from your stomach and oesophagus and getting into your lungs. It will take around 30 seconds for you to fall asleep. Once you are unconscious, an endotracheal tube will be passed into your mouth and down your throat to make sure that oxygen can be delivered to your lungs and to prevent food and fluid from coming back up. You will be injected with other medication to relax your abdominal muscles and the anaesthetist will monitor levels of anaesthetic and anti-nausea medication throughout.

Delivery

The operation will then be performed quickly and your baby should be delivered within minutes. You will be asleep for 45 to 60 minutes, because of the time required for stitching and you will be woken about five or 10 minutes after that. Once the operation is over, you will be given pain relief and possibly a morphine-based medication for a few days afterwards (see page 250).

A note for dads

You will not be allowed into the operating theatre while your partner is having a general anaesthetic, but normally your baby will be brought out to you for skin-to-skin contact or a cuddle as soon as possible after the birth.

You may intend to have a completely natural childbirth, with no interventions, but be prepared to discuss pain-relief options all the same.

PAIN RELIEF: PROS, CONS & AVAILABILITY

Pain relief	Pros	Cons	Availability
Entonox (gas and air/ oxygen)	Can be effective, especially in first-stage labour, and can be used throughout. It is administered by you, so you remain in control. Fast-acting and wears off quickly, so it doesn't affect your baby. Can be used in conjunction with a birthing pool and during home births.	Although it takes the edge off your perception of pain, it doesn't stop it altogether. It may not be enough to cope with very strong contractions or induced or augmented labour (see pages 226–9). Can make you feel nauseous and disorientated.	Can be used during home birth, in birthing centres and hospitals.
Pethidine and diamorphine	Pethidine alters your perception of pain, though you are still aware of what is going on. Diamorphine can give some women a sense of well-being, so this may help you to relax.	Opioids are less effective in dealing with pain than epidurals or spinal blocks and can cause nausea and vomiting, dizziness and disorientation. Opioids can depress breathing during labour and so reduce the amount of oxygen in your body and that which is sent to your baby. These drugs cross the placenta and so can affect your baby's breathing after delivery and make him sleepy and less responsive. Opioids can make your memory of labour and delivery less clear and can cause difficulty with opening your bowels. This means that if you have to have an emergency procedure the risk of regurgitation is marginally increased. Pethidine can make you feel as though you are no longer in control of your body.	Can be administered by midwives, so (with an advance prescription from a doctor) it can be used in home birth, birthing centres and hospitals.
Epidurals	Give complete pain relief for 90 per cent of women and the remaining 10 per cent have a marked improvement in their levels of pain. The procedure removes pain, but leaves you alert. They work for extended periods of time as they can be topped up as and when needed. Epidural anaesthetics do not cross the placenta, though they can raise the baby's temperature – a factor that should be taken into account if the baby is born with a raised temperature (i.e. it is likely to have been caused by the epidural rather than by an infection). With an epidural in place, if further intervention, such as forceps/ventouse delivery or a Caesarean section (see pages 284–9) become necessary, the medication can be topped up, reducing the likelihood of a general anaesthetic having to be administered.	About one in 10 women do not achieve complete relief from pain with an epidural. This will mean having some, or continuous, foetal monitoring (see pages 278–9) and you will be given a urinary catheter. If you have a high-dose epidural you may not be able to use your legs, so you will be unable to get out of bed or stand. High-dose epidurals can also make it more difficult for you to be able to know when to push in labour. A few women develop a headache afterwards or their blood pressure can fall (see page 246). There are some very rare risks: infection (around one in 100,000); blood clotting in the epidural space (one in 170,000); unconsciousness caused by the epidural tube intruding into the spinal fluid (around one in 100,000); and some form of paralysis (one in 250,000 chance).	Can only be administered by an anaesthetist, so it is not available at home births or in birthing centres. Therefore you need to be sure that your hospital has 24-hour anaesthetic cover for the labour ward. You should also inform the hospital on your arrival that you want to have an epidural.

PAIN RELIEF: PROS, CONS & AVAILABILITY (continued)

Pain relief	Pros	Cons	Availability
Spinal block	Offers complete pain relief. Enables you to remain alert during labour, without pain and is fast-acting. It is given for third- or fourth-degree tears, which are repaired in the operating theatre.	May be uncomfortable during the administration. Can cause loss of bladder control, so you will be given a urinary catheter (see page 246). May cause feelings of nausea and light-headedness. In rare cases it can cause a decrease in blood pressure and therefore lower levels of oxygen to your baby. May interfere with your ability to push (possibly leading to further intervention).	Can only be administered by an anaesthetist, so it is not available at home births or in birthing centres. You need to be sure that your hospital has 24-hour anaesthetic cover for the labour ward.
Pudendal block	Provides effective local pain relief in the lower part of the vagina and anus when no other pain relief is being used. Blocks are given for forceps or ventouse births when no other pain relief is used. It rarely causes any side-effects for you or your baby.	Will not relieve uterine contractions, but it can sometimes decrease your urge to push.	Can be administered by a doctor, so it does not require an anaesthetist, but is only available in hospitals.

Your birth partner's presence is invaluable – he (or she) can give you plenty of help and support.

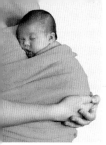

NATURAL PAIN RELIEF

You don't have to rely on conventional medicine to help pain in labour and childbirth. There are natural methods that you can use to manage pain that can either be used exclusively, without drugs at all, or to complement medical pain relief.

If you are expecting your first baby, the particular pain of labour will be completely unfamiliar to you. Therefore it can be hard to predict how you will react to it. If you have a good knowledge of the pain-relief options available it can help you approach your pain management with greater confidence and work out your strategies for dealing with it.

One of the simplest ways to help your labour progress and make your contractions more hard-working and effective is to keep as active as you can. Lying down is likely to make you feel rather helpless and it may actually increase the length of your labour and the pain that could come with it. However, it is perfectly natural to want to rest and you may have no choice but to lie down if your labour turns out to be more complex as time goes by.

TYPES OF NATURAL PAIN RELIEF

These can be divided into two main groups:

1 Pain relief that involves the use of equipment, such as a TENS machines, or the skills of expert practitioners who will administer hydrotherapy or water-births, acupuncture, acupressure, hypnotherapy and reflexology

2 Natural methods that are within your control (or your birthing partner's) such as homeopathy, massage, breathing and relaxation techniques, hypnobirthing and aromatherapy

Most women find that if they can move about while being supported by a birth partner in the early stages of labour it can help to take their minds off the pain and it allows their baby to work with, rather than against, gravity. If you keep moving around, you are also more likely to discover positions that are helpful and useful to you, which you can change according to whatever stage you are in (see pages 266–9 and 278–81).

If you understand what is happening to your body and why (see pages 230–3) knowledge and being informed can help you to deal with contractions as normal and helpful sensations rather than feeling that the pain is a signal that something is amiss. Relaxation is one of the most important ways you can deal with the challenges of labour and birth and if you already have all your complementary remedies selected and organised, it will be easier for you to focus on the different stages of labour and birth.

Transcutaneous Electrical Nerve Stimulation (TENS)

This is a portable, battery-operated device that works by stimulating the body to produce more natural painkillers and by interrupting or reducing the pain signals to the brain. It has small wires attached to electrodes stuck to your back, on either side of your spine (usually two are placed under your bra straps and two above the knicker line, though it varies).

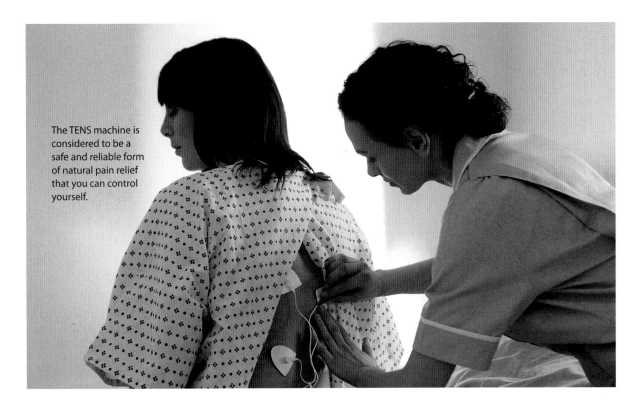

The TENS machine is considered to be a safe and reliable form of natural pain relief that you can control yourself.

HOW THE TENS MACHINE WORKS

The TENS machine sends small electrical impulses through your skin (which feel rather like the tingling sensation of pins and needles) to stimulate the production of endorphins and encephalins (the body's natural painkilling hormones). It also sends messages along nerve roots to the pain pathways in the brain to interrupt pain signals. TENS is probably most effective in first-stage labour and because it takes a while for the endorphins to build up, it is important that you use it right from the beginning of labour. Start at a low setting and increase the frequency and strength of the signals as your contractions become more intense. Or use the booster button for an extra surge of power when you need it. A qualified acupuncturist may also be able to show you how to use it on your acupressure points.

A TENS machine can be used in conjunction with many other forms of pain relief and it is considered to be very safe, with no side-effects, so it will not harm your baby. Many women report that it is useful in early labour, but that it is not sufficiently strong as a form of pain relief

for the intense contractions of established labour. Having the electrodes in place on your back will also mean that it is more difficult for your back to be massaged – if you were planning to do this. However if you find that the TENS machine is not helping, you can remove the electrodes and stop using it at any time.

It's important to learn how to use the TENS machine before you actually need it, but it is easy to master and is a popular form of pain relief, as it is under your personal control. It can be used at home or in hospital and you can walk about with it. However you cannot use it in a birthing pool and you might have to stop using it during electronic foetal monitoring. You also should not use it if you are less than 37 weeks' pregnant or you have a pacemaker. Consult your doctor first if you have epilepsy or heart disease as TENS may not be suitable for you. You will need to buy or hire a TENS machine well before labour and you should purchase extra batteries in case you need them.

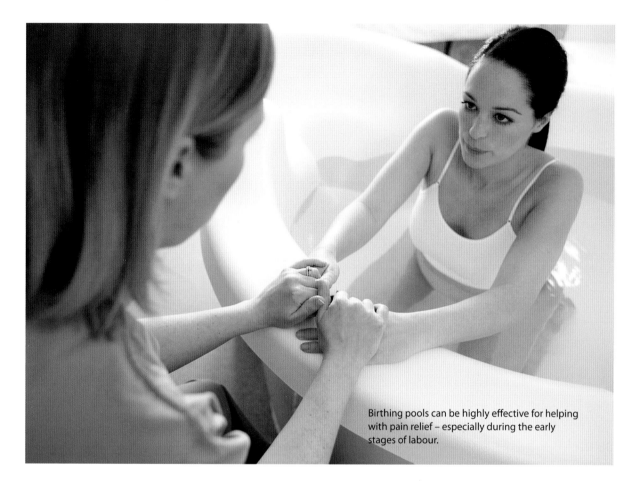

Birthing pools can be highly effective for helping with pain relief – especially during the early stages of labour.

Hydrotherapy & water-birthing

Spending time in warm water can be very soothing during labour – especially during the early stages – and it may even help to progress it. The warmth of the water can help relax your muscles and its buoyancy can relieve pressure on your pelvis. However you need to ensure that the water is no hotter than 37°C/98.6°F). As long as your membranes haven't ruptured (see page 232), you should be able to immerse your bump in water for a little while. While you are still at home you can use your normal bath, even if your membranes have ruptured.

Availability

If you are having a home birth you can use your ordinary bath during early-stage labour or hire a birthing pool to use throughout. Many hospitals and birthing centres now have birthing pools to use during labour and for giving birth in. Water-births are now becoming very popular.

Discuss water-birth with your midwife

Whether you are having a home or hospital birth, you also need to check that your midwife is experienced in using a birthing pool and is quite happy to assist you with it. These days water-birthing is far more common than formerly and most hospitals are happy to facilitate them, though there may be some private obstetricians who are not used to them. You will remain in the pool to give birth, since babies are born with a reflex that prevents them from breathing until they are in the open air. However, the baby does need to be brought to the surface as soon as he is born.

NATURAL PAIN RELIEF Q&AS

"My friend managed throughout her labour with just gas and air (entonox). I want to do things as naturally as possible and my partner thinks I should only use natural pain relief, but what if I can't do it?"

Everyone's labour is different and no one can predict how they will react to pain. Why not put together a 'package' of natural methods that you feel comfortable with and enlist your partner's help so that he knows what you want to use and when? You may find that using a TENS machine (see page 252), or spending time in warm water, using homeopathic remedies (see pages 256–7) and entonox (see pages 244–5) will help you a great deal during early labour. The key is to have confidence in what you are doing. Fear and anxiety increase pain, which makes you breathe more shallowly, meaning that your muscles receive less oxygen, which in turn means experiencing more pain (see page 238).

Practise visualisation and relaxation exercises (see page 239) and try not to worry. Discuss concerns with your partner, but make it clear that if you find you need help to cope with pain, you will ask for it. Remember that the aim of labour and birth is to have a healthy baby – it's not an endurance test.

"I've heard that some midwives offer acupuncture for pain relief during labour. Does it really work?"

There is an increasing interest in this method of pain relief and many midwives have seen its benefits to women and are being trained to use it. Rather like TENS (see page 252) it is thought that the acupuncture needles can interrupt the pain signals to the brain and so lessen them. It also helps to relax and calm many women – it is the fear of pain that often makes the pain worse.

If you want to find out more about this method, you should ask your midwife or hospital whether any of the staff are trained and experienced in using it during labour. If not, you could consider asking a qualified acupuncturist to attend you at the hospital (or in your own home if you are having a home birth).

You will need to consult your midwife or hospital, though, and bear in mind that it will be difficult to predict when your labour will begin, so your acupuncturist will need to be flexible about dates and times.

Acupuncture & acupressure

Acupuncture is safe to use during your labour (although you should consult your doctor or midwife first if you have any complications or existing health problems). However you will need to speak to your hospital, birthing centre or midwife before making arrangements to find an acupuncturist who is willing to attend you. If this is not possible, you and/or your partner may be able to learn basic acupressure by learning how to apply pressure to specific points on your body using fingers, knuckles or palms. By doing this you may be able to release endorphins to ease the pain and reduce stress.

Hypnotherapy

You may be able to emplay a hypnotherapist to attend you during labour, but you will need to check that

this is possible at your chosen hospital or birthing centre and if you are having a home birth you will need to ask your midwife out of courtesy. If you have attended classes you will have learned self-hypnosis, relaxation and breathing techniques (see pages 110, 144 and 239). Hypnosis doesn't mean that you will be in a 'trance' – the aim is that you should be relaxed and calm, but in control. This should help you to cope with the pain and encourage your body to release endorphins to replace the stress hormones that make your body more tense.

Reflexology

Gentle pressure should be applied to specific points on your feet, which are thought to correspond to certain parts of your body. Reflexology is popular as a remedy for common complaints in pregnancy

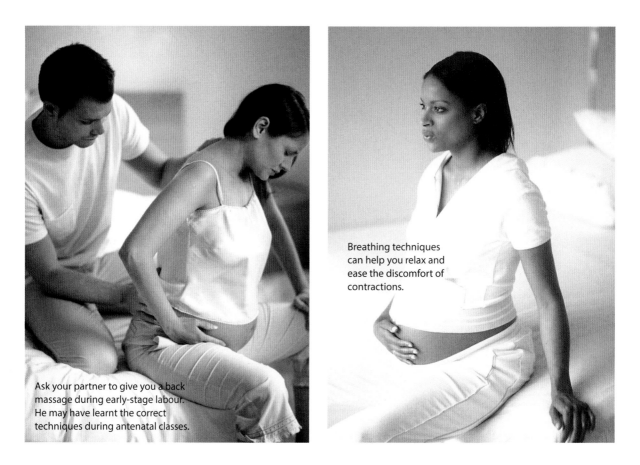

Ask your partner to give you a back massage during early-stage labour. He may have learnt the correct techniques during antenatal classes.

Breathing techniques can help you relax and ease the discomfort of contractions.

(see page 41), but if you wish to use it as pain relief in labour you and your partner will need to learn the correct techniques in advance and/or book a reflexologist to attend you during it. Again, you will need to check with your midwife that this is possible and find a reflexologist who is able to spend time with you during labour. Reflexology is particularly well suited to early labour, but if you want to keep moving about, it may be more helpful and effective between contractions.

Homeopathy

This is based on the principle of treating like with like, in order to prompt the body's own healing processes into action and accelerate recovery. Homeopathy can be used in conjunction with other forms of complementary and conventional medicine, but in common with all forms of complementary

therapy, it is not a replacement for medical treatment in the case of a serious medical condition. Although there is no scientific evidence to demonstrate how it works or why, many women feel that it is helpful throughout pregnancy and labour. Homeopathy is safe to use at any time during labour as it uses low-potency remedies that have no side-effects.

You can consult a qualified practitioner for specific remedies or buy a pregnancy and childbirth kit with remedies that are specifically intended for use during pregnancy, childbirth and for postnatal symptoms. All the remedies in these kits are supplied in 200c potency and instructions are included on how and when to use them. However, if you intend to self-prescribe (or take remedies supplied by a homeopath) you should speak to your midwife or doctor first. Whenever you take any homeopathic remedies you should avoid eating half an hour before and after the dose and do not use or take strong substances such as mint toothpastes as they can interfere with the potency of the remedy.

Massage

Massage can be helpful in many ways during labour, but your birth partner should bear in mind that at certain stages you might not want it, so he must take care to be sensitive to your needs. Stroking or kneading the muscles in your back and thighs can help to improve your circulation – which in turn helps to deliver more oxygen to the contracting muscles of the uterus and to your baby – and it also helps to relax you. During your contractions you may find that firm massage helps to distract you and between contractions you may find that it helps to refresh you (especially if you use uplifting essential oils such as geranium or neroli, though you need to check their suitability first – see pages 40–1). If you have a lot of back pain during labour, your partner should use the heels of the palms to make large circles over the sacrum, which is the place where your spine meets your pelvis.

Breathing & relaxation

A really good supply of oxygen is essential to labour and so it is very useful to try to concentrate on your breathing. Your muscles will work more effectively when you have your contractions and the effort involved in focusing on your breathing may also help you to use visualisation (see page 239) and create a distraction from the pain. In early labour it can be helpful to try to slow your breathing slightly – try breathing in for a count of five and breathing out for a count of seven. If you feel panicky you may breathe too quickly and hyperventilate, but neither should you hold your breath for long periods either. You may have learned some specific techniques at your antenatal classes, but even if you have not, taking slow, deep breaths at the beginning and end of each contraction will help to ensure that you and your baby receive plenty of oxygen.

Aromatherapy

Essential oils are highly concentrated oils derived from plants and are used in aromatherapy to stimulate, revive or relax you. Some oils, such as lavender, are particularly useful for easing anxiety and so these may help you to deal with the pain of contractions. You may also find that hot and cold flannels that have been dampened with water containing diluted essential oils are soothing.

Essential oils can be used in a vaporiser, but if they are to be applied to your skin – and they are particularly useful for massage – they should always be diluted in a carrier oil (see page 41). Again, you should check with your midwife or doctor before you use them and preferably consult a qualified aromatherapist.

Alternatively purchase a pregnancy and childbirth aromatherapy kit containing all the suitable oils and detailed instructions for their use. If you want to use other oils, it is important to check their suitability and safety first (see pages 40–1). During labour you should not use aromatherapy oils of nutmeg, rosemary, jasmine or sage.

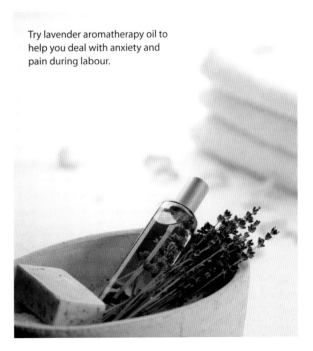

Try lavender aromatherapy oil to help you deal with anxiety and pain during labour.

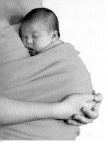

AM I IN LABOUR?

How will you know when you are in labour? You may experience all, or only some, of the symptoms detailed here, but rest assured, when you really are in labour – you'll know.

If you are having your first baby, your body may begin preparing for labour several weeks before it actually starts (preparation may occur closer to the birth if this is your second or subsequent pregnancy). You may find that you have more vaginal secretions, episodes of diarrhoea or shivering and if you notice these changes in conjunction with more frequent or intense Braxton Hicks' contractions you may think that labour has begun. However the practice contractions are usually irregular, they do not usually build in intensity and they may taper off. Unlike labour contractions, too, they feel more 'cramping' than 'tightening' and pain may also shoot up from your cervix. You may find that a warm bath makes them cease. This is not 'false' labour, but

'pre'-labour and is all part of your body's preparations. Chances are that if you are unsure whether labour has started, it probably hasn't, but it might be wise to call your midwife for advice. You may even get to the labour ward and find that you are not yet in labour, but don't be too disappointed and certainly not embarrassed – health professionals on labour wards are used to it – false alarms don't matter as long as you and your baby are safe.

The nesting instinct

As one of the signs that labour is under way, you may feel a tremendous urge to 'nest', with a sudden desire to clean and organise your home. Try to resist this if you think that your labour is really beginning as you

ARE YOU IN TRUE OR PRE-LABOUR?

You are in true labour if:

Your contractions have a regular pattern and rhythm

Your contractions are becoming progressively stronger and are accompanied by abdominal tightening or pain

Your contractions persist, no matter whether you are walking, bathing or resting

Your contractions are accompanied by a 'show'

Your cervix is dilating (see pages 231–2)

You are in pre-labour if:

Your contractions are irregular – coming, for example, at first every five and then slackening off to every 10 minutes

Your contractions do not become progressively stronger and are not accompanied by abdominal tightening or pain

Your contractions abate completely

Your contractions are not accompanied by a 'show'

Your cervix is softening and becoming thinner, but it is not yet actually opening (see pages 231–2)

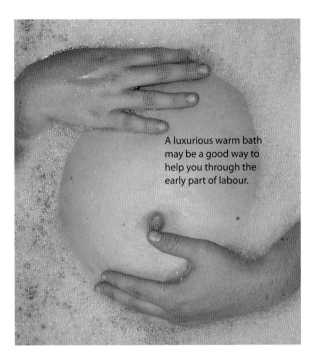

A luxurious warm bath may be a good way to help you through the early part of labour.

will need to conserve energy and strength for the hours to come. Even when your contractions begin, try to ignore them for as long as you can. Have something to eat, get some rest and do things that will distract you. Try to remain upright and mobile, but don't do anything too strenuous. If it is night time, try to get some sleep. Studies show that, in general, the longer women remain at home when labour starts, the quicker and easier labour and birth will be. By staying at home in familiar surroundings you will have more distractions at your disposal.

Progression

It is useful to know that many women have several symptoms of labour having begun, which are then followed by hours of no progression at all. Labour contractions generally progress so that they gradually increase in intensity and frequency, but not always. If you are in considerable discomfort, however, and your contractions have been coming about every 10 minutes, lasting around a minute and preventing you from carrying on a conversation, you may want to get to the hospital soon.

Possible signs of labour

The most sure sign that labour has begun is when your cervix dilates (see pages 231–2), but there are other symptoms that may indicate imminent labour:

You may have a 'show' (see page 232). This is a sign that the cervix is softening and is when the mucus plug that has sealed the cervix and protected your baby from infection is expelled. It is jelly-like and may be pinkish-brown and blood-stained. (There should only be a little blood, so if there is a lot, call your midwife or doctor). Some women do not notice the expulsion of the plug, so if you have other symptoms without this, you could still be in labour.

Your membranes may rupture (see page 232). The membranes or 'waters' are the amniotic fluid that your baby has been cushioned in, and when it is time for him to be born, the amniotic sac breaks and the fluid drains out. It may happen as a slow trickle or a sudden gush, so wear a sanitary pad (important for monitoring the fluid's colour). Amniotic fluid should be clear and a pale straw colour. If you are losing blood, or the liquid is smelly or coloured yellow, green or brown it means that the fluid contains meconium. Contact your midwife and get to hospital as soon as you can. Hospitals expect you to come in straight away once membranes have ruptured, night or day. The midwives will monitor the baby and then, if all is well, you can go home to await events. If you are in established labour you will remain in hospital. (Note: You must avoid intercourse once your membranes have ruptured.)

Your contractions become regular (see page 233). Labour is a different journey for each woman, but if your contractions have a rhythmic pattern and they build in intensity and length, you are likely to be in labour. They usually start by lasting around 30 seconds and gradually build so that they continue for up to 60 seconds. They tend to feel like a 'tightening' over your pubic bone or a rhythmic aching in your back. If they last for 60 seconds and occur every three to five minutes if you are in established labour. Call your midwife and set off for the hospital.

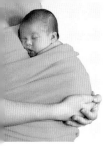

HOW PARTNERS CAN HELP

If you are going to be present during labour and birth (and even if you are not) you need to be prepared. Your partner will require your help with the practicalities, her physical comfort, pain relief and perhaps, most of all, she will need your emotional support and love.

If you have been at all anxious about your own role during labour, those concerns will probably recede into the back of your mind when D-Day finally arrives. Your priority must be your pregnant partner now and you must focus on, and be sensitive to, her needs. Being a birthing partner and supporting someone through labour and birth is not an easy job – but it comes with incredible rewards.

If you have attended some antenatal classes and read at least part of this book you will have gained some useful advice on holding and supporting your partner throughout labour. She will need you to do physical things such as help her to get into certain positions (see pages 270–1) and massage her back, but you will also have to be flexible and understand that as labour progresses the massage she found soothing in the first stage might merely irritate as labour progresses.

Changes in emotions

Be prepared for unexpected changes in your partner's emotions, too. When women reach the stage of transition (see page 269) it is common for them to react angrily and 'blame' the partner for their present predicament. If this does happen, it is usually best if you actually retreat to another part of the room and quietly remain there, but *do* remain. If she has reached this point, the baby is likely to be born sooner rather than later and neither of you will really want you to miss out on this momentous event. However, some women fret about their partners – worrying that they are all right.

As the baby moves down the birth canal, the bad temper that your partner may be exhibiting could now turn to fear and she will need you to reassure and comfort her. Do not be surprised, therefore, if you find that you are in demand again within just a few minutes of being banished – this is simply a reflection of the enormous physical, mental and emotional challenges that she is facing.

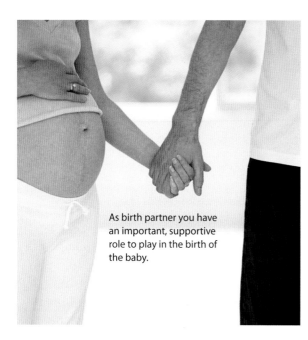

As birth partner you have an important, supportive role to play in the birth of the baby.

THINGS YOU CAN DO

Familiarise yourself with what happens during labour (see pages 230–3), what kind of equipment may be used (such as for electronic foetal monitoring – see pages 276–7), what methods of pain relief may be available and how it works (see pages 244–57) and what may happen if your partner is induced (see pages 226–9), has a Caesarean (see pages 286–9) or if your baby needs extra help (see pages 298–301)

Make sure that your employer knows when your baby is due and negotiate your parental leave – remember that few babies arrive exactly on time, so yours may come some time earlier or later than the EDD. Keep a note of the progress of your ongoing work projects so that you can hand over responsibilities to colleagues quickly and easily

When you are at work or away from home, make sure that you keep in regular contact with your partner in the two or three weeks before the EDD. Keep your mobile phone fully charged, switched on and within earshot at all times

Make a list of contacts with the telephone numbers of your partner's midwife, doctor and the nearest hospital (even if you are planning a home birth). Add the names and numbers of all the relatives and friends you will want to phone once your baby has been born. Forgetting people accidentally may cause unnecessary upset

Work out the best way to get to the hospital or birthing centre. If you are driving there, make sure that your car always has plenty of fuel on board and know the route. Check that you have money to pay for parking. If you plan to use a taxi, make sure that the company is reliable, that they know the nature and importance of the journey and have an alternative company on stand-by just in case

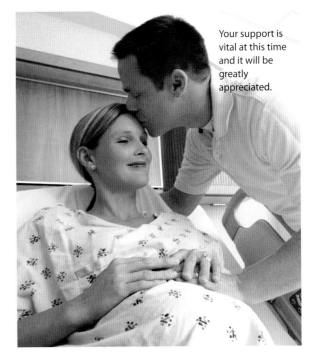

Your support is vital at this time and it will be greatly appreciated.

Supporting her decisions

If you have practised breathing and relaxation techniques together and have a homeopathic kit ready, do not be disappointed if your partner now rejects all of this. Perhaps she hoped to use only natural methods of pain relief, but now finds the contractions stronger than she anticipated and all she wants is an epidural. If that is so, support her decision and do all you can to make sure that the hospital staff comply with her wishes – if possible.

You may worry that you will be sick or faint at an important moment – but this is very unlikely. As your baby is born, you are more likely to be excited and fascinated. There's no need to look at the 'business end' of things; focus on your partner's face and concentrate on telling her how well she is doing. If you feel light-headed, leave the room temporarily, sit with your head between your knees and take slow, deep breaths until you feel better. The best way to deal with anxieties is to find out as much as you can beforehand. Talk to other fathers and research as much you can. If you are unsure of anything, ask the doctor or midwife. The more you understand, the more supportive you can be. Your partner requires you to act as her advocate, so you need to be well informed and stay in tune with what she wants.

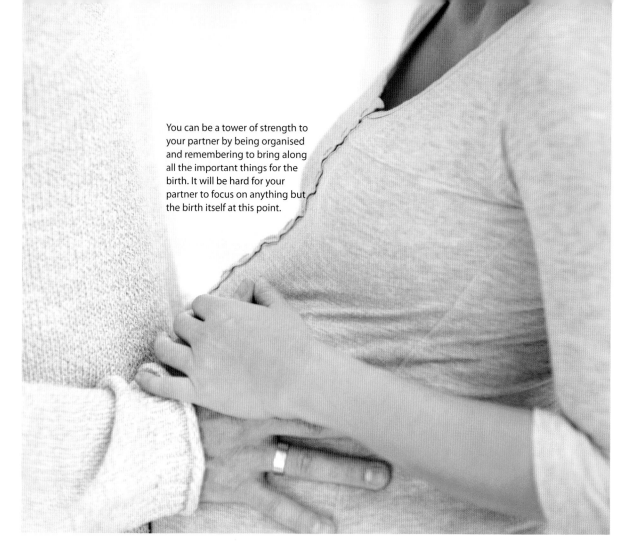

You can be a tower of strength to your partner by being organised and remembering to bring along all the important things for the birth. It will be hard for your partner to focus on anything but the birth itself at this point.

Ways you can help

Deal with the practical matters:

- Call the midwife or hospital when necessary.
- Time her contractions. You can use an app to do this. However, it may be best to ignore timing in the early stages and focus on distracting your partner (make her laugh and keep her comfortable). It will soon become clear when contractions are regular, which is what is needed before you phone the hospital. Ignore irregular contractions if you can.
- Assemble the packed bags for your partner and new baby (see pages 218–21).
- Pack a bag for yourself with a clean shirt, toiletries and bathing trunks (if a birthing pool might be used for pain relief or for the birth itself).
- Bring a camera, your mobile phone, list of contacts and change for a public phone (if mobiles can't be used in the labour ward).
- Pack nutritious snacks and plenty of cold drinks for you both (see page 241).
- Bring your partner's list of birth preferences and antenatal notes to give to the midwife when you arrive (but keep a copy of the birth preferences for your own reference).
- Help your partner to use the TENS machine and/or pack it (plus extra batteries, too).
- Bring all the complementary remedies and labour aids (such as a birthing ball or personal music) that your partner might need.
- Remember to put your baby's car seat in the car and bring the instructions to make sure you know how to secure it properly.

Your partner's physical needs

- In early labour, encourage your partner to remain reasonably active, though movement shouldn't be too strenuous. If contractions start at night and they are not too severe, try to make sure that you both get some sleep (or at least a good rest) – it may be quite some time before your baby arrives – so you both need to conserve your energy.
- Stay close to her and touch her if she wants you to.
- Support her if she wants to stand or walk and her legs feel tired or unsteady.
- Encourage her to stay upright and lean forwards if she can, to change positions frequently and give her physical support to do so if she needs it.
- Plump up her pillows or give her rolled-up blankets or towels if she needs more back support.
- Her contractions may give her back pain or cramp. Use a warm compress or flannel to soothe the muscles in her back.
- Remind her to pass urine frequently (a full bladder can slow labour).
- If she is hot, cool her face or other parts of her body with a clean, damp flannel.
- Tempt her with small amounts of her favourite snacks.
- Keep her well hydrated and hold cool drinks for her while she takes sips through a flexible straw.
- If she is sick, try not to react negatively (nausea is common during labour). Help to tidy her up quickly and assist her with cleaning her teeth.
- Help her to breathe steadily, slowly and deeply.
- Massage her lower back, shoulders, thighs or feet (see page 257).
- Ensure that her privacy is respected and if she doesn't want to wear clothes during labour then don't pass comment.
- Try to ensure that her surroundings are as stress-free as possible. If it is not necessary to have all the lights on in the delivery room, turn some off and encourage her to relax and rest whenever she can.
- If intervention is suggested, make sure that you both understand what is going on and why.

SUPPORT HER NEED FOR PAIN RELIEF

Help her to relax and to stay calm. If she breathes properly she will be getting plenty of oxygen, which will help her contractions to be more productive and less painful

If she says it hurts, don't try to reason with her or be critical, just sympathise and encourage her – she doesn't expect you to solve everything for her – she just needs you to listen and be on her side

Supply her with any homeopathic remedies that she needs (keep the midwife informed of anything she intends to take)

If she wants medical pain relief, support her and make sure that the staff do all they can to provide what she needs

WHAT IF YOU CAN'T BE AT THE BIRTH?

You may have decided not to be present at your baby's birth – perhaps for cultural reasons. If this is the case, there are still plenty of practical preparations you can assist with. These can include, most importantly, making sure that your partner has everything she needs and getting her to the hospital or calling the midwife to your home.

You can deal with the practicalities of getting your partner to the delivery room and you could also support her during her labour and just withdraw at the final stage. But make sure that she has someone she knows and trusts to be her birth partner. Some women prefer to have a close female friend or relative to attend them in labour, or a doula (see page 201).

If your partner has decided that she would rather you were not there, it may be because she is concerned that she might feel inhibited in front of you. Try to discuss these issues and respect her wishes. Although being present at your baby's birth can be a wonderfully enriching experience, if it is not suitable for you as a couple, it will not affect the bond between you and your baby.

Emotional support check list

- In early labour try to distract your partner with music, massage or by keeping her moving.
- Remind her why this is happening and that each contraction brings her closer to meeting the baby.
- Keep things light and make her laugh.
- Don't get upset if she is irritable.
- Don't try to talk to her or expect her to reply when she is in the midst of a contraction, but help her to breathe through it.
- Between contractions encourage her and use repetition to help her get into a state of relaxation. Say things like: 'Let it go', 'Soften', 'Drop your shoulders', 'Open your hands', 'Well done' or 'That's fantastic.'

- If she's heard enough from you she will tell you so and as labour progresses she may need complete silence. Just holding her hand may be all that she wants at this point.
- Keep out the way, if necessary, but don't move too far away from her.
- Don't strike up a conversation with the midwife. Your partner won't appreciate you chatting over her head. Respect her wishes and try to keep the room quiet and relaxed.
- Don't forget to look after yourself. Make sure that you take short breaks, if you need them. Eat and drink and try to get a little rest. You can support your partner better if you recharge your batteries now and then.

Just meeting your new son or daughter will make all the preparation and waiting worthwhile.

HOW TO COPE WITH AN EMERGENCY BIRTH

It is extremely unlikely that your partner will give birth suddenly or on the way to hospital (especially with a first baby), but many partners worry about being unable to cope, so here are some points to help you:

Keep calm. If you are at home and the birth seems imminent, stay there. If you are driving, pull over somewhere safe and telephone or get help, but do not leave your partner alone

Call an ambulance straight away. Tell the operator exactly where you are and what is happening. They will need to know the EDD, the name of the hospital you are going to and whether there are any special medical needs or complications with the pregnancy

If you are at home, unlock the door so that the midwife and ambulance crew can access your home when they arrive. Put lights on, inside and out, to help them to find you

Try not to worry. If your baby is coming quickly, it may be because he is finding it easy to make his way out, so it is likely to be a relatively easy and uncomplicated birth

Try to get your partner into a comfortable position so that her bottom is near to the floor and put some towels, sheets or blankets under her

If you have access to soap and water, wash your hands and lower arms thoroughly

Don't let her push. If she feels the urge to push or bear down. Get her to pant or blow at an imaginary feather. Once your baby's head has 'crowned' and you can see it she should push at the start of each contraction as you count to 10

Place your hand very gently on your baby's head as he emerges and let it come out slowly. Do not pull on his head (or any other part of his body)

As his head emerges, tell your partner to stop pushing – you need to check that the umbilical cord is not around his neck. If it is, either the baby can be born 'through' it or you could turn the baby to unravel it

Clean away any mucus or fluid from your baby's nose with a towel or soft cloth

Now (if it is possible) deliver the rest of your baby by placing your hands very gently on either side of his head and direct him down towards the ground rather than up towards you – until his shoulder emerges. Once his shoulder is out, you need to support his head and shoulder and direct him upwards. The rest of his body may be delivered quite quickly, so be prepared to 'catch' him as he comes out. If your baby does not emerge quickly or his shoulder does not appear, encourage your partner to push, but do not pull at the baby

If your baby looks slightly blue and is floppy, cover him immediately to keep him warm. You need to rub him gently with a towel to stimulate his breathing. Talk to him and blow on his face. You may need to stroke the sides of his nose from the bridge to the nostrils to expel mucus or fluid. Place him skin-to skin across his mother's stomach so that his head is slightly lower than his legs and feet to help any fluids drain from his nose and mouth and gently rub his back

If within a minute or so of birth, he is still not breathing, wrap him up to keep him warm and put him on his back. Support his head and shoulders. Then cover his mouth and nose with your mouth and, taking in fresh air, give him five of your breaths for two or three seconds each time. Check his chest is moving up and down as you breathe into him. Most babies will respond to this and begin breathing independently

Place him back on his mother's stomach. If the cord is long enough, put him to his mother's breast so that he can nuzzle her. Dry him thoroughly and wrap him up warmly. Wrap your partner in blankets or towels.The drying will stimulate the baby to breathe. Ensure there are no draughts in the room

Do not pull or cut the umbilical cord. Wait for professional assistance

Do not wash your partner, but keep her covered and warm

If help still hasn't arrived, you may have to deliver the placenta yourself. Your partner may need to push it out with a contraction. Elevate it for a few minutes once it is delivered, so that the blood drains into the baby. Don't throw it away, but put it in a plastic bag near by because the midwife or doctor will need to examine it and deal with your baby's cord

Remain absolutely calm and stay with your partner and baby until help arrives

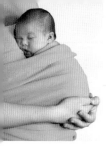

FIRST-STAGE LABOUR

The first stage of labour has two phases: early, or latent, labour and active, or established, labour. Your uterus must contract regularly to make your cervix dilate and only when it is fully dilated can your baby pass into the birth canal ready for her birth.

Early labour

The early, or latent, phase of labour can last more than a day – especially if this is your first pregnancy. The contractions in this phase gradually become stronger and more uncomfortable, and usually increase in frequency, although they may be

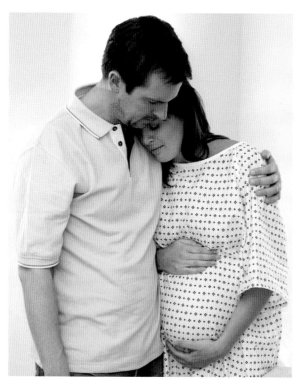

Walk around as much as you can during early labour and ask your partner to support you when you need it.

irregular for some time (see page 233). During this part of your labour, your cervix is shortening and thinning – a process known as 'effacement' (see page 231), you may have a 'show' and your membranes may rupture early on or later (see page 232). As early labour continues, the contractions will cause your cervix to gradually dilate (see pages 231–2) and when you reach 3–4 cm (1–1 ½ in) dilated and your contractions are stronger and occurring regularly, you will be considered to be in active, or established, labour. This can take quite some time, however – it is often the longest part of labour and it commonly takes longer to progress from 1–2 cm (⅓–¾ in) dilated to being 5–6 cm (2–2⅓ in) than it does to reach full dilatation at 10 cm (4 in).

Mild contractions

In this latent phase, the contractions will generally be milder, unless you have had induction or augmentation (see pages 226–9), so the discomfort will probably be manageable. However, if you do find it too much, you will probably be encouraged to take paracetamol, use a TENS machine or entonox, which enables you to be upright and active for as long as possible and encourages descent of the baby's head. Using a variety of positions in early labour can be helpful. If you are not yet in established labour but feel you need further pain relief, pethidine may be offered, but you will then be immobile.

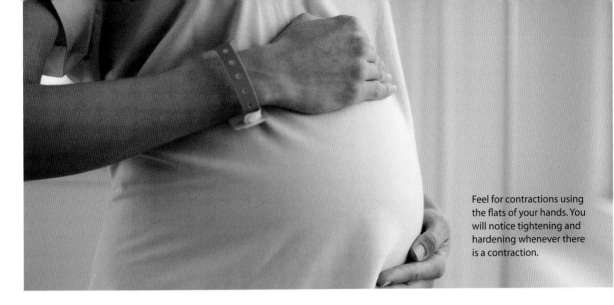

Feel for contractions using the flats of your hands. You will notice tightening and hardening whenever there is a contraction.

Established first-stage labour

Established labour will be said to have begun once you have reached around 4 cm (1½ in) dilatation, and your midwife may perform an internal examination (see box right), but she will also be able to tell by feeling the contractions across your abdomen. At this stage your contractions can be felt with the flat of your hand around the centre of your abdomen and you will also notice a tightening and hardening of the muscles there.

Changing contractions

Your contractions will gradually become longer and more painful. They will occur more frequently, in a definite rhythm. You will also be able to feel them at the top of your abdomen and spreading downwards and across it. This is a sign that they are pushing your baby's head down on to your cervix, encouraging it to open further. In first labours around 90 per cent of women will dilate at about 0.5 cm (¹⁄₂₀ in) per hour, but with subsequent babies this usually happens more quickly.

The timing of contractions is calculated from the start of one contraction to the start of the next. At first, contractions may occur every 15 or 10 minutes and last for around 30 to 45 seconds. Then they will probably increase, to come every five minutes, then every two minutes. By the time you have reached this last phase of established first labour, called the 'transition' (see page 269), your contractions may be between four and two minutes apart and probably last for 60 to 90 seconds, so there will be little respite between them. During this established stage you will need to reassess your pain relief (see pages 244–257).

INTERNAL VAGINAL EXAMINATIONS

In a first labour you can expect to have two or three internal examinations, which will be carried out by your midwife. She will usually use her forefingers to do this, but if she needs to check whether the amniotic fluid is leaking, she may also use a speculum.

The vaginal examination will be used to check a number of aspects of your labour, including: the effacement of the cervix, the cervical dilatation, the part of the baby presenting and the position, whether the membranes are intact and the level of the presenting part in the pelvis.

Hopefully during a subsequent examination, the midwife will confirm progress as regards further effacement, dilatation and lower level of the baby's head brought on by good, effective contractions. If progress is slow, your midwife will try to establish why this is and whether anything should be done to augment labour.

THE ENGAGEMENT

When you go into labour you may hear your midwife talk about your 'station' (also called the 'engagement'). This simply means the level at which your baby's head is situated, or 'engaged', in your pelvis (see page 214) and is noted on a scale of fifths. The midwife will talk about the baby being so many 'fifths palpable'. If the baby is four-fifths palpable then most of the baby's head can be felt abdominally. If the baby's head is deeply engaged then only a very small part of it can be felt abdominally (one-fifth).

During labour the baby's head is referred to as being -3 to +3 in relation to the ischial spines. When you are fully dilated the baby should be level with the ischial spines or below. The baby will then descend as you push.

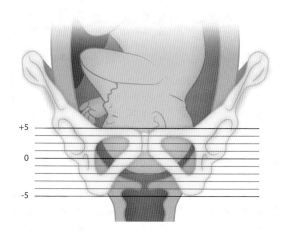

+5

0

-5

WHAT HAPPENS IF YOU GO TO HOSPITAL

If you think you may be in labour and are planning a home birth, call your midwife or midwife team. However, if you are going into hospital, call ahead and let them know you are on your way, so that a room can be prepared.

When you arrive, give your personal details and hand over your antenatal notes plus your list of birth preferences. You may then be shown to a labour room. Your EDD will be checked and the midwife will probably try to find out whether you have had a 'show' (see page 232) and/or if your membranes have ruptured. You will be asked about your contractions and will probably be asked to produce a urine specimen. The midwife will take a history of what has happened so far, such as the frequency of your contractions. You will also have your abdomen felt and palpated and you may have an internal examination (see page 267). Your baby's heart will also be listened to after a contraction, to be sure that she is coping well.

If you are found to be in early labour, you may be sent home. If this happens it doesn't mean you shouldn't have come to the hospital – it is better to be there to be checked

that all is well. However, most early labours progress more quickly when the woman can take advantage of the distractions of her own home, so it is usually the best place to be until labour becomes established.

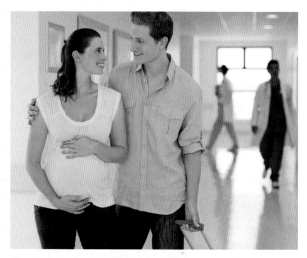

When you arrive in hospital you may experience a feeling of 'this is it!' Let your partner take care of your hospital bag so that you don't have to worry about it – it's one less thing to think about.

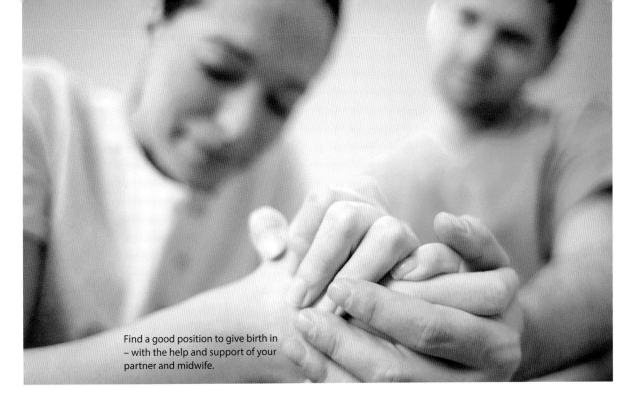

Find a good position to give birth in – with the help and support of your partner and midwife.

The transition phase

First-time mothers are usually unaware of the transition phase; it is far more common in subsequent labours. This is the stage when most women want to give up, run away or even demand a Caesarean section. The birth is very close, but it feels out of reach, due to the intensity of the contractions. Transition may start from 7 cm (2¾ in), but full dilatation is usually reached soon. On average transition lasts for about 30 minutes, although it can be quicker – or slower – and take up to two hours.

A challenging time

Transition can be one of the most challenging phases of labour and your contractions are likely to intensify and become more frequent, so that they arrive every 30 to 90 seconds and may last up to 60 or 90 seconds. This can make contractions feel almost continuous, which can be alarming. Labour will have developed a momentum of its own and will not stop until your baby is born, but transition is also a sign it is nearly over and your baby will be born soon. You may feel a strong pressure in your lower back (even if you have an epidural) and have an almost overwhelming urge to push, but you must wait until your midwife has ascertained that your cervix is fully dilated. It is common to shake and perhaps even vomit at this stage and you may also experience hot flushes, but this will pass quickly.

At this stage you may need extra support. You are likely to feel very tired and perhaps overwhelmed by the sense that your body seems out of your control. Your birth partner now needs to stay close by and encourage you (even if you are irritable – see page 260). Accept your midwife's help and find the best position to give birth in. You may want to lean against the raised back of the bed or be on all-fours, with your bottom raised, to relieve some of the pressure on your pelvis. You may need to delay pushing and so your midwife may encourage you to pant or blow to resist the urge to bear down. It is unlikely you will be able to have pain relief, such as pethidine, at this point (see pages 244 and 250) because it would make your baby too sleepy at birth, but if you have an epidural in place, you may want to have a top-up now – before your baby is delivered. An epidural is the best remedy when you are pushing on an undilated cervix because it is so hard to stop.

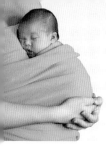

FIRST-STAGE POSITIONS

The key to progress during the first stage of labour, as long as it has been confirmed, is to keep active and to use different postures and positions to encourage your baby's descent. Try to practise these in advance and you'll feel more confident when your labour begins.

There are two main kinds of position you can use during first-stage labour (as long as it has been confirmed): active positions to progress your labour and supported positions to help you relax and conserve your energy. Labour can be a long, drawn-out process, so although it is good for you to keep as mobile as you can, it is also important that you get some rest, so you need to alternate your activities. This is where your birth partner can give you plenty of support and encouragement. Try to 'listen' to your body and relax as much as you can. Breathe deeply and trust in your body's ability to do what comes naturally.

Active positions

Research shows that women who remain active during labour generally have more effective contractions and experience less pain. Perhaps because of this, their labours also tend to be shorter. Therefore it makes sense to keep moving around for

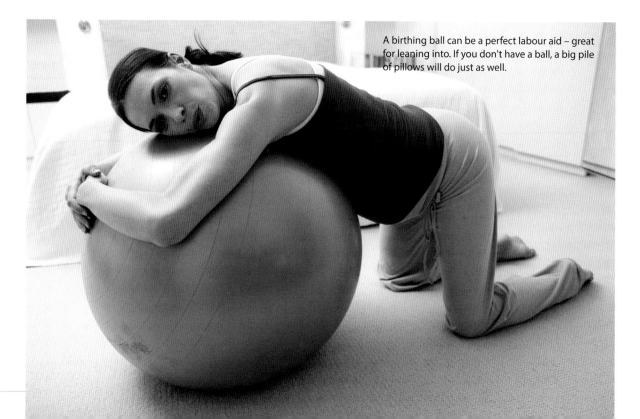

A birthing ball can be a perfect labour aid – great for leaning into. If you don't have a ball, a big pile of pillows will do just as well.

An ideal position for resting during first-stage labour – place pillows under your head, beneath your bump and between your legs. You will feel well supported and comfortable.

as long as you can. You may feel like lying down in search of comfort, but this is likely to slow things down, so try to use labour aids such as birthing balls or piles of cushions that will both ease discomfort as you lean into them, but also allow you to move – or at least keep an upright posture. Rocking back and forth can be both comforting and distracting during a contraction and you can try combining the rocking with hip rotations as you lean over a birthing ball. You can also try going on all-fours on your hands and knees and rotating your pelvis in a clockwise, then anti-clockwise, direction.

Supported positions

Lean against your partner as a contraction comes; try marching on the spot as you do so, or simply make a noise – whatever helps you. Inhibitions sometimes hold women back during labour, but the sooner you can lose yours, the more painkilling hormones (endorphins) will be released. Try sitting on a birthing ball and rocking backwards and forwards. Sit astride a chair and place a plump cushion against the back of it, so that you can lean forwards with

your abdomen against it – this will help your pelvis to open up, support your pelvic muscles and give you the benefit of gravity.

Snacks are good

Eat small snacks from time to time to keep your blood-sugar levels stable and your energy levels high (see page 147). Make sure that you remain well hydrated, too, and drink plenty of water, watered-down fruit juice or slow-release isotonic drinks. Kneel and lean over a pile of cushions and get your partner to massage your back (especially the lower part) – you could use a carrier oil mixed with an aromatherapy oil such as lavender, neroli, marjoram or jasmine.

Taking a rest

If you are feeling very tired and need to re-energise, lie on your side with one leg bent and put some large pillows or cushions under your head, bump and leg (see picture above). If you have access to a bath or a birthing pool, sit upright or kneel and use the warm water to support the weight of your body.

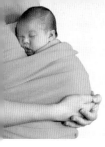

WHEN LABOUR IS SLOW

If your labour seems to be moving along unusually slowly your midwife will make an assessment to find out why – and what, if anything, can be done to help you on your way.

I f you don't seem to be making much progress in labour, there may be several reasons why. It could be that your contractions are inefficient and dilatation of your cervix is slow, so they are not making your cervix open up enough, or it may be because your baby's head is too large to fit through your pelvis (this is known as cephalopelvic disproportion or CPD). Or it could be because your baby is in a posterior position, with his back facing yours (see pages 212–15). However, there might be some other reason why labour is not progressing.

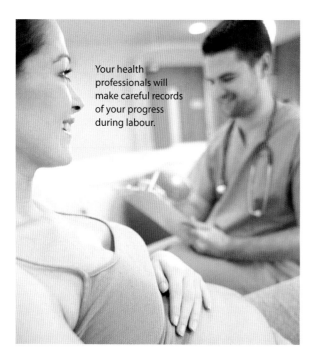

Your health professionals will make careful records of your progress during labour.

AUGMENTATION OF LABOUR

If labour began spontaneously, but has now slowed or even stopped, your midwife will use a partogram (see page 274) to make an assessment of the nature of the problem and whether or when augmentation should be used. If your contractions seem to be reasonably efficient, but your membranes have not yet ruptured, then the midwife may decide to rupture them artificially (ARM – see page 228) and this may then accelerate your labour sufficiently.

If your contractions are infrequent, irregular or weak and your membranes have already ruptured, you may be given syntocinon via an intravenous drip in the same way as for an induction (see pages 226–9). The dose should be fairly small at first and be gradually increased so that you have strong contractions occurring every three minutes or so.

With both ARM and syntocinon, your contractions will be more powerful and more painful, so that you may need another, stronger form of pain relief (see pages 244–51). If you do have syntocinon, you will need to be carefully monitored and your baby will require continuous monitoring (see pages 276–7) to ensure that she does not become distressed.

You will be re-examined every two hours to check on how you are progressing and the results will be plotted on the partogram. If there is still little, or no, progress, then a Caesarean section may be recommended as the safest form of delivery.

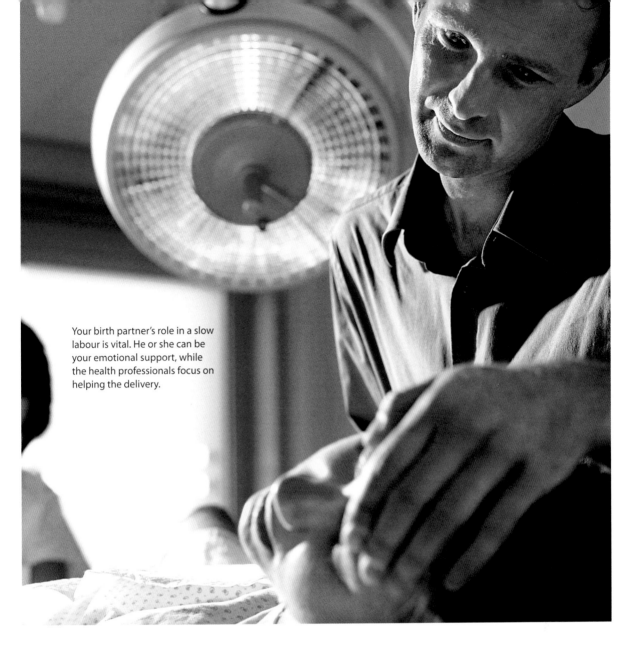

Your birth partner's role in a slow labour is vital. He or she can be your emotional support, while the health professionals focus on helping the delivery.

Inefficient contractions

Your labour can only progress through the necessary stages if contractions are productive and move downwards over your whole uterus – to dilate your cervix and push your baby through it. If your contractions are inefficient, get up and walk about and work with gravity. Inefficient contractions are classified as underactive (hypo) or even overactive (hyper) and they occur in around 5 per cent of first-time labours and 1 per cent of all labours. Underactivity will usually respond to stimulation by

an intravenous injection of the synthetic oxytocin hormone, syntocinon (see page 228), in a procedure known as 'augmenting' labour (see box left). The hyperactive form is also called 'incoordinate uterine activity' because it is characterised by different parts of the uterus contracting independently. This type of contraction will not dilate the cervix properly and can be painful. If the woman has an epidural it may be difficult to assess where the contractions are taking place and how strong they are, so a partogram can be used to record uterine activity (see page 274).

THE PARTOGRAM

The partogram is a large chart on which the midwife will record the foetal heart rate, the dilatation of your cervix and the engagement reached by your baby (see page 214). It also records the results of your urine analysis, the amount of fluid that you have taken orally, any intravenous fluids you have received, the amount of oxytocin (if it is administered) and whether you have been given any medical pain relief, including entonox (see pages 244–5).

It also shows a graph of the frequency and severity of your contractions and plots your blood pressure and pulse.

The partogram usually shows guidelines for first-time and subsequent labours for the midwife to compare yours with (though, of course, these are only guidelines), and they can be a useful sign when things are progressing too slowly, so that action can be taken, if necessary.

This is an example of a typical partogram. It documents all the observations that the midwife makes. This one shows a normal labour. The foetus's heart rate is recorded at the top, while the dilatation of the cervix, contractions per 10 minutes, drugs given plus blood pressure and urine are shown in sections below. Partogram forms may vary in the way the information is laid out.

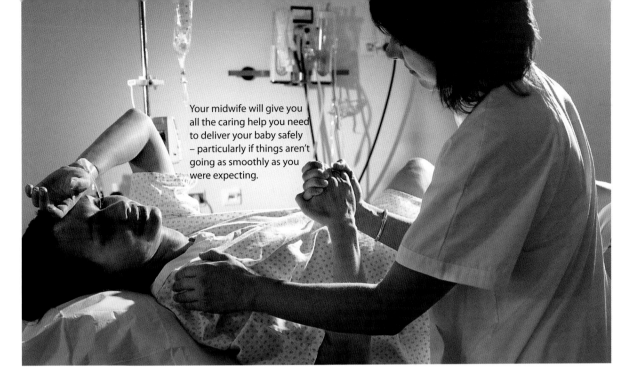

Your midwife will give you all the caring help you need to deliver your baby safely – particularly if things aren't going as smoothly as you were expecting.

CEPHALOPELVIC DISPROPORTION (CPD)

This means that the baby's head is too large for the mother's pelvis. If you have this had problem once, it doesn't mean that future babies will be too large for you, but you may be advised to have a Caesarean section (see pages 286–9) if it is suspected. For most women, CPD is something that will have been detected earlier in the pregnancy and if your height is less than 150 cm (5 ft) tall and your shoe size three or smaller, then you may have a small pelvis. This doesn't mean that vaginal delivery is impossible, but you may choose to have a 'trial of labour', where your progress will be carefully monitored using a partogram (see left).

If progress is too slow, or your baby's head has not engaged sufficiently, then a Caesarean section may be the best option for you. Very occasionally, labour does not progress because of an obstruction. This may be because the baby is lying transverse (see pages 214–15) or her shoulder or another part of her body has caused a difficult presentation. Even more rarely it may be due to ovarian cysts or a congenital abnormality in the baby. Unless the obstruction can be easily cleared, it is most likely that a Caesarean will be the best way to deliver the baby.

OCCIPITO-POSTERIOR PRESENTATION

Your labour is more likely to be quick and less complicated if your baby is in the optimum position of occipito-anterior (OA). If the back of her head is against your spine (occipito-posterior/OP – see pages 214–15) it can be more difficult for her to turn and come through the birth canal. Some babies presenting in this position may be straightforward to deliver and are born normally. They are sometimes called 'star-gazers': looking up to the skies. A baby with a large head may be more difficult to birth and an episiotomy may be required. Babies that present with their back to their mother's back are commonly called 'back-to-back' deliveries. If your baby is in this position it puts more pressure on your back and is often known as 'backache labour'. Your midwife may suggest all-fours position and rocking forwards. Stay upright for as long as possible and avoid lying on your back, as the weight of your baby will be thrown towards your back and it will be much harder for her to turn. Around 10 per cent of babies begin labour in this position, but most change position by the end of the first stage (see pages 266–7). If this does not happen, manual rotation using forceps or ventouse (see pages 284–5) may be needed, with pain relief. If this is not an option or does not succeed, then a Caesarean is necessary.

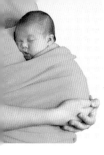

finding out about your progress

MONITORING

Once you are in established labour, your progress will be monitored. Your baby's heartbeat and your contractions will be assessed in a number of ways – to ensure that all is well.

Your baby's heartbeat is a very good indicator of how well she is coping with the contractions and labour. In straightforward labours her heartbeat will be monitored intermittently with a hand-held device known as a Doppler sonicaid. If a difficulty is suspected, your labour has been augmented (see page 272) or you have a high-risk pregnancy (see pages 32–5) then you may be advised to have external electronic foetal monitoring (EFM). This involves your baby's heartbeat and your contractions being continuously tracked on a cardiotocograph machine (CTG – see opposite), which receives messages from devices strapped to your abdomen. The CTG then produces a continuous printout of the readings and the results may be plotted on a partogram (see page 274). A baby who is doing well should have a heart rate of between 120 and160 beats per minute and this should alter by about five or 15 beats almost continuously. This is known as 'good variability'. A lack of variability between contractions indicates that the baby may not be coping so well and may be in distress, as does a heart rate that is either 100 beats per minute, or less, or 180 beats per minute or more.

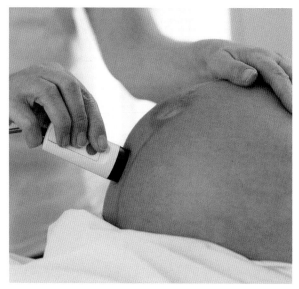

The midwife may use a hand-held monitor to assess your baby's heart rate.

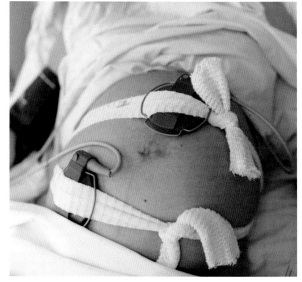

Two monitors may be attached to your bump so that monitoring can be assessed continuously.

EXTERNAL FOETAL MONITORING (EFM)

A cardiotocograph (CTG) is a printout of readings produced by devices that are strapped to your bump. They tell your midwife how many beats your baby's heart is beating per minute and what the intensity of your contractions is.

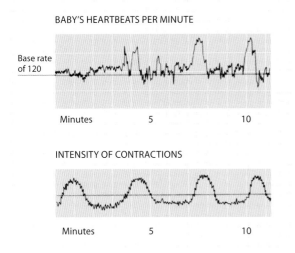

BABY'S HEARTBEATS PER MINUTE

Base rate of 120

Minutes   5   10

INTENSITY OF CONTRACTIONS

Minutes   5   10

SCALP ELECTRODE

To perform internal heart monitoring, an electrode must be attached to your baby's head, or whichever part of her body is presenting. This will mean that a more accurate reading is possible.

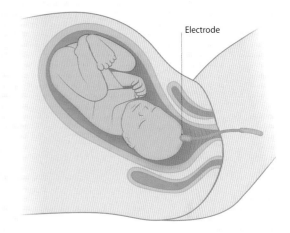

Electrode

How monitoring is done

Electronic foetal monitoring (EFM) can be carried out in two ways: external EFM (see above) and internal EFM using a scalp electrode (see above right). With most external devices strapped to your abdomen you should be able to stand, squat or sit, but unless your hospital has the type monitored by a radio signal, you will be unable to walk around or move far from the machine.

If there are concerns about your baby's heart rate, it may be suggested that internal monitoring is necessary. This means that a small electrode is clipped to your baby's scalp (or bottom if that is what is presenting). This picks up the electrical impulses from the baby's heart and is a more accurate way of monitoring her heart's activity. It can only be positioned if your cervix has dilated to 2 cm (¾ in) and your membranes have ruptured. Once the clip is attached, the wire linked to the machine comes out through the cervix and vagina and you will be unable to move far from the monitor. Your midwife should discuss exactly why this form of monitoring is being done. It may be uncomfortable for your baby, and because it pierces the skin on her scalp there is a small risk of mild infection, which will be treated with antibiotics after birth. However if you have a serious transmittable disease, such as hepatitis B or C or HIV, a scalp electrode should not be used.

If your baby is in distress

If this form of monitoring indicates your baby is in distress, then the medical team may take a small foetal blood sample (FBS). If this shows a high level of acidity it indicates that your baby is short of oxygen, so intervention will be necessary. What happens next will depend on how close you are to delivery. If you are only partly dilated emergency Caesarean will be best. If you are 10 cm (4 in) dilated, then it may be possible to deliver your baby with forceps or ventouse (see pages 284–5).

progressing towards the birth

SECOND-STAGE LABOUR

The second stage of labour will begin when your cervix is fully dilated. It will involve a good deal of energetic pushing and although it will be tiring – and you will need plenty of mental, emotional and physical support – the result will be the birth of your baby.

As you progress from established first-stage labour to the advanced, or transition, stage there are likely to be some noticeable changes in you. Your contractions will be more intense and probably so close together that they feel almost indistinguishable from one another.

As you approach transition, which heralds the start of the second stage, you may become less chatty and perhaps lose your sense of humour for a while.

You may want to focus on what you are doing and it will help if you can visualise what is happening to your cervix as it opens fully and visualise your baby as she descends. To do this you will need plenty of understanding and support from your partner, who should try to be sensitive to your needs and refrain from unnecessary conversation.

Your partner can help you by coaching you through your breathing techniques.

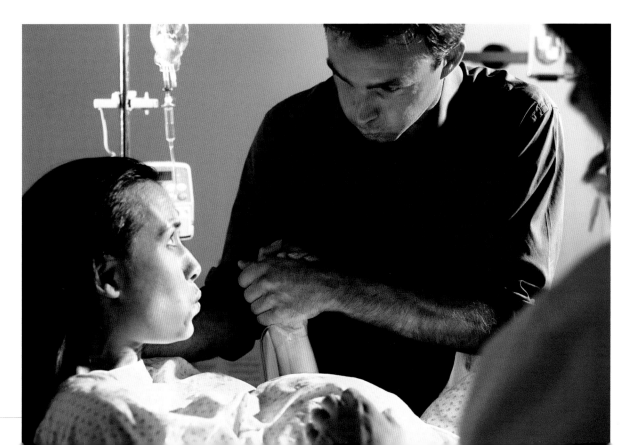

Getting through transition

As you reach transition, when the cervix becomes almost fully dilated, you may become shaky and feel nauseous. If you feel panicky, there is a chance that you might hyperventilate. This means that your partner and your midwife will need to keep you firmly focused on your breathing. You might feel emotionally vulnerable, too. Perhaps you want to 'give up' and feel either frightened or angry (or both). This is the part where many women shout and swear at their partners – or even at the midwife. The medical staff will be quite used to this, so if it should happen, don't worry – either now or later on.

Your partner should remain close by, but stay in tune with your needs and not take offence at what you say in the heat of the moment. One of the most important things they can do during transition and second stage is to make you feel safe and keep reassuring you. It is helpful if they maintain eye contact – helping you focus on your baby.

Second-stage labour

The second stage will start when you are 10 cm (4 in) dilated – for a first baby this usually lasts between 45 minutes and two hours, and as little as 15 to 45 minutes in subsequent labours. Although your contractions may be even stronger, they will be less frequent in the second stage (occurring usually every two minutes). You may need a drink or a snack to boost your energy before you get to the pushing stage. The atmosphere in the room may change – your journey is nearly over.

It may help if you change position now. Go with your inclinations and ask your partner to support you in trying out positions to encourage the baby to drop down. An upright position is helpful to try to avoid tearing (see pages 282–3) because it allows the pressure of the baby's head to be evenly distributed over the opening of the vagina. It also reduces the force on the back wall of the vagina and the perineum. Spending time in warm water may help the tissue to stretch and make the delivery easier.

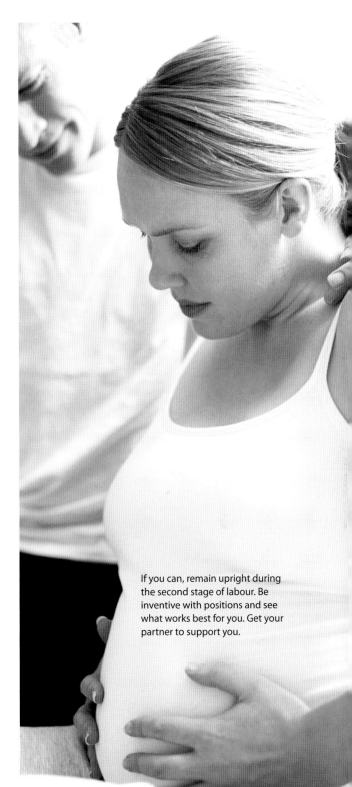

If you can, remain upright during the second stage of labour. Be inventive with positions and see what works best for you. Get your partner to support you.

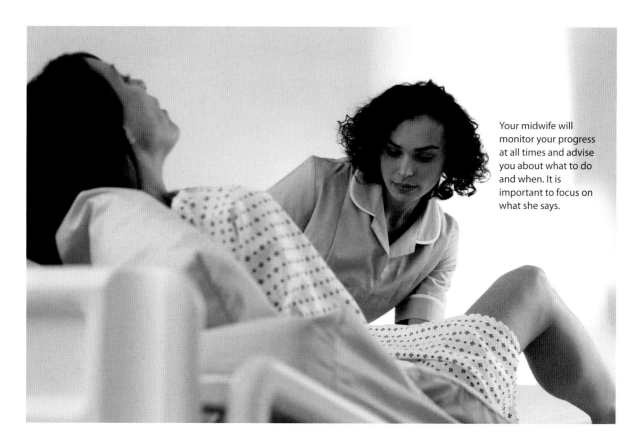

Your midwife will monitor your progress at all times and advise you about what to do and when. It is important to focus on what she says.

Listen to your midwife

You may have a sensation of fullness and a strong urge to push, but you may also be anxious that you might open your bowels, which can make some women hold back in this second stage of labour. Be assured that should this happen, your midwife will not be at all shocked and will clean you up quickly and efficiently.

Once second stage has been confirmed the midwife may guide you, encouraging you to push with the contractions and not waste valuable time and energy.

If you do feel like pushing before the midwife advises you to, do so, but since the cervix is not yet fully dilated, try raising your bottom up while on all-fours and try to blow instead of pushing (imagine you are blowing candles out). This is useful, also, when the baby is coming quickly and you are in transit to hospital or are unattended at home.

Ready to push

By now, you are likely to feel the excitement in the room as everyone becomes aware that the baby is close to being born. You may feel a sudden surge of energy. As you get ready to push, you may feel like roaring or you may withdraw and focus on what your body is telling you. Notice that these second-stage contractions feel different and are expulsive. You may not be able to help bearing down, as the baby's head on the pelvic floor puts pressure on your back passage. Don't be afraid to go with it. The midwife will guide you – especially as the head crowns.

As your baby rotates her head and shoulders to navigate the birth canal you will probably feel the urge to bear down and once your midwife tells you to, you can begin to push. Now you can work with your contractions, which will feel 'thrusting'. You may want to squat or kneel upright or get on to all-fours. Being upright while your partner and

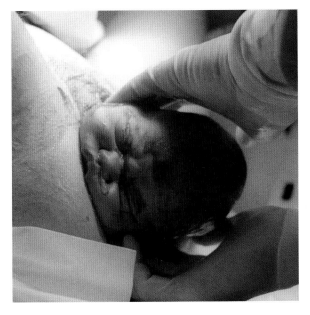

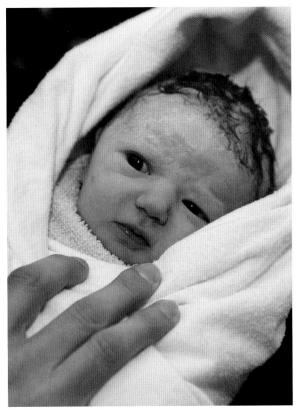

ABOVE Her amazing journey almost over, your baby emerges at last. At this point her head is turned to one side, so that her first shoulder can be delivered.

RIGHT Cosily wrapped up, you can now have the chance to look at your new baby more closely. Newborns sometimes look squashed, but this effect goes in a day or two.

midwife support you on either side makes your contractions more productive, maximises your pushing efforts by using gravity and opens the pelvic cavity. Your midwife may encourage you to push, but it is more likely that this will happen involuntarily, the strength of these second-stage contractions making you bear down naturally. Try to make the effort last. Rather than making little pushes, push really hard to move the baby further on with each step. Take big breaths, filling your lungs before each effort. Direct your pushing as far into your bottom as you can, while your chin rests on your chest. A birthing stool can be very helpful.

'Crowning' & delivery

The baby moves down the birth canal as you push, but slips back when you relax. She may take 'two steps forwards and one step back' – she rocks as she stretches the perineal muscles. It's a bit like pushing

your foot into a tight rubber boot – it takes time. Try to make the pushes effective. Being upright allows gravity to give you a helping hand.

Eventually your baby's head is visible – known as 'crowning'. It may then be covered briefly once more, but as it appears again and stays there, your vagina stretches wide and you may feel a stinging sensation. Your midwife may tell you to stop pushing to allow your perineum to stretch more slowly and you may be able to feel or see the top of your baby's head. If your baby is in the optimum position for birth (see pages 212–15), her face will be towards your back and her neck will be flexed. If the baby's heartbeat has given cause for concern, your midwife will check that the cord is not around her neck and if it is will unhook it (or the baby can be born 'through' the cord). Then she will turn to the side to allow her shoulders to be delivered. The rest of her body then emerges and you will see all of her at last.

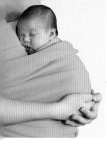

what you should be aware of

INCISIONS & TEARS

You may be fortunate enough to give birth without tearing or the need for an episiotomy (incision), but should you be one of the many women who are likely to tear during delivery, your midwife or doctor will discuss whether it is best to allow a small tear or whether an incision would be a better option.

Episiotomies

An episiotomy is a cut that is made in the perineum (the area of skin between the vagina and anus) to assist the birth of the baby. If you feel particularly strongly about an episiotomy – that you want to avoid having one or that you prefer to have one instead of risking tearing – you should tell your midwife early on in labour.

Episiotomies were once routine in UK hospitals – it was thought that they prevented uncontrolled tearing and later vaginal prolapse. However that has since been disproved, so episiotomies are only likely to be performed for one or more of the following reasons: to ease the delivery of a baby by forceps (see pages 284–5); for a breech birth (see page 213) – although most breech babies are now delivered by Caesarean; to deliver a very large baby; because the perineum is too tight to stretch sufficiently; to protect the head of a premature baby; because the baby is in distress and swift delivery is necessary; or to prevent a more serious tear.

Permission & procedure

Your midwife or doctor should explain why they think an episiotomy is necessary and obtain your permission before they carry it out. Your lower area will then be cleaned with antiseptic and you will be injected with a local anaesthetic in the perineum (unless you have already had an epidural – in which case the anaesthetic will be topped up). You will then be cut, with the incision usually made at an angle, down and away from the vagina (medio-lateral cut) rather than straight down from the vagina towards the rectum (midline cut). The reason why the medio-lateral cut is favoured is that it avoids the rectal area and this is particularly important if you have a forceps delivery because it may extend the cut. Although the midline cut is easier to repair, if it does tear further it may tear into the rectum.

After the birth

Once your baby has been born and your placenta and membranes have been delivered, your midwife or doctor will repair the incision. You may be asked to place your legs in stirrups/footrests and you will be given a further injection of anaesthetic or an epidural top-up, if necessary. The midwife or doctor will then suture the different layers, drawing together the posterior wall of your vagina, your perineal muscle and your skin. The stitches will be dissolvable and so will not need to be removed later. Immediately afterwards you may be offered a painkilling suppository and it will be recommended that you take paracetamol or anti-inflammatory painkiller.

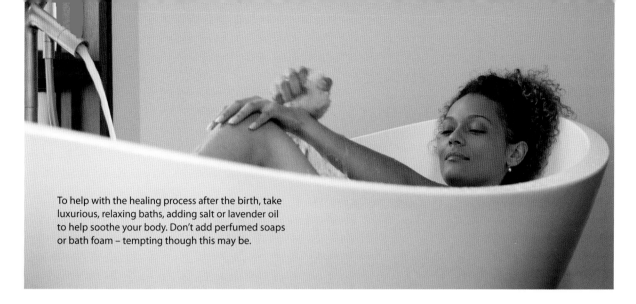

To help with the healing process after the birth, take luxurious, relaxing baths, adding salt or lavender oil to help soothe your body. Don't add perfumed soaps or bath foam – tempting though this may be.

Things you can do

In the next day or so the area will be sore and may feel tight as your skin swells. Bathing in warm water with a cup of sea salt or a few drops of lavender oil (diluted in a carrier oil) added to it can be soothing. You do not need to add any disinfectant to your bath water, though, and you should avoid using highly perfumed soaps or bath foam. Cooling packs applied to the area can also help. Try to keep yourself as clean and dry as possible by gently patting the area dry after bathing and changing your pads regularly. You should heal within a couple of weeks.

There are several natural remedies, such as arnica, that may help (see page 320). Once you have recovered it is unlikely you will suffer any lasting effects from the episiotomy, but occasionally women do experience a certain amount of discomfort during intercourse. Massaging yourself with unscented oil or cream may help, but if the problem persists seek advice from your doctor.

Perineal tears

Tears are particularly common in a first labour, but vary in their degree of severity. The most minor will heal by themselves, but even second-degree tears, which may require stitches, tend to heal more easily than an episiotomy. You will be given antibiotics after third- and fourth-degree tears to prevent infection. Tears are classified by the tissue layers involved:

First-degree tears

Classified as minor tears, first-degree tears are superficial as they only affect the skin around the vagina. Most heal quite easily by themselves.

Second-degree tears

Second-degree tears involve both skin and muscle, but the anal sphincter is unaffected. They usually need to be stitched for the layers to repair properly.

Third-degree tears

Third-degree tears are relatively unusual and involve the skin, muscle and anal sphincter being torn, but the mucous membranes of the rectum usually remain intact. These tears need to be repaired very carefully, layer by layer.

Fourth-degree tears

Fourth-degree tears are very rare and occur in only 1 per cent of births. The rectal mucous membranes are also damaged, along with all the skin and muscle tissue of the vagina, perineum and the anal sphincter. They must be repaired carefully to avoid a permanent opening remaining between the vagina and the anus. They are more likely to occur with a forceps delivery, an occipito-posterior presentation (see pages 212–15) or a very large baby being delivered to a small mother, though such babies are more likely to be born by Caesarean section.

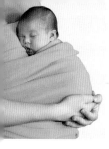

why you might need

ASSISTED BIRTH

Even with the best preparations in place, some births just do not go according to plan and you may find that you need some extra assistance to bring your baby into the world.

In the UK, around one in eight babies need an assisted birth. The purpose of using this procedure is to mimic a normal birth, with the minimum risk to you and your baby. To do this, an obstetrician or midwife will use a vacuum extractor (known as a 'ventouse') or forceps to assist your baby to be born in time with your natural contractions.

Both ventouse and forceps are safe and will only be used if absolutely necessary. Assisted deliveries are usually carried out by obstetricians, but some senior midwives are trained in their use. So if you have a home birth, your midwife may have them with her. If you are in hospital, it is likely that there will also be a paediatrician present to check your baby's health as soon as she is delivered.

If you really do not want an assisted delivery, the only safe alternative is an emergency Caesarean. However, the consequences of having one at a late stage can be problematic and it may take longer to deliver your baby than by forceps. If you need an assisted birth with your first baby, it is unlikely that you will need one in a subsequent birth.

Why assisted birth may be necessary
• Your baby is becoming distressed and needs to be delivered quickly.
• You have been pushing for a long time, but are too exhausted to deliver your baby.
• Your contractions are too weak and your baby is not making progress through your pelvis.

THE BIRTH CANAL

Your baby has to move down through the birth canal to be born. However, it is not a straight passage and with the aid of your pelvic floor muscles she has to make a number of rotational manoeuvres known as the 'mechanisms of labour'.

It is thought that the human birth canal is curved because we evolved from creatures that walked on all-fours to being fully upright humans. This gradual change caused the human spine to curve and the pelvis to tilt, which gave us the 'curve of Carus', as the bend in the birth canal is known. During a forceps or ventouse delivery, the doctor or midwife must ease the baby out, following this curve.

• You have a medical condition, such as a heart condition, and can only push for a limited time.
• Your baby is being born prematurely.
• You are having a very large baby.
• Your baby is in a difficult position, such as occipito-posterior (see pages 212–15).
• Your baby is in the breech position (although most breech babies are now delivered by Caesarean – see pages 286–9).
• Your pelvis is very small or shaped in a way that makes delivery difficult.
• You are expecting twins (if the second twin is becoming distressed, the first one will need to be delivered quickly).

Ventouse

A ventouse (vacuum extractor) is an instrument that uses suction to pull the baby out of the birth canal. Small, hand-held ventouses are frequently used and these are not attached to a suction machine – the suction is created by a pumping mechanism. A soft plastic cup is placed on your baby's head and once in place, suction is applied so that a vacuum is formed. As you have a contraction and push, the midwife gently pulls, to help deliver your baby. Most babies are delivered within three pulls.

Occasionally, the cup will come off and need to be replaced. If delivery has not been successful after a few pulls, the obstetrician may decide to use forceps or deliver your baby by Caesarean section. In a successful ventouse delivery, as your baby's head is born the vacuum is released and the cup is removed. The rest of your baby should then be delivered normally. She will have some swelling and redness where the cup has been positioned, which may take a few weeks to disappear. Rarely, a larger bruise may form, which is a collection of blood under the scalp. This will also disperse, but it may take a few weeks longer. Ventouse is generally less painful and causes less damage to the mother than forceps might, but it may still require an episiotomy or cause tearing (see pages 282–3). A ventouse will not be used if you are giving birth at less than 34 weeks because your baby's head is too soft and vulnerable.

Forceps

Forceps are smooth metal instruments that resemble large tongs curved to fit around your baby's head. During a normal head-down delivery, the forceps are carefully positioned around your baby's head and joined together at the handles. With the aid of your contractions and pushing, the obstetrician or midwife will then gently pull to deliver your baby.

Forceps can cause more discomfort to the mother than ventouse, but they protect your baby's head. They can leave marks or bruising on the head and face and her head may seem slightly misshapen, but

these effects will usually disappear within a week or so (see pages 302–5). It is useful to remember that a baby's head always undergoes some moulding through pressure during any vaginal birth. Rarely, some slight facial palsy is caused to the baby, but this usually resolves itself after a few weeks.

How assisted births are carried out

Before your assisted birth starts, you will be asked to put your legs in stirrups or rest them in leg supports (the latter are more common now), so that the medical team has the best visibility and access to your baby. Your obstetrician will then examine you to make sure your baby can be safely delivered vaginally and if so, he or she will choose the most appropriate instrument to help you.

If the practitioner is using ventouse the procedure will usually be done in the delivery room, but if forceps are required, your obstetrician may decide to do this in the operating theatre in case an emergency Caesarean is necessary (see pages 287–9).

You may then be covered with sterile drapes and given a local anaesthetic injection inside the vagina (a pudendal block – see pages 248–51) if you do not already have an epidural in place (see pages 246–51). A small sterile tube will be passed into your bladder to empty it – to prevent damage to it. The ventouse or forceps will then be applied to your baby's head and as a contraction comes you will be asked to push. As you do so he or she will pull firmly but gently to help your baby to be born.

Afterwards

You may feel a little sore and if you have had an episiotomy or tearing this will have been stitched – so you may find that it stings when you urinate (see pages 318–19). Your vaginal and perineal tissues will be swollen, but will heal within a few weeks. Pain relief, such as paracetamol, will help and there are several complementary remedies you can use (see pages 318–20). You may be prescribed antibiotics as a preventative against the small risk of infection.

CAESAREAN SECTION

There are several reasons why a Caesarean section may be performed – it may be carried out as an emergency procedure or an elective one, depending on individual circumstances.

A Caesarean, or C-section, involves making an incision in your abdomen and through the wall of the uterus. Your baby is then delivered through the incision. There are two main types:

- An elective Caesarean, when a medical need for the operation becomes apparent during pregnancy.
- An emergency procedure, when circumstances during labour call for urgent delivery of the baby.

Elective Caesarean

An elective Caesarean is one that takes place before labour begins. You will usually have had time to discuss the procedure in advance with your midwife or doctor and will know the scheduled date.

ASSESSING URGENCY

The urgency of the Caesarean will be assessed and graded by a doctor according to the following criteria:

Grade 1 There is an immediate threat to the life of the baby or mother

Grade 2 There is concern for the mother's or the baby's health, but no acute threat to life

Grade 3 There is no immediate threat to the mother or the baby, but an early delivery is considered safest

Grade 4 The procedure is planned to suit the mother or the hospital

Reasons for an elective Caesarean

- You are expecting twins, triplets or more – one or more of the babies may be in a breech position, with bottom or feet first, or two or more of the babies may share a placenta. This means that a Caesarean is necessary to prevent the babies being deprived of oxygen.
- Your baby is in the breech position. Although it is possible to give birth to breech babies vaginally, it is usually more difficult and may require assistance in the form of forceps (see pages 284–5). Some hospitals have a policy of elective Caesarean section at 38 weeks for all breech babies.
- Your baby is in the transverse position (lying horizontally across your uterus). This may mean that her shoulder will enter the birth canal first and could cause an obstruction.
- You have a medical condition, such as heart disease, diabetes or high blood pressure that makes vaginal delivery too risky.
- You have placenta praevia, so the placenta is covering part, or all, of your cervix and therefore the birth canal (see page 209).
- The placenta is no longer functioning efficiently, so your baby is not getting an adequate supply of oxygen and nutrients.
- You have experienced heavy bleeding (antepartum haemorrhage) during your pregnancy.
- You have a transmittable disease, such as HIV or hepatitis, so a Caesarean may be the best way to

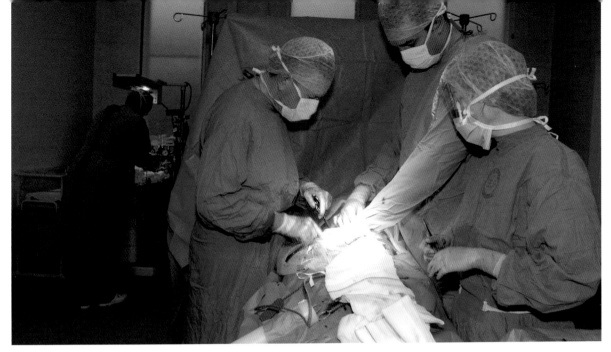

When you are having your Caesarean, you will be shielded from what is going on by a screen.

deliver your baby with the least amount of risk to her (see page 73).

- You have severe pre-eclampsia (see pages 208–9).
- Your baby is very large or your pelvis is small or so shaped that a vaginal birth may be too difficult (see page 284).
- Your baby is very small or failing to thrive in the uterus (see pages 192–3).
- You may have previously given birth by Caesarean section and it has been decided that it will be safer for you to do so again (although this is not always the case).
- You have had a serious vaginal tear that may open up again during a vaginal delivery (see pages 282–3).
- If you are over 35 years old you are more likely to need a Caesarean because of increased risk of complications during pregnancy (see pages 72–3).

Emergency Caesarean

An emergency Caesarean is one that takes place during labour because of complications. Occasionally it is necessary to deliver the baby within minutes, but most often an 'emergency' Caesarean is simply one that is not planned ahead of time.

Reasons for an emergency Caesarean

- Your baby is in distress (perhaps because she is not receiving enough oxygen) and needs to be delivered quickly.
- Your labour is failing to progress and move your baby down the birth canal, causing distress to her.
- You have placental abruption (the placenta is beginning to peel away from your uterus wall) and so there is a risk of severe haemorrhage.
- You have undergone an unsuccessful assisted delivery using forceps or ventouse.
- Your baby has not progressed into the birth canal, perhaps because of an obstruction or because she is too large for your pelvis.

ENTITLEMENT

You are not automatically entitled to a Caesarean section in the UK (NHS) if you do not have a clinical (physical or mental) need for it. If you do request a Caesarean, you will be asked to give your reasons and you will be provided with information about the risks and the benefits. If, after discussion, you still want to have the operation, you should be allowed to have a Caesarean.

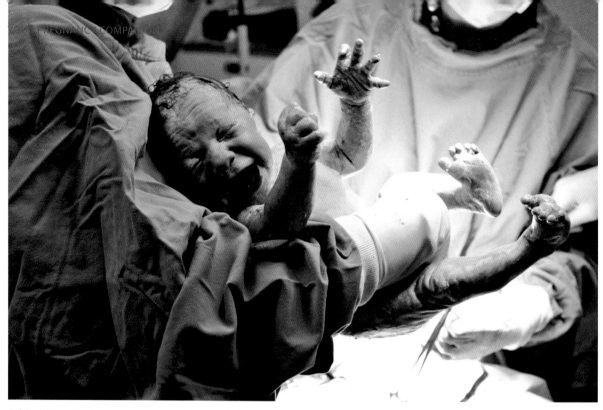

Safely delivered by Caesarean, your baby takes her first breaths and gives her first cries.

The procedure

Most Caesarean sections are carried out using regional anaesthesia such as epidurals, spinal blocks or CSE (see page 248) these days, but in rare cases, general anaesthesia may be necessary. If you have regional anaesthesia you will be awake throughout, but pain free. Normally your partner is allowed to be there with you.

Even though Caesarean sections take time to perform, the actual delivery is usually quick. If you are awake it can be rather nerve-racking, but generally you only feel a few tugs and you are well shielded visually from what is going on. The moment you receive your baby in your arms you are distracted and most of the remaining time is taken up with suturing, which can take a little while.

Caesareans usually take between 30 and 45 minutes to perform. In an emergency, the whole operation can be carried out within 30 minutes. If yours is an elective procedure (or there is time), you will probably be offered antibiotics to reduce the risk of developing an infection after the operation. You

may walk into theatre or be taken there. An intravenous drip will be sited in the back of your hand or your arm so that you can be given essential fluids and extra pain relief, if necessary. If you do not already have an epidural in place you will need to

POST-OPERATIVE WARNING SIGNS

Caesarean sections are considered to be safe and are used in around 24 per cent of births in the UK, however there is an increased risk of infection and thrombosis (blood clot), so you need to be aware of the signs. You should contact your midwife or doctor at once if you have the following symptoms afterwards:

Severe abdominal pain

Leaking urine

Painful or severe vaginal bleeding

Swelling or pain in your calf

Shortness of breath or a sudden, unexplained cough

VAGINAL BIRTH AFTER A CAESAREAN

It used to be said that 'once a Caesarean always a Caesarean', but this was when vertical incisions were the most common type given. Doctors were often reluctant to allow a woman to try for a vaginal birth after a previous Caesarean delivery (VBAC) in case it put too much pressure on the scar.

Now that most Caesareans are carried out using a smaller, horizontal, incision the risk of rupture is much less likely. In this lower region of the uterus the muscle wall is thinner and so heals more easily. Many women are encouraged to have a 'trial of labour' and the chances of successfully achieving a vaginal delivery are as high as 70 per cent. It is also untrue that women can only have a maximum of two Caesareans, although the wall of the uterus is inevitably weaker. It all depends on individual circumstances.

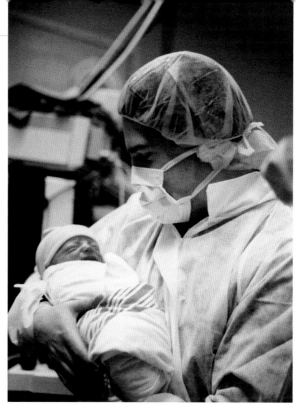

Your partner will be able to hold the baby straight away.

have one inserted or be given a spinal block. Once the anaesthetist is satisfied that your pain relief is complete, you will have a catheter inserted into your bladder. This will be left in place for a while after the operation, so that you do not have to get out of bed when you are recovering. Some of your pubic hair may be shaved along your bikini line and your abdomen will be cleaned with antiseptic. You will then be covered with drapes and a screen will usually be placed across your abdomen so you do not have to see anything. However, you can ask to have the screen lowered to see your baby being born or you can request a mirror. The operating table may be tilted to an angle of around 15 degrees to take the pressure off your uterus and abdomen and reduce the risk of your blood pressure dropping suddenly.

Horizontal or vertical

Most Caesarean incisions are made across the top of the pubic bone in a horizontal line. This is because the uterine muscle heals better here than in a vertical incision and the scar is less visible. However, vertical

C-sections are sometimes used for babies that are in an awkward position or for premature babies when they need particularly delicate handling. In most cases, the surgeon will make an incision of about 20 cm (8 in) across your lower abdomen (along the bikini line) and then a second cut into your uterus.

Assessment

Your baby will be assessed by a paediatrician using the Apgar score (see pages 294–5) and if all is well, she will be handed to you (or your partner) and you will be encouraged to have skin-to-skin contact (see pages 292–3). If there are concerns, she will be taken to the special care baby unit (SCBU). You will probably be given an injection of oxytocin to encourage your uterus to contract and reduce blood loss. The surgeon will deliver the placenta and close the incision, using dissolving stitches.

You will probably be encouraged to get up the next day and you may be home as soon as three days afterwards. You will need some painkillers and plenty of time to gently recover at home (see pages 322–3).

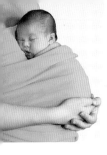

TWINS & MORE

Giving birth to twins, triplets, or more, undoubtedly increases the risk of complications, but you and your babies will be closely monitored and will receive close attention and special care.

Multiple pregnancies naturally occur in around one in every 90 women, but with the increased use of fertility treatments, multiple pregnancies in the UK have increased over the last 20 years. Such pregnancies are considered high risk (see pages 32–5), so if you are expecting more than one baby you will have experienced careful monitoring throughout the nine months. When it is time for your babies to be born, the type of delivery you have will depend on the position of your twins and a number of other factors. So although more than half of twins, and almost all triplets, are born by Caesarean section, vaginal delivery is possible, though hospital birth is advised. With twins, vaginal birth generally comes about as a result of going into labour prematurely or if your cervix is already dilated.

Going into spontaneous labour

You are twice as likely to go into labour early if you are having twins (around week 37 is the most common time) and if you are having triplets it is more likely to happen at 34 weeks – and 32 weeks if you are having quads. At 34 weeks, babies' systems are fully formed, but not completely mature, so they will need help with respiration, temperature control and blood-sugar levels (see page 147). The average birth weight for multiple babies is less than for single babies, with 2.5 kg (5.5 lb) for twins, 1.8 kg (4 lb) for triplets and 1.4 kg (3 lb) for quads, but no matter what their birth weight, multiple babies are far more likely to be admitted to the Special Care Baby Unit (SCBU) because they tend to need help with breathing and feeding. Provided there are no other complications, once feeding has been established and your babies are putting on weight their stay in hospital should be short.

Vaginal delivery

If you have a vaginal birth, your obstetrician's main concern will be the health of the second twin. Even if your 'first' twin is in a good, head-down position, it is difficult to predict how the second baby will cope. You will be in a large delivery room because there will be one professional assigned to each baby (one or two obstetricians, two midwives and two paediatricians, plus an anaesthetist). Continuous foetal monitoring is likely and as well as the bands being around your abdomen (see pages 276–7), the first baby may have a clip attached to her head (see page 277) so that both babies can be monitored without confusion. When the first baby is delivered her cord will be clamped in two places. This is to prevent the transfer of blood from the second twin, who may take a while longer to be born.

Delivering the second twin

If the first twin is born without difficulty, ultrasound may be used to find out how the second baby is positioned. If all is well, then she should be delivered

Twins need particular care and attention to make sure all is well.

within about 30 minutes, but if things take longer, an emergency Caesarean may have to be performed. This is why you may be advised to have an epidural in place, so that it can be utilised quickly if you should need assisted delivery of either baby (see pages 284–5) or a Caesarean. This is also why so many twin births take the form of Caesarean deliveries – few obstetricians want to deal with this level of unpredictability and mothers do not want to go through labour and vaginal delivery of one twin if they then have to have a Caesarean for the second.

It is common for contractions to decrease after the vaginal delivery of the first twin, so many obstetricians then use a syntocinon drip (see page 228) to stimulate further, stronger contractions. If

the second baby does not progress through the birth canal fairly swiftly, then forceps may be used to aid her passage (see pages 284–5). If this is unsuccessful, then a Caesarean is the only option.

Managing the third stage

If all is well and the second baby is delivered vaginally, the third stage of labour will be actively managed because the risk of haemorrhage is higher in twin births. As soon as the babies have been delivered the syntocinon infusion will be increased and you will also be given an injection of syntometrine to encourage your uterus to contract. Your placentas should be delivered within five to 15 minutes – a swift result is preferable as it minimises the risk of heavy bleeding.

Delivering multiples by Caesarean

There are a number of reasons why you may be advised to have an elective Caesarean delivery of your babies (see box below). If you have them by Caesarean, you can expect an even larger team than usual to be caring for you in the theatre. The procedure for Caesarean birth of twins is virtually the same as for single babies (see pages 284–9), but you can expect to stay in hospital a little longer while your babies' progress is monitored.

WHY HAVE AN ELECTIVE CAESAREAN?

You are expecting three babies or more

In the case of twins, the first twin is not presenting head-first

You are expecting identical twins (who share a placenta) and who have, or are at risk of developing, twin-to-twin transfusion syndrome (TTTS – see page 197)

Placenta praevia (see page 209) has been diagnosed

Intrauterine growth restriction (IUGR – see pages 192–3) has been diagnosed

Your second twin is estimated to weigh 500 g (1 lb) less than the first

Your babies are 36 weeks, or less, but labour has begun and they are too delicate for a vaginal delivery, so an emergency Caesarean is the safest option

You have been diagnosed with pre-eclampsia (see pages 208–9)

One or both of the twins has an abnormality

The babies are conjoined ('Siamese') twins

It is considered that you are at greater risk of complications developing after 37 weeks, so an earlier delivery is preferable

You have requested a Caesarean section

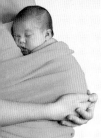

YOUR BABY'S ARRIVAL

Congratulations! You did it and no matter how you achieved it – whether it was with or without the aid of pain relief or assistance, whether it was a vaginal delivery or by Caesarean, you carried your baby, nurtured and nourished her for up to nine months and you have now delivered her into the world.

What your baby needs from you now is love and in those precious first minutes after birth that can be best expressed by putting your baby's bare skin next to yours.

The importance of skin-to-skin

Skin-to-skin contact is now expected of all new mothers, whether they intend to breastfeed or not. Babies get cold quickly after delivery and the most effective way of regulating their temperature is via skin-to-skin contact. If you are unable to hold your baby immediately (perhaps you feel sick or shaky, or you have had a Caesarean and feel you cannot hold her yet) your partner can do so. Men can wear front-buttoning shirts, so that a few buttons can be undone to slip their baby inside. She will be comforted and calmed by the warmth of his body and the thump of his heart and he will begin the process of forming an unbreakable bond with her.

The first minutes

In the first minute after your baby's birth, the midwife or doctor will examine her to check that all is well and she will be given an Apgar score (see pages 294–5). This assessment will be repeated at five minutes after birth, but if all is well after the first score your baby will be given to you to hold. She will have to cope with a flood of new sensations. She is breathing air for the first time and noise is no longer muffled by your abdomen. The light in the delivery room may seem very bright, but if you are able to dim it, she may relax. Your baby's vision will be blurred, but if you hold her close (within 25–30 cm/10–12 in), she can focus on your face. Hold her and talk softly to her – she will be comforted by the sound of your voice, which she will easily recognise (see pages 188–9). She may have cried loudly when she was delivered and might take time to calm down, or she could have been quiet. By holding her close and gently reassuring her, you send a strong message of love and protection. As she begins to absorb this, you may notice her fists unclenching so that her palms and fingers rest on your skin.

Rooting reflex

Newborn babies have an extraordinarily strong, natural rooting reflex and if your baby is placed on your abdomen she will instinctively wriggle towards your breast. Whether you intend to breastfeed or not, your baby is comforted and kept warm if resting against her mother's chest. She may need a little more time to master the skill of breathing before she starts to suck, but even if she just nuzzles at your nipple it will be doing you both good. Your baby will benefit

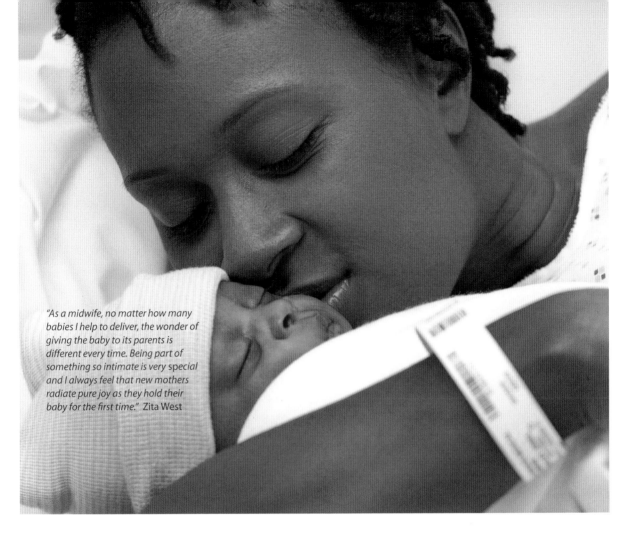

"As a midwife, no matter how many babies I help to deliver, the wonder of giving the baby to its parents is different every time. Being part of something so intimate is very special and I always feel that new mothers radiate pure joy as they hold their baby for the first time." Zita West

by practising her feeding and as she touches your nipple, your body will release oxytocin that will help your uterus to contract and return to its normal size (see pages 318–19). Once your baby begins to suck she will get the benefit of your colostrum, which is rich in nutrients and antibodies and will help to protect her from infection (see pages 328–9). Suckling will also help to stimulate your body to release prolactin, which will help your breast milk to come in (see pages 328–9).

A wakeful time

Your newborn may stay awake for a while after birth as she takes in her new surroundings and becomes familiar with the sight of her parents. If she does not feed straight away, do not be alarmed. She may be tired after labour and birth and if she was born at full term she will have some energy stores. Premature babies will need to be given bottle or drip feeds of expressed milk or formula because they will have fewer reserves. If they are born before 35 weeks their sucking reflex will not yet be properly developed.

Your baby is here

While you and your partner gaze at your newborn, there will be plenty of activity in the room. The placenta has to be delivered during the third stage of labour (see pages 296–7) and if you had an episiotomy or tearing (see pages 282–9) you will need to be stitched. Your midwife may help you get cleaned up and soon you will need food (see page 314). You may be unaware of all these things, however. The waiting is over and your beautiful baby is here.

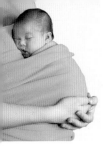

IMMEDIATE CHECKS

Immediately after your baby's birth, she will receive a good deal
of medical attention to make sure that all is well. These checks are
carried out on all newborns, so try not to worry – if all is well your
baby will soon be in your arms.

As soon as your baby has been born (or even as she emerges), your midwife or doctor will clear away any mucus or blood from her nose and mouth.

Apgar checks

Just one minute after your baby's birth, the midwife or doctor will assess your baby's overall health and condition using the Apgar scoring system. This is named after Dr Virginia Apgar, the American physician who devised it, but the letters also form an acronym for the functions being assessed (see chart opposite):

Appearance (skin colour)
Pulse (heart rate)
Grimace (or reflexes after certain stimuli)
Activity (muscle tone and movement)
Respiration (breathing)

The maximum score is 10, with a possible two points for each of the signs that are assessed. A score of seven or higher in the first check means that the baby seems to be in good condition; a score between four and six usually indicates that the baby may need some help (most probably with breathing, so airways may need to be properly cleared); and a baby with a score of less than four will require resuscitation and life-saving procedures. Apgar scores are very useful

for assessing babies immediately after birth, but a low score at this time does not necessarily predict long-term health problems. Most babies improve their scores at the second check, which takes place five minutes after birth. If they do not, they may be checked again at 10 minutes after delivery, but are likely to need some extra attention in the Special Care Baby Unit (SCBU – see pages 298–301).

Further checks

As the Apgar scores are being assessed, your midwife will be cleaning away blood, mucus, fluid or meconium (see page 178) from your baby's skin. Babies lose heat very rapidly after birth, partly because they have a relatively large area of skin in proportion to their body weight and also because their bodies are unable to regulate their temperature efficiently at first. Being wet can exacerbate the effects, leaving the warm environment of the uterus and being exposed to the relatively cold air of the delivery room. This is why it is so important to dry the baby and for her to have skin-to-skin contact with her mother or father (see pages 292–3). She will also be encouraged to feed if she shows signs of being interested. Your baby will also be weighed and her head circumference will be measured after a while. Your midwife or doctor will also examine your baby's face and tummy, and run her fingers over her spine. Your baby's anus will also be briefly checked to

APGAR SCORE CHART

Apgar sign	2	1	0
Appearance (skin colour)	Normal pink colour all over (hands and feet are pink in dark-skinned babies)	Body pink, but hands and feet are bluish	Pale or bluish grey all over
Pulse (heart rate)	Normal (100 beats per minute or over)	Below 100 beats per minute (BPM)	No pulse detectable
Grimace (or reflexes after certain stimuli)	Lusty, strong cry, pulls away, coughs or sneezes in response to stimulation	Only makes facial (not bodily) movements with stimulation	No response to stimulation
Activity (muscle tone and movement)	Spontaneous, active movement	Some movement of extremities (arms and legs may be flexed)	No movement detectable, or weak, floppy movement
Respiration (breathing)	Normal, regular rate and effort with a good cry	Irregular or slow breathing with a weak cry	No breathing

Note: Black or Asian babies may have their skin colour (and therefore the efficiency of their circulatory systems) checked by having the insides of their mouths examined and the palms and soles of their feet checked.

make sure that it is open and all her fingers and toes will be counted.

With your permission, your baby may also be given an injection or oral dose of vitamin K to help her blood to clot (see page 186). Then she will be given an ankle or wristband with her surname, date of birth and hospital number. This should be in place before she leaves the delivery room, to ensure that there can be no confusion later on. Your baby's hospital cot will also be labeled.

Within 48 hours of your baby's delivery she will be given a thorough assessment by a paediatrican (see pages 306–7). This will involve examining her head, eyes and ears, mouth, heart, lungs, genitals, hand and feet, spine, hips, reflexes and skin. If your baby's appearance is not quite as you expected, try not to worry (see pages 302–5). Most common problems, such as swollen facial or body features, will change over the next 24 hours and a misshapen head (perhaps after an assisted delivery – see pages 284–5) will gradually become a 'normal' shape.

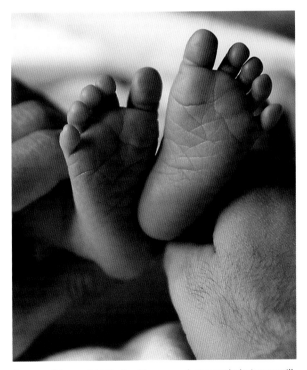

As part of the post-birth checking procedure, your baby's toes will be counted.

THE THIRD STAGE

The third stage of labour is when your placenta is delivered. By the time this has happened you may be so occupied with your new arrival that you will not be aware that it's even happening.

Clamping & cutting the cord

After your baby has been delivered, she will probably be placed on your abdomen – if all is well. Her umbilical cord will still be attached at this point, and unless she has been in distress during her birth, it can be left to pulsate for a few minutes more. This will allow more nutrient-rich blood from the placenta to be available to her, but if you have opted for stem cell collection (see page 200), the cord will need to be clamped quickly.

If your baby has suffered from any distress during delivery it may be necessary for the cord to be clamped and cut promptly, too, so that the medical team can attend to her. Be assured that although it can be a good thing to delay cutting the cord for a little while, if it has to be done immediately it will not harm your baby. However if she has had a difficult time during delivery it is much more important that the medical team should be able to give her the expert care that she needs straight away.

Procedure

A plastic cord clamp is placed about 1 cm (⅓ in) away from the baby and a metal clamp from the delivery pack is clamped 3 cm (1 in) from that one. Most partners want to cut the cord, but if they do not the midwife will do it. It is cut between the two clamps, the plastic one remaining on the baby. As the cord shrivels, it comes away from the abdomen and should fall off between seven and 10 days later.

Delivering the placenta

Once the cord has been cut, it is time for the third stage of labour – the delivery of the placenta. After your baby has been born your uterus will continue to contract and shrink, so that the placenta begins to come away from the uterine wall. This takes place through the blood vessels rupturing, or tearing, creating a clot, which further aids the placenta in peeling away from the wall. Once separation is complete, the uterine walls contract further to encourage the torn blood vessels to clot.

The decision whether to have an active third stage or a physiological one is an individual choice based on the type of labour you have had and past birth history. Both have advantages and disadvantages. In a physiological one the blood loss may be heavier, but the midwife will assess this. Most hospitals and midwives advise active management if you have had any intervention, a long labour, an epidural or concerns that make the third stage high risk.

Active management

The active management process is more controlled, so most hospitals advise it. You will normally have had an opportunity to discuss this in advance with your midwife. If you have opted for this approach you will be given an injection of syntocinon or syntometrine in your thigh as your baby is delivered. Syntocinon is a synthetic version of oxytocin – the hormone that encourages contractions and syntometrine is syntocinon combined with ergometrine, which makes the contractions more effective. As your uterus contracts, your midwife will then perform controlled cord traction (CCT), which means that she will place one hand above your pubic bone on your abdomen, while she gently pulls the umbilical cord with the other. This is designed to make sure that the placenta and membranes are delivered soon.

Physiological third stage

If you opt for a physiological third stage then once the cord has stopped pulsating and has been clamped and cut, it lengthens and as the placenta moves into the lower segment of the uterus you may feel some pressure. Being upright will help to expel the placenta easily – normally with one push. Just holding your baby, at this time, will encourage your body to produce more oxytocin to help deliver the placenta. Nature intended the cord to be just the right length to bring the baby up to the breast, so this is what you might try now. As long as there is

no excessive bleeding, you may wait up to an hour for the placenta to deliver physiologically, but usually this happens within minutes. If you have a normal birth then the third stage should follow normally, too. It is usual to have a physiological third stage with a water birth. By the time the woman gets out of the pool the placenta is often already on its way. Some hospitals deliver the placenta in the pool.

EXAMINING MEMBRANES/PLACENTA

Once the membranes and placenta have been delivered, they must be checked to make sure that they are complete and undamaged. If any of the placenta remains inside the mother it can cause further bleeding or infection after the birth. The dinner plate-sized disc will be weighed and measured and results recorded. A healthy placenta normally weighs around one-sixth of the baby's weight and measures 20–25 cm (8–10 in) in diameter and unless you have requested to take it away with you, the hospital will dispose of it. If there is anything unusual about it (see below), it will be sent to the path lab for analysis.

WHEN THINGS GO AWRY

Most third-stage deliveries proceed quite smoothly, but occasionally things can go wrong. Problems may include:

Retained placenta This only affects around 1 per cent of deliveries and is when the placenta remains in the uterus for more than an hour after the baby has been born. It is more common in premature births (because the cord may be thinner and therefore break off). If the placenta remains *in utero* there is a strong risk of postpartum haemorrhage (see right), so it will need to be removed quickly. This is usually done by an obstetrician in the operating theatre under epidural pain relief or general anaesthetic (see pages 246–51).

Primary postpartum haemorrhage (PPH) Around 6 per cent of UK deliveries may be affected by this complication – when the woman loses 500 ml (1 pt) of blood, or more, in the first 24 hours after giving birth. It is more common with difficult deliveries, where forceps or ventouse have had to be used,

or when an emergency Caesarean has had to be performed, although preventative action, such as active management of the third stage, has greatly improved the chances of avoiding such a problem. If you need treatment it will be readily available. Making sure your iron levels are good prior to going into labour will help with recovery if this occurs.

Secondary postpartum haemorrhage This can include any sudden loss of blood that takes place from 24 hours and up to six weeks after the delivery and is usually caused by pieces of the placenta or membranes being left behind in the uterus. These can become infected and, in turn, result in more bleeding. It is usually quickly detected when the delivered placenta is examined, but if it is not, then the mother will usually feel unwell and have an unpleasant discharge. She should be treated with antibiotics and surgical removal of the retained matter.

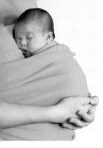

SPECIAL CARE

If there are any concerns about your baby's health she may be taken to the Special Care Baby Unit (SCBU) or neonatal intensive care unit. Around 10 per cent of all babies born in the UK need some assistance once they are born and although this can be upsetting, try to remember that your baby will be getting the best care possible.

There are a number of reasons why your baby may need special care – the most common one being premature birth (see page 194). Premature babies are classified as those born before 37 weeks. After this number of weeks, depending on the degree of prematurity, how early your baby has been born, the more complications to her future

health there will be and the higher level of intensive the care she will need. Many babies need help to breathe and are ventilated to facilitate this. Often the lungs are immature and the baby cannot breathe on her own. If you go into premature labour you will be given steriod injections to help her lungs mature. Babies born at 34 weeks, or earlier, may also need

AFTER THE BIRTH

Once your baby has been born, she will be assessed (see pages 294–5) and given help with breathing, if necessary. You may have the opportunity to hold her briefly, but she is most likely to be taken to the SCBU as soon as possible. If your hospital does not have a unit, she will be transferred to one that does by ambulance.

This experience can undoubtedly be distressing for you as it can feel as if your baby has been 'taken away' from you, but try to remember that although your baby needs specialist help at this crucial and delicate time, she also needs you and there will be plenty of things that you can do to help her become stronger (see page 301). In the SCBU she will be receiving the best possible medical care and this, combined with your love and attention, is most likely to help her to develop into a strong, healthy child.

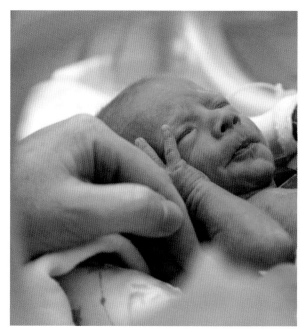

Your baby is in the special care unit, but she needs your loving attention just as much – if not more – than a 'normal' baby.

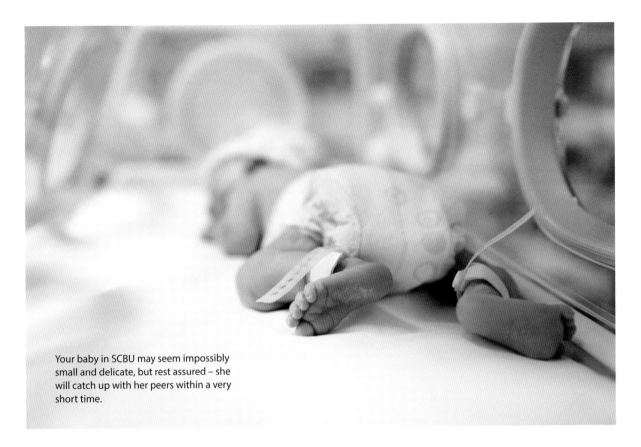

Your baby in SCBU may seem impossibly small and delicate, but rest assured – she will catch up with her peers within a very short time.

help with regulating body temperature and feeding because their sucking reflexes have not yet developed and their tiny stomachs cannot cope with large quantities of liquid, so feeding has to be controlled. Twins or multiple babies are also often admitted to the SCBU, not only because they are often delivered early but also because they tend to be smaller and weigh less than single babies (see pages 194–5).

Other reasons

Your baby may also be admitted to the SCBU if you have had a difficult delivery or if you or your baby has an existing health condition that makes it difficult for her to thrive without help. Babies with severe jaundice – a build-up of bilirubin in the blood, which can result if the newborn baby's immature liver is unable to break down the excess number of red blood cells that most newborns are born with – may be treated with phototherapy lamps. A low

Apgar score, infection and you being diabetic are also reasons for admission.

What happens in the SCBU

The number of visitors admitted to the unit will be limited, depending on how ill the baby is, to prevent exposure to infection, but you and your partner should be able to visit at any time. There is a high ratio of staff to babies and they will be highly trained (see page 300). You may be able to spend time with your baby before she is taken to the SCBU, but if she needs to be on a ventilator, she may be taken there straight away. Your partner may be able to go with her while you complete the third stage of delivery, and in many hospitals you are given a photograph to look in the meantime.

While your baby is in the unit she will be constantly monitored and staff may have to carry out a number of basic tests. She will most probably be

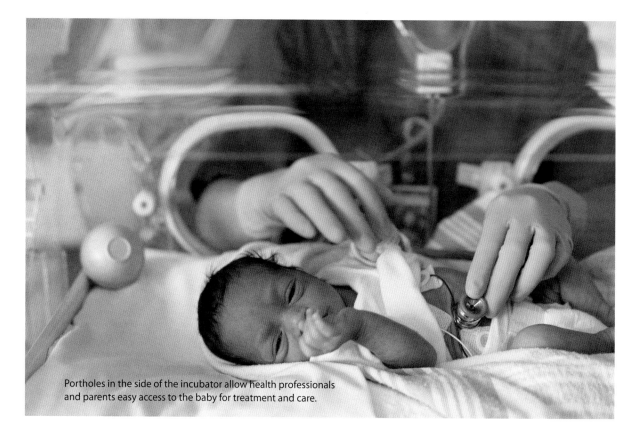

Portholes in the side of the incubator allow health professionals and parents easy access to the baby for treatment and care.

WHO'S WHO IN THE SCBU?

There are different levels of special care, from Level 1 to Level 3. Not all hospitals have Level 1, so your baby may need to be transferred to a different one. Ask staff to explain what they are doing and why and what the equipment is for (you will soon get used to it and the daily routine and will be encouraged to help and be involved). Most care will be carried out by neonatal nurses. Ward rounds with doctors may occur each morning, with extra rounds during the day. Some hospitals allow parents to stay for these visits.

The doctors have three tiers of seniority:
Consultants who are paediatricians have overall responsibility for the care of your baby and the decisions that need to be made. The doctors in his/her team will be senior registrars and senior house officers. The nursing team is headed by neonatal nurse specialists, who are highly skilled

Registrars supervise SHOs and will have a minimum of five years' medical school training followed by at least five years in practice as qualified doctors. Registrars also stay in the hospital, so that they can provide emergency care for babies if it is needed

Senior House Officers (SHOs) will have at least two years' experience of working as a doctor following a minimum of five years' training at medical school

The unit is likely to have a number of other members of staff, which may include pharmacists, dieticians, physiotherapists and healthcare assistants as well as psychotherapists, who can offer help to parents.

placed in an incubator, but most of these have openings in the sides so that you can touch her. She may also be given IV fluids, blood and possibly antibiotics and she is likely to be attached to various monitors. She may also have fine tubes in her nose to help her to breathe and receive enough oxygen. All this may be upsetting for you, but the staff will do their best to answer your questions and involve you in your baby's care. It may seem at first as though you cannot do much to help your baby, but your contribution (and even just your presence) is invaluable to your baby's progress (see right).

Coping & going home

Some babies only need to stay in the SCBU for a few days, but others remain there for weeks or even months. Going home without your baby can be a difficult thing to do, and although it is natural to want to be at the SCBU with her, try to spend time at home rebuilding your strength by resting and eating well (see pages 318–21).

Keep expressing your milk. You need to keep stimulating your breasts to produce more. Breastfeeding works on a supply-and-demand system, so if you don't, your supply will dwindle and be inadequate when your baby is well enough to take more (see page 328). Special-care babies are usually able to go home once they can feed properly. Your baby will need to weigh at least 2 kg (4 lb 7 oz) and is likely to be kept in the SCBU until she has reached at least two or three weeks beyond her original EDD (if she was premature).

Some hospitals have facilities for mothers to stay with their babies, so that they gain confidence caring for her. It is helpful to remember that although premature babies can have a difficult start, with attention from the SCBU and plenty of loving care from their parents, most babies catch up quickly, though their future health does depend on how premature they were. By the age of two there is usually no difference between them and children who were born full term.

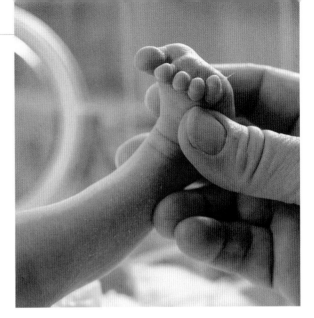

WHAT YOU CAN DO

If your baby is tiny or delicate you may only be able to practise 'still-holding', which means you can place your hand very lightly on your baby's body for a few seconds. Her skin may be too thin and fragile to cope with more just yet, but you can also talk to her and the familiar sound of your voice will soothe her.

You should also be able to express milk for her and although she will only be able to manage limited quantities, it can be frozen and stored. As she becomes stronger, you should be able to feed her, change her and clean her and perhaps stroke and hold her. Many hospitals encourage parents to practise 'kangaroo care', which means that you tuck your baby inside your shirt and place her skin-to-skin. She will be able to smell you and be reassured by your heartbeat and voice. This technique promotes bonding and research has shown that it has a remarkable effect on the progress of special-care babies.

Don't underestimate how exhausting this time will be for you as parents – if your baby is very sick, the first few weeks are a roller-coaster ride of ups and downs. The bonds you form with the medical staff and other parents are vital and will help you through this difficult time. Look after your relationship with your partner and make sure that you both rest and build up your reserves of strength.

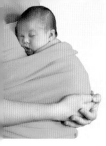

BABY'S APPEARANCE

During the months of pregnancy, you will naturally have wondered what your baby will look like and may have formed a vivid mental image of your new son or daughter. Newborns naturally reflect their birth journey, but, rest assured, it will only take a few days for adverse signs to disappear for good.

Your baby's head shape

If your baby was delivered vaginally she is likely to have a slightly pointed head shape. This is due to it being squeezed as she travelled down through the birth canal. Her skull bones are soft and overlap to allow her to pass through the bony passageway as smoothly as possible. She may also have a soft tissue swelling known as a 'caput', which can be caused by her head pressing against your cervix as it dilates or

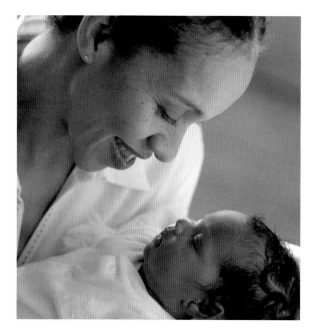

by the vacuum action of a ventouse delivery (see page 285), but this, too, will subside in a few days or so. A haematoma swelling may also result from vacuum extraction, but this will soon disappear. If she had a foetal monitoring clip attached to her head (see page 277), she may have a small cut and bruising and if she was delivered with the aid of forceps, she may have bruising and some indentations in the sides of her head. However, these will disappear in a short time and her head will return to its normal shape. If your baby was born by Caesarean section she is more likely to have a rounder head and less puffy face (see right), but even some babies born in this way may have some degree of head moulding if they have been in the 'engaged' position within the pelvis (see page 214).

On the top of her head you may notice a pulsating spot, which is known as the anterior fontanelle (one of two on her head). This is where your baby's skull bones have not yet fused and it is thought that they are there to allow the baby's head to grow rapidly during the first year of life. The fontanelles tend to look very vulnerable, but are, in fact, composed of quite tough, fibrous tissue, so gentle touching there should do no harm.

Now you can examine your baby's face as closely as you like – after all these months of waiting.

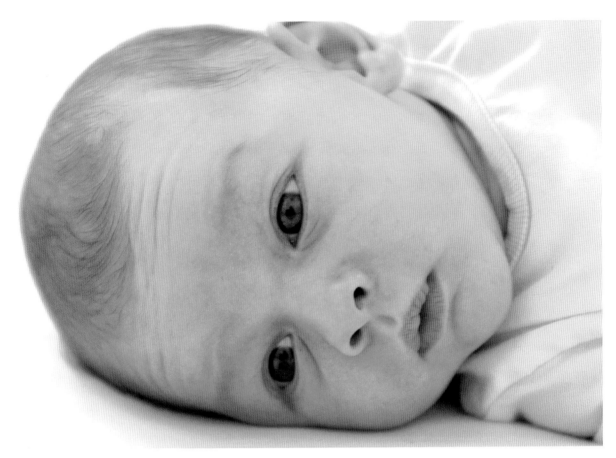

Whatever colour your baby's eyes may turn out to be later, they may start off being dark blue.

Your baby's face

Every mum finds their baby beautiful, but unlike the 'perfect' examples you see on television advertisements and in magazines, newborn faces straight after delivery can display traces of blood, the baby may be pale, red or grey, a little puffy or show forceps marks, depending on the style of delivery. Newborns frequently have puffy faces as a result of the position they may have been in while still inside the uterus and the pressure they have undergone during the second stage of labour.

You may notice that your baby's nose seems flattened or even squashed to one side. Again, this is quite common and temporary – as a result of the impact of birth. Her eyes may be very puffy and she may only open one eye, or neither, for a while. Do not try to force her; it may be that the swelling is preventing her eyes from opening wide, but you could try raising her above your head – you may be able to see her eyes open a little as she looks down.

Eye colour & condition

Your baby's eye colour at this early stage is most likely dark blue (even if her eyes are eventually brown). This is because the body's natural pigment (melanin) is not present in the baby's irises at birth, but as the amounts increase, so her eye colour will alter. By the time she is a year old it is likely that it is established. If she has been born with yellow discharge around her eyes she may have 'sticky eye', which is a common newborn condition and is not serious, but does require treatment from a doctor.

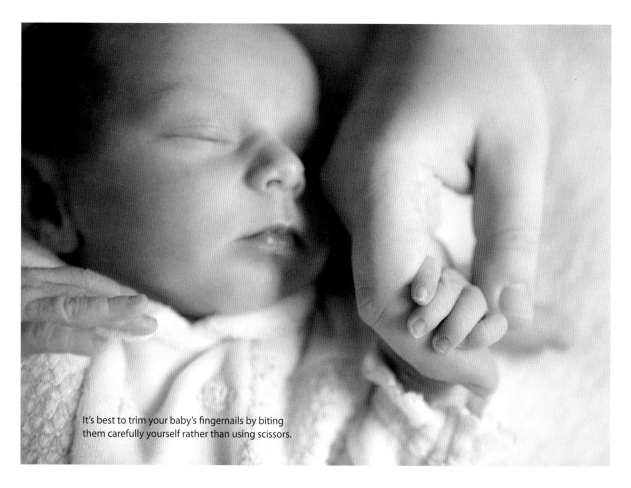

It's best to trim your baby's fingernails by biting them carefully yourself rather than using scissors.

DIFFERENT TYPES OF BIRTHMARK

Most birthmarks are simply collections of blood vessels under the skin and will not require any further treatment. If your baby has them, try not to worry and remember that most fade or disappear within a year or so. A few may not disappear, but there are treatments to help to deal with them when your child is older. Different types may include:

'Stork bites' or 'salmon patches' are pink skin patches that may appear on the baby's forehead, nose and eyelids or on the back of the neck. Most fade quite quickly and disappear within a year. They are affectionately known as 'angel kisses'

'Strawberry' marks usually begin as small red dots and are collections of blood capillaries. Although they may increase in size during the baby's first year, they usually disappear by the time the child is five years of age

'Mongolian spots' are common to darker-skinned babies and appear as dark, bluish patches on the skin around the baby's bottom, tops of thighs or on the back and shoulders. They are due to there being clusters of pigmentation, but they usually fade within a year

'Café au lait' patches are usually permanent, light brown or coffee-coloured flat patches on the skin

'Port wine' stains are the rarest form of birthmark and are dark red or purplish marks on the skin (usually on the face, neck or head). They will not fade with time, but can often be successfully treated in later life with laser therapy or plastic surgery by an experienced dermatologist

Your baby's skin

Most babies are born with a covering of vernix on their skin. This is the thick, white, waxy substance that protects the skin from the watery environment of the uterus. Premature babies have a thicker coating of it, while overdue babies have little. This vernix, nature's natural moisturiser, is best left to be absorbed into the skin naturally. It does so very quickly and keeps your baby's skin super-soft. Babies may also be delivered with blood and mucus on their skin or meconium (their first bowel movement – sometimes passed during delivery). If this is the case, your baby may have the greenish-black meconium under her finger- and toenails and so she is likely to be bathed after delivery.

Tiny spots on the face, known as 'milia', or 'milk spots', may be visible, but they are nothing to worry about as they are simply blocked sebaceous glands. Your baby may have quite a pink body, but bluish hands and feet. This is due to immature circulation, which should improve over the next few days. Your baby may also have one or more birthmarks (see left), but your paediatrician may be able to identify what kind they are when your baby has her first thorough check (see pages 306–7)

Your baby's hair & fingernails

Some newborns (especially those who are born prematurely) may also have a covering of fine, downy hair, especially on their arms, back and shoulders. This is not a permanent feature and it will wear off during the first few months. If your baby has any hair on her head, it is likely to be extremely fine and soft, but it may be quite a different colour and texture to the hair that will replace it during the next few months. If your baby is born already possessing long fingernails she could scratch herself, but it is wise not to try to cut them with scissors because you might accidentally damage the nail bed. The best solution is to nibble them very gently yourself, or you could try putting soft, cotton 'scratch mittens' on your baby's hands.

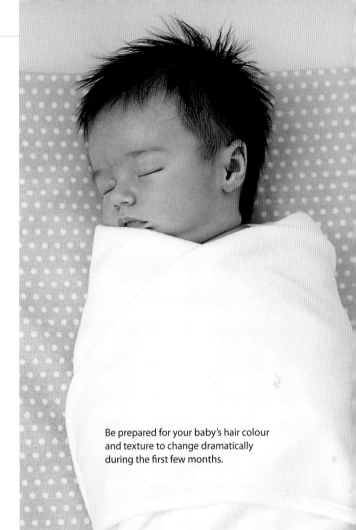

Be prepared for your baby's hair colour and texture to change dramatically during the first few months.

Swollen breasts & genitals

You may be surprised to see that both boys and girls may have swollen breasts and genitals at birth. This is due to your pregnancy hormones, which remain in your baby's body for a short while after birth.

Your baby girl might discharge a tiny amount of blood because her uterus is temporarily thickened and then broken down with the waxing and waning of your hormones.

Boys may have swollen testicles immediately after the birth, but these will settle after a few days. Sometimes the testicles will not yet have descended from the abdomen, but this, too, will usually correct itself in time.

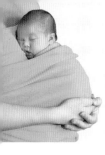

FIRST MEDICAL CHECKS

Within 48 hours or so of your baby's birth she will have her first full medical check, where a series of tests will be carried out to ensure that all is well.

These first checks will cause your baby no pain, but she may protest a little. You will be present throughout, and (if you are not too tired to concentrate) it may offer a good opportunity for you to ask the paediatrican about anything that may concern you.

If you stay in hospital for more than 24 hours you will probably have these checks carried out before you and your baby are discharged home. If yours was a home birth your doctor will probably visit you there. The six main checks are as follows:

Head
Beginning at the top of your baby's head, the doctor will check the fontanelles (see page 302) and look at the shape of her head, to ensure that it is consistent with the nature of her birth.

Mouth
Your baby's mouth will be examined to be sure that her palate (the roof of her mouth) is complete and intact. Her tongue will also be checked to make sure that it moves freely and is not 'tied'.

Heart, lungs & major organs
The doctor will use a stethoscope to listen to your baby's heart and lungs. This is to detect any signs of a heart murmur (although these are reasonably common in newborns and usually right themselves in time – so if a mild murmur is detected at this

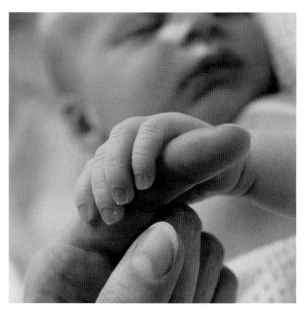

Grasping is one of the main reflexes to be checked for during the all-important post-birth checks.

point, there is probably no cause for concern). The pulse in your baby's groin (known as the femoral pulse) will also be checked. Your baby's lungs should be free of any fluid and the doctor will listen to make sure that they sound completely normal.

With one hand on your baby's back and the other on her abdomen, the doctor will feel to make sure that her kidneys, liver and spleen are all where they should be. Your baby's genitals will also be examined and if your baby is a boy his testes will be checked to see whether they have descended.

YOUR BABY'S REFLEXES

Your baby will be born ready-equipped with a number of reflexes that will help her to survive outside your uterus. These, too, will be checked by the paediatrician (or doctor or midwife if you have a home birth). Sometimes these reflexes may seem less strong than expected, but this may be due to medication if yours was a long labour.

The grasping reflex

This is tested by gently touching your baby's palm with a finger (or some other object). Her fingers will instinctively curl around the adult finger (as you may have already noticed when you first held her after birth). This reflex will stay in place until she has reached about six months of age.

The rooting reflex

From almost the moment of birth until about four months of age, the rooting reflex will cause your baby to turn her face whenever her cheek is touched. She will then open her mouth and expect to feed, so when breastfeeding you simply press her cheek to your breast to encourage her to open her mouth to latch on (see page 333).

The Moro reflex

If your baby's head is allowed to drop backwards unsupported (though this should never happen), she will be likely to fling out her arms and legs – as if her whole body is falling. This reflex disappears by the time she is around two months of age, but it should never be put to the test as it could cause damage to her neck. So if you ever see your baby responding in this way, you need to make sure that she is held more securely in future (see page 327). (Warning: never let anyone who has been drinking hold your baby.)

The plantar grasp

If you stroke your baby's foot along the sole, her toes will splay out and her foot will turn inwards. This is a reflex action that lasts a little longer than some of the other newborn responses and can be seen in children of up to two years of age.

The sucking reflex

This reflex is designed to help the baby feed from birth and if you gently put a small (clean) finger into your baby's mouth and touch the roof you will find that she can suck surprisingly strongly. By about two months she will have got the hang of feeding and the reflex will fade.

The stepping reflex

This is an interesting reflex to observe: if you hold your baby upright and let her feet touch a flat surface she will appear to take deliberate 'steps'. However, you should take care not to put any pressure on her feet, as her body is nowhere near ready for walking yet. The reflex does not last long and will have completely disappeared by the time she is four months old.

Arms, legs, hands & feet

Your baby's limbs will be extended to make sure that they are of an equal length, that the legs and feet are properly aligned, that there are the correct number of fingers and toes and that there is no sign of any webbing between them.

Occasionally, the doctor may also look at the baby's palms because if there are fewer than two creases on each hand there is a small possibility that the baby has Down's syndrome.

Hips

Your baby's legs will be opened wide and then bent and unbent to check the stability of the hip joints or any sign of dislocation.

Spine

The doctor will check the vertebrae to see if they are in place and aligned. The base of the spine is checked for a sacral dimple – a deep one could indicate a problem with the lower part of the spinal cord.

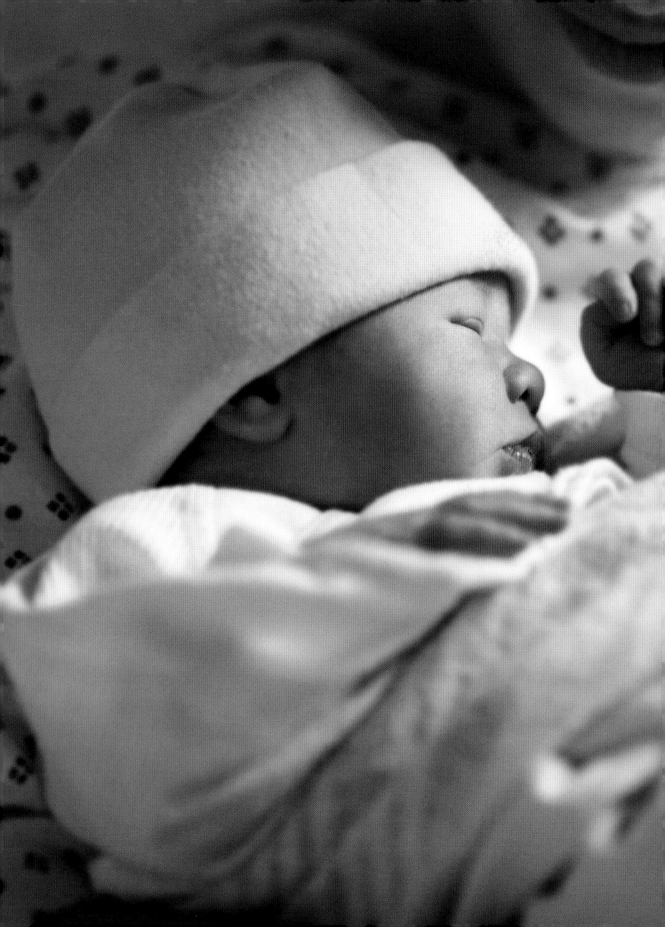

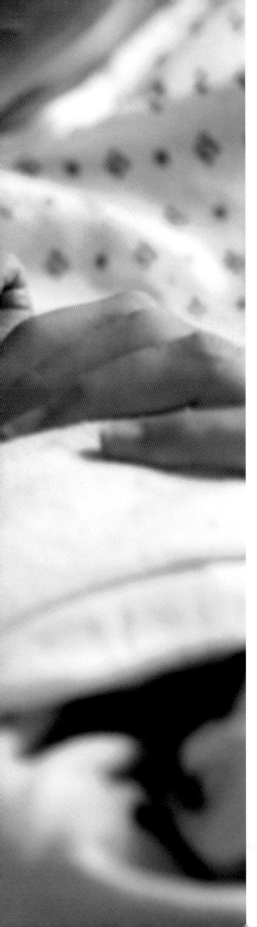

chapter 7

your baby's
EARLY DAYS

Whether this is your first baby, your second or your third, now you can start to care for her and get to know this long-awaited new addition to your family. Take the time to introduce her to other family members and enjoy this special time together.

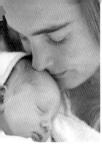

PARENTING HORMONES

Now that your baby is here, you are a family and your baby needs to feel the same love and protection that you gave her while she was inside you. Trust your instincts – you will find that you are 'ready-programmed' for parenting.

Despite being equipped with a set of instinctive reflexes (see page 307), such as the rooting reflex that helps babies to find their mother's nipple and take the first of many feeds, human babies are relatively helpless when they are born. But fortunately they are also innately lovable to their parents and everything about them, from their round faces and relatively large eyes to their first mewling cries and even their smell, is designed to trigger their parents' protective instincts.

Chemical reactions

When you look into your baby's eyes and hold her skin-to-skin an extraordinary chemical reaction takes place. Your body releases a huge surge of oxytocin that has already been present in your body in high levels during labour and birth. Not only does this hormone stimulate contractions and effectively 'orchestrate' your baby's birth, but it also acts as a chemical messenger that encourages bonding and physical contact. That physical contact stimulates both

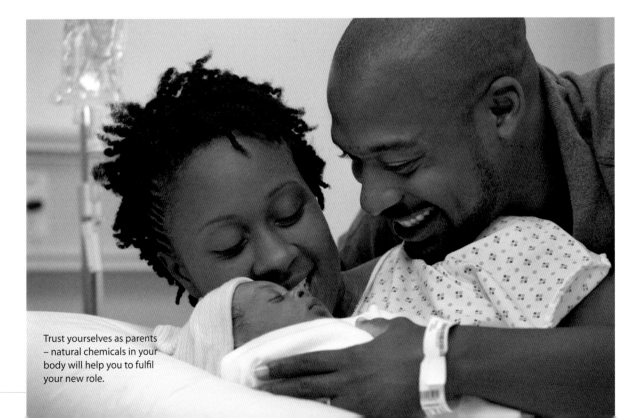

Trust yourselves as parents – natural chemicals in your body will help you to fulfil your new role.

your brain and your baby's to want even more affection and contact and so those first few moments together, when your newborn rests on your tummy or breast, really do work wonders for you both.

Important smells

High levels of oxytocin also enable you to become familiar with the unique smell of your baby. You will be quite unaware of it, but nature has programmed you to prefer that smell to all others. Likewise, your baby has had your smell 'imprinted' on her brain from her time in your uterus, when she swallowed some of the amniotic fluid. Although its smell was slightly different to that of your body (and particularly your breasts), she can divine the underlying signature scent of her mother.

Studies have shown, too, that once placed to the breast after birth, even babies who were subsequently fed with formula recognised and actively preferred the scent of their mother's breasts. This is partly why, if you can get the technique going well (see pages 332–4), breastfeeding will feel natural and right – it constantly reinforces that chemical bond between you and your baby. Even if you do not manage to actually feed your baby in the first hour after birth, any attempts you make thereafter will prompt a huge surge in the levels of oxytocin in you both.

Lowering stress levels

If, however, you are unable to breastfeed your baby in this short window of opportunity (perhaps you or your baby has been unwell and you required extra medical attention) do not worry. Although you may have missed this first natural 'high' you will continue to release oxytocin every time you hold and breastfeed your baby (it is also contained in your breastmilk) – and the more you do this the higher the levels of oxytocin you will release. Not only does this make you feel good, but, crucially, it calms your baby and lowers her stress levels, too (see pages 328–9 and 335). The very action of suckling at your breast helps your baby's brain to make connections

that ensure that she will want to continue to feed in future – thereby helping to ensure her survival. If these early experiences of breastfeeding and holding are accompanied by other pleasurable sensations, such as singing, rocking, stroking or the touch of a soft blanket, they can also become part of a baby's sense of secure attachment and provide comfort even in your absence.

Fatherly hormones

Your baby's father will not be excluded from this hormone exchange. Towards the end of your pregnancy his body will have oxytocin in higher quantities than it usually does and once you have given birth and he is able to hold his baby skin-to-skin he will release even more. Again, the more he holds and interacts with his baby, the more 'parenting' hormones are released in his body, including vasopressin, which both encourages bonding between him and you and prompts his brain to activate protective instincts towards you and his baby.

Trusting your instincts

Babies are exquisitely sensitive to their environment at birth and can detect smells or chemical signals that their parents emit, but are quite unaware of. Pheromones are manufactured in our skin and babies are programmed to respond to them so that they can tell when their parents are calm and relaxed or anxious and stressed. This may be why some very stressed mothers seem to have particularly fretful babies – one anxiety feeds into another.

Understanding what these chemical messages mean and why they are released helps to remind us that on a very basic level, parenting really is an instinctive activity. By responding to your baby's needs for love and protection you hold her close, which then triggers greater maternal and paternal feelings in you both, while your baby 'rewards' you with increased eye contact and, eventually, that first amazing smile.

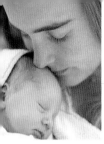

THE FIRST 24 HOURS

Once you have had some time to get to know your new baby and enjoy the first few hours as a family, you may want to freshen up, have something to eat and get some rest. If you are in hospital you may be going home very soon, but there are a few things to do first.

As your uterus contracts after giving birth, you will feel some after-pains and will pass more blood and tissue, known as 'lochia', from the lining of your uterus. This will be quite heavy at first and is likely to last for around 10 days or so, although it will gradually change from being very red to becoming pinker and lighter in colour and quantity. After your baby has been born and the third stage of delivery has been completed you will probably be given a large pad to soak up further blood. After some time holding your baby and getting to know her, you may stay in the delivery room or be moved to the postnatal ward. You will be monitored for a while longer and your temperature and blood pressure will be taken at regular intervals.

Visiting the bathroom

If all is well, you may then wish to go to the bathroom and perhaps even have a shower. If your partner is no longer at the hospital with you, you may need to put your baby in her bedside cot. This sudden loss of contact may disturb her, however, so it may be a good idea to wrap her in a soft cotton blanket so that she has the sensation of still being held (see right). You may feel a little anxious about leaving her while you visit the bathroom, but be assured that maternity units have strict security rules and systems in place. If you are still worried, you could ask one of the nurses or another new mum to watch over your baby – or perhaps you could even wheel her cot to the bathroom with you.

It is very common to feel a little wobbly after giving birth. If you are not catheterised (see page 246) and able to get up to go to the bathroom you may need someone to lend you a supporting arm. When you urinate, you may find that it stings because you have stretched your perineal region and may have some tearing or stitches from an

Don't forget to look after yourself, too. You can make use of the hospital baby cot when you need to put your baby down.

SWADDLING

Swaddling used to be routine practise in maternity hospitals, but there was debate over whether it might contribute to sudden infant death syndrome (SIDS –see page 340).

Old-fashioned swaddling involved wrapping the baby securely in a blanket so that her arms and general movements were restricted. This is not thought to be a good idea these days, but some gentle, loose wrapping will give your baby the comfort and reassurance of being able to feel contact and keep her warm, too. You can purchase ready-made 'swaddle pods', though a large baby blanket is just as good.

It is useful to try to think about what a baby experiences during pregnancy: she is enclosed in a warm, dark environment, but one that has 'walls' she can touch. Once she has been born her world seems to lack the security of known limits (unless she is held in your arms), so loose swaddling may help her feel safe and 'held' by the blanket.

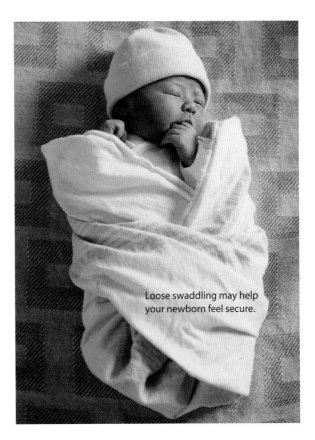

Loose swaddling may help your newborn feel secure.

episiotomy. To prevent this, it is a good idea to pour a cup of tepid water over your vulva as you urinate. This will dilute the acid in your urine and lessen the stinging sensation. You may also wish to have a shower (check with your midwife that this is all right first) and once you are feeling fresher, put on a maternity nursing bra for comfort. When you are back at your bed you may want something to eat and drink, if you have not already been able to do so. Take things gently and ensure that you and your baby get some rest. You have certainly earned it.

Going home

If you have had a Caesarean section or any complications during labour and birth you may have to stay in hospital for a few days, but it is likely that your midwives will try to get you up and out of bed within 24 hours of giving birth to keep your circulation working efficiently and prevent the risk of thrombosis. It is good to move around as much as you can, but you will be sore after a Caesarean and you will need to take care of yourself once you get home (see pages 322–3).

Ready to be discharged

When you are ready to go home (if the birth was complication-free, this may be as little as six hours after delivery), you will need to be formally discharged from hospital. If there are any concerns raised as a result, they will be passed on to your doctor. Your baby will be examined by the midwife at home within 48 hours of the birth or you may have an appointment to come back and see the doctor. Your community midwife will also be notified of your discharge from hospital and visit you at home on the first, fifth and tenth days. Arrangements will also be made for your baby to have a Guthrie heel-prick test around five days after her birth. This

POST-BIRTH NUTRITION

In Traditional Chinese Medicine (TCM – see pages 38–9) it was traditional after the birth for the mother to rest and just focus on the baby. The ancient Chinese believed that if you didn't pay attention to the new soul it would leave. Warming, healing and nourishing foods, such as soups and iron-rich foods, were believed to build up qi energy.

In many European countries it is traditional to offer the new mother some warming chicken soup, but this is unlikely to happen in the UK. This is why it is important to plan what food to take to hospital when you go into labour (see pages 240–1) and to have plenty of good-quality ingredients stored in the fridge and kitchen cupboards to tide you over the first few days at home.

Although your diet in the third trimester should have helped to build up your energy levels (see pages 184–7), you will probably feel very hungry once you and your baby find time to rest after all the excitement of her arrival.

You will need a nutrition-packed, balanced diet to help your body to heal and as your milk 'comes in' during the next few days (see pages 328–31). However right now you need something warming, comforting and not too demanding to eat and digest easily.

What you eat after you have given birth may depend on the time of day (or night). There may be something that you crave in these first few hours and perhaps your partner can bring it for you, but don't forget that you should still avoid certain foods that may cause illness because of your lowered immune system (see page 87).

If you have given birth at home, you may well be able to eat a good home-cooked meal if you have someone to make it for you, but in hospital it may be a little more difficult. However, you may be able to at least have a flask of warm soup and perhaps some more of the snacks that you or your partner prepared for labour (see page 241) – or some fresh supplies. You will certainly need to drink plenty of fluids and water and watered-down pure fruit juices are both hydrating and refreshing.

You will need to avoid becoming constipated in the next few days as your perineal region will be tender and you should avoid straining to pass stools, so a fresh smoothie made from a variety of fruits would be a good idea, along with any chunks of fresh fruit that you can manage.

---

involves taking a tiny sample of blood from her heel to check that she is not affected by phenylketonuria (a rare metabolic disorder), cystic fibrosis or a thyroid deficiency.

You will also need to have a postnatal check and you can expect to have your blood pressure and temperature tested again. The midwife will feel your abdomen to make sure that your uterus is contracting. She may examine your breasts, your perineum and your calves and ankles to make sure they are not swollen. You may have your haemoglobin level checked with a blood test and if you are anaemic you should be given iron tablets.

If you are not already immune to rubella (see page 71) you will also be given a vaccination. You may be surprised to be asked about contraception, too. This is because most women resume ovulation just six to eight weeks after giving birth, so another pregnancy so soon is usually best avoided.

Useful advice

Before you leave hospital you should also have had some advice and help with holding your baby (see page 327), feeding her (see pages 328–39), keeping her clean (see pages 344–5) and changing her nappies (see pages 346–7). You will also be given a

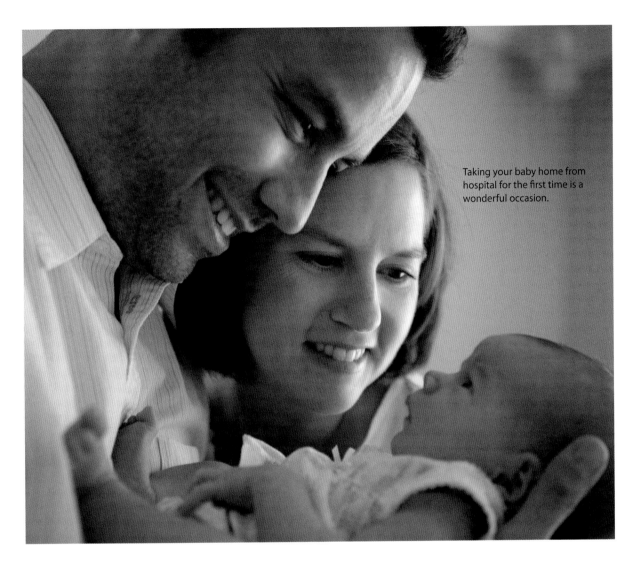

Taking your baby home from hospital for the first time is a wonderful occasion.

list of contacts should you feel worried about your baby's progress (although you will also receive visits from your community midwife at home, where it may be easier to discuss any concerns you have. Your midwife will be keeping a close eye on your physical and mental recovery too – see pages 360–1). You may also be reminded that you should register your baby's birth, and you'll be given the address of your local registrar's office. Registering your baby's birth is a legal requirement and you will need to have decided on her name by then. You have 42 days from the date of delivery to register, however, so you will still have a while to decide.

Travelling home

If you are taking your baby home by car (whether your own or a taxi) you will need to have your baby's rear-facing car seat with you. This is a legal requirement (see pages 168–9). The seat must not be placed on the car's front seat (especially if it is fitted with airbags). Cover your baby with a cotton blanket as you leave hospital (and put on a soft cotton hat), but remove layers once she is in the car to avoid overheating. You will not feel like driving, and if you have had a Caesarean you will not be able to drive for some time yet, either. However you should check with your insurers to find out the timescale.

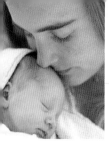

WHAT YOUR BABY FEELS

Some babies sleep easily after meeting their parents and greeting the outside world for the first time, while others find it harder to settle. Your new baby's first few hours will be full of 'firsts' and it will help all of you if you can try to understand how she may be feeling.

I f you had been happily living in warm, moist environment where you were never hungry or bothered by too much light or noise, how would you feel if you were forcefully expelled from it, squeezed through a twisting, tight tunnel and out into cold, dry air – then bombarded with light, noise and unfamiliar sensations? This is roughly what babies have to go through as they are born – so,

really, is it any wonder that so many of them seem a little distressed? Once your baby has been placed on your tummy or breast, gently held and softly spoken to in a voice that she can recognise, perhaps she will begin to relax.

The cranial osteopathy option

Many babies cope with prolonged, and even difficult, births well, while others seem hyper-alert and difficult to soothe. Some cry for long periods, yell when they are put on their backs to sleep or they may find it hard to latch on and feed. Such problems may sort themselves out in time, but many parents take their new babies to cranial osteopaths, who may be able to detect lasting pressure or tension in the baby's body and relieve it (see right).

Quiet time

Every baby's brain is working hard at birth, absorbing the nature of their new surroundings and processing the information that their eyes, ears and skin are telling them about their parents and other individuals. However, some babies seem more able to cope with these sensations than others and learning to recognise what your baby can tolerate is one of the first challenges of being a parent. Spending quiet

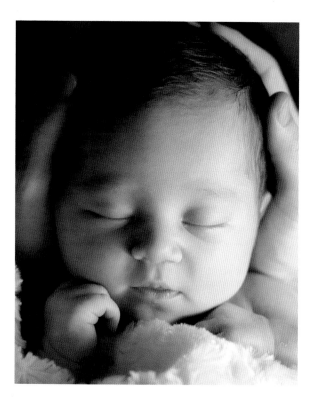

The nature of your baby's birth may have had a noticeable effect on the way she reacts to the outside world.

ABOUT CRANIAL OSTEOPATHY

Some mothers will already be familiar with cranial osteopathy because they may have visited one in the latter stages of pregnancy. It can offer help if pregnant women suffer from backache or painful hip joints as ligaments are softened in readiness for labour and birth (see page 174).

Cranial osteopaths treat all parts of the body, but are particularly skilled in subtle manipulation of the skull's bones, muscles and tissue. This is especially appropriate for newborn babies whose heads have undergone a great deal of squeezing and moulding during delivery.

Many cranial osteopaths believe that birth can be stressful for babies and that the forces that the baby feels on her head and body as she twists through the birth canal can affect all parts of her body. They argue that not only can the nerves in the lips, cheeks and tongue be affected by birth compressions, which can greatly influence a baby's ability to latch on and her level of comfort during feeding, but that these can also influence the future development of her teeth. It is also thought that compression and tension in the skull can affect the nerves and muscles that support the function of the eyes and compromise effective drainage of the Eustachian tube in the ears, which may make the baby more susceptible to infection.

Even babies who were not delivered vaginally, but by Caesarean section may have a slightly odd-shaped or sore head because of the way they were lying in the uterus. Sometimes new babies have difficulty latching on, seem unable to open their mouths wide or are reluctant to feed on one side. This is more common in babies who have been delivered with the assistance of forceps or ventouse, but the problem is always worth investigating because it may be that the nature of the delivery caused their jaw to be slightly misaligned. A cranial osteopath will very gently and delicately feel the baby's skull and face and if there is a misalignment they will slowly and almost imperceptibly massage it back into place.

It is essential to find a registered cranial osteopath who is experienced in treating babies – and particularly newborns (see Resources). A really good one will be sensitive to the baby and proceed slowly and gently. The treatment room should be warm and although you may find it a little too warm yourself, it is important that your baby should feel comfortable and hardly notice being undressed. If the lighting is dim, too, your baby will relax even more and may even fall asleep.

time with your new baby, holding her skin-to-skin, looking into her eyes and smiling and talking softly (see page 366) is the best way to help her adjust to life outside your womb. If all is well, she will be equipped with all her senses functioning (see pages 180–1), but she will not yet be able to 'turn down' some of the messages that she is receiving – and that is where you and your partner can help.

While you are in hospital, you can ask for lights to be dimmed, minimise noise and keep her close to you. When you hold her at your breast you have her at the exact distance from your face at which she can best focus, so you are enabling her to see you as clearly as she can at this early stage.

What may happen

In the next few hours your baby will have her first feed (see page 332) and pass her first bowel motion in the form of greenish black meconium (see page 178). She may be bathed and clothed for the first time and will have her first checks by the midwife.

Be sure to keep her warm at all times and be aware that she loses heat from her head very easily. If she needs extra medical help she may be in the SCBU (see pages 298–301) and have tests each day, be attached to monitors or have tubes in her nose. By gently touching her and talking to her you can help her to cope with these new experiences. You can be her advocate and her refuge.

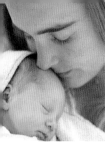

YOUR POST-BIRTH BODY

Your body has been through a momentous event and has probably worked harder than it ever has done before. Now is the time to rest and allow it to heal. In the immediate period after delivery you may experience a number of common after-effects.

The process of labour and giving birth stimulates your body to release nature's natural painkillers, which are called endorphins, and for a while the elation of meeting your baby for the first time may have taken your mind off any aches and pains.

However, it is common to feel rather battered after delivery is over, particularly once the tiredness sets in. Take things gently. It is important to realise that although many of the changes your body went through when you were pregnant will come to an end quite abruptly, it will take a while for it to return to its pre-pregnancy state.

Postnatal discomforts

If you had a Caesarean section you will have a particular set of after-effects to cope with (see pages 322–3). No matter what kind of labour and delivery you went through you are bound to experience a number of discomforts such as after-pains, perineal tenderness (especially if you tore, had an episiotomy or stitches – see pages 282–3) as well as increasingly heavy and aching breasts when your milk starts to come in (see pages 328–9).

Although all these symptoms are absolutely normal, talk to your midwife or doctor if you are concerned or are finding it especially hard to cope. There are a number of natural remedies that you can use (see page 321).

Your perineum

You will probably find that your perineum is most sore in the first three days after delivery and if you had stitches they may feel very tight as the traumatised tissue swells around them. Many midwives recommend sitting on an inflatable ring for the first few days so that the perineum is not under any pressure from direct contact with hard surfaces. Cool packs and arnica cream may help and if you take a bath, you can try adding a cupful of sea salt to assist healing and/or a few drops of pure lavender oil diluted in a carrier oil or a cup of milk.

Taking homeopathic remedies such as arnica tablets is also commonly recommended and many women start them before labour begins (see page 211). Even if you didn't tear you are most likely to feel a dull ache in your perineum as a result of the stretching and pressure during the second stage of labour. You may also find that the area stings when you urinate (see pages 312–13). Bathing your vulva in lukewarm water may help.

After-pains & bleeding

You will also have some postnatal bleeding, known as 'lochia' (see page 312), which may be heavy at first, when the blood is mixed with mucus and tissue. This may last 10 days, or more, but will gradually lessen. Take a good supply of maternity pads to hospital plus comfortable cotton knickers.

Your abdomen will seem soft and flabby after so many months of being stretched and, if you are having your second or subsequent baby, you will have after-pains that will feel like mild contractions. They will last for three days or so after delivery and may become stronger as you breastfeed because your baby's sucking on your nipple prompts your body to release oxytocin (see page 328). As you have after-pains, more lochia may be expelled and you may feel quite uncomfortable, but try to welcome the pains because they are helping your uterus contract and return to its normal size and shape. If you find them hard to cope with, speak to your midwife or doctor.

Your bladder

Your bladder will have undergone some stress during labour and delivery, too, and you may find that you have difficulty in passing urine, but this will be noted when you are examined after delivery. You may need to be catheterised to allow the muscles around your bladder to rest and recover. The physical strain of labour may also make your bladder more susceptible to infection, so you should drink plenty of water as a preventative measure. If you do get an infection, it will require prompt treatment with antibiotics. More commonly, you may have some temporary stress incontinence and leak urine when you cough, sneeze or laugh. This should pass, but the sooner you resume your pelvic floor exercises (see page 141) the better. If the problem does not improve over time contact your doctor – you may need specialist help.

Your breasts

Immediately after delivery your breasts will contain colostrum, the nutrient-rich, yellow liquid that is full of antibodies to protect your baby (see pages 328–9). Your breasts will be soft at first, but within three or four days your milk will start to come in and they may feel quite hard, hot, swollen and tender. You can try some complementary remedies and cooling packs that may help, but the best solution is to feed your baby as much, and as often, as you can.

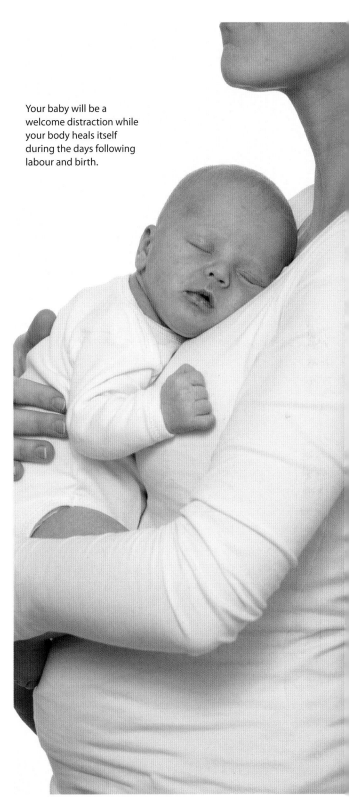

Your baby will be a welcome distraction while your body heals itself during the days following labour and birth.

Caring for your perineum
Nutrition

After the blood loss of delivery you will need to replace vital nutrients. Try eating foods that are rich in vitamin C and zinc:

• Vitamin C is good for tissue repair and iron absorption. Good sources include oranges, grapefruit, lemons and limes, kiwi fruit, strawberries, blackcurrants, tomatoes and broccoli (see page 84).
• Zinc is good for the production of hormones and to assist healing. Good sources include wholegrain foods, fish, poultry, beef, nuts, sweetcorn and bananas (see page 85).

Complementary therapies for perineum care

Consult your midwife or doctor before you try any complementary therapies and make sure that your practitioners are fully qualified and accredited.

Acupuncture An acupuncturist may treat you by positioning needles around your ears to stimulate the genital area and promote healing. You could also use your TENS machine by placing the pads on either side of your coccyx (but you should ask an acupuncturist to demonstrate how to do this first).

Aromatherapy A few drops of essential oil of lavender, calendula or tea tree, diluted first in some carrier oil (such as sweet almond or grapeseed oil) can be added to your bath water.

SELF-HELP TIPS FOR PERINEUM CARE

Eat healthily and include plenty of fresh fruit and vegetables to assist healing

Keep your perineum clean (especially after visiting the bathroom), but avoid using perfumed soaps, oils and shower or bath foams. Pat the area dry with soft loo paper or a soft, clean towel

Change your sanitary pads as often as you can and try to allow the area to 'breathe' now and then

Homeopathy Take care to follow the manufacturer's dosage instructions, but remedies are best prescribed by a professional homeopath to match your precise symptoms. Kits are available for labour. Contact a registered homeopath.

You could try these remedies and take them in the following dose: after delivery take one tablet every two to three hours for the first day and then take a dose two or three times a day for the next two or three days, as needed.

• **Arnica 30c** The number-one remedy for pain and bruising after birth. Ideally you should start taking it before you go into labour (see page 211).
• **Hypericum 30c** For relieving pain in areas rich in nerve endings, such as the intense pain that may follow an episiotomy, a forceps or ventouse delivery. It may also help to ease shooting pains and pain in the coccyx or perineum.
• **Staphysagria 30c** To help severe pain and sensitivity of the genitals, feeling worse after sitting.
• **Bellis perennis 30c** For deep, aching pain and bruised soreness in the pelvis following a forceps delivery or similar trauma, if arnica doesn't help.
• **Calendula** This can be taken orally in the 6c or 30c strength, but it can also be directly applied to the sore area in the form of a cream, gel or tincture.

Flower remedies If you have a sore perineum try crabapple to soothe it.

Breast problems in the early days
Complementary therapies for breast problems

Consult your midwife or doctor before you try any complementary therapies and make sure that your practitioners are fully qualified and accredited.

Acupuncture Your milk will probably come in about three days after delivery, but occasionally (sometimes after a Caesarean) it may be delayed. If you are anaemic or exhausted it may also affect the amount of milk that you produce at first. Then anxiety over the issue can make things worse – so you need to keep feeding your baby to stimulate your breasts to produce more. Acupuncture or acupressure may help

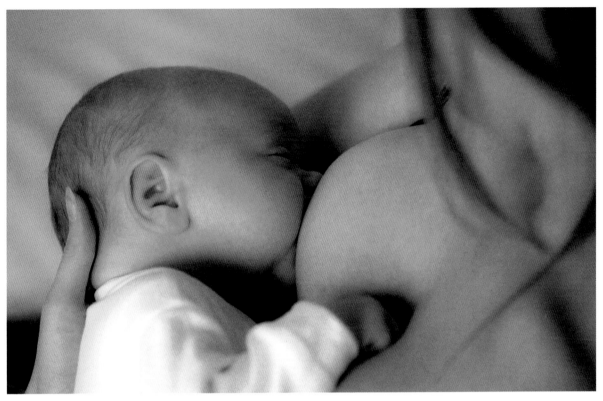

There are plenty of self-help remedies available to you to get breastfeeding going and to keep any problems at bay.

to ease your anxiety and stimulate the flow of milk. Consult a qualified, experienced therapist.

Homeopathy Take care to follow the manufacturer's dosage instructions, but remedies are best prescribed by a professional homeopath to match your precise symptoms. Contact a registered homeopath. Try:

- **Calendula cream** Use this for cracking nipples, both as a preventative and to help healing (though cracked nipples are a sure sign that the baby is not latching on properly and you need help and practice with your technique – see pages 332–4).
- **Phytolacca 30c and belladonna 30c** If your breasts become hard and engorged and for mastitis (see page 335). Take one tablet every two to three hours for the first day and then take a dose two or three times a day for the next two or three days, as and when needed.
- **Urtica urens 30c** To improve milk amount/flow.

Western herbalism For insufficient milk supply try drinking fennel tea or chewing fennel seeds.

Note: If you have a sudden fever, chills and flu-like symptoms, red or inflamed areas on your breasts consult your doctor as you may have mastitis and require prompt treatment in the form of antibiotics that are safe for your baby.

SELF-HELP TIPS FOR BREAST PROBLEMS

Get plenty of rest

Drink lots of water

Make sure that your baby latches on properly (see page 333)

Feed as often as your baby wants to (it may seem a lot at first, but things will settle down after a while – see page 329)

AFTER A CAESAREAN

Within 48 hours, or so, of your baby's birth by Caesarean section she will have her first full medical check, where a series of tests will be carried out to ensure that all is well.

How you may feel after a Caesarean will very much depend on the circumstances surrounding it. If yours was an elective Caesarean you may have had a relatively straightforward delivery, but if it was an emergency procedure, after a long labour, you may be feeling rather shocked and sore.

Recovery time

It will take longer to recover from a Caesarean section than a vaginal delivery, but you should be able to get out of bed soon after the operation (at least within 24 hours) and you'll be encouraged to rotate your ankles regularly, even while you are lying down – to help to prevent thrombosis. You should also do some deep-breathing exercises to clear any congestion from your lungs. Most women stay in hospital for three to four days afterwards, but if you and your baby are well and want to go home earlier, you may be able to leave sooner and have some of your follow-up care in your own home.

Light postnatal lochia

Your postnatal bleeding (lochia – see page 312) is very likely to be less heavy than it would be after a vaginal delivery because the surgeon will have cleaned the inside of your uterus after removing the placenta. However you will have some bleeding for 10 days or so and you may also experience some after-pains as your uterus contracts.

Pain-relief options & recovery

You will need some strong pain relief at first and if your operation was carried out with an epidural this may be topped up for a while. You will probably still have some IV fluids and a catheter, but once this is removed you will be checked to see that you can urinate normally.

You may be offered patient-controlled analgesia (PCA) by means of a small hand-held pump that allows you to control small doses of pain relief intravenously. Alternatively, you may be given anal suppositories or tablets (the latter will work slowly and be generally less effective, so it is more effective when the most acute pain has worn off).

Your surgical wound will be tender and covered with a dressing for at least 24 hours. You will be given specific advice on how look after it and prevent infection, but it's good advice to wear loose clothing, cotton underwear, and to clean and dry the wound daily. Your midwife or physiotherapist will also give you advice about postnatal exercises that will help you in your recovery.

Your stitches may be dissolving ones, but if not, they will probably be removed after about five days and should only be mildly uncomfortable. The scar will still be quite red, raised and a little sore, so try to avoid wearing clothes that may rub. Allow the scar to be exposed to the air from time to time. You should be able to shower and bathe, but avoid using scented soap, oils, bath or shower products and dry the scar carefully by patting it gently with a clean towel. After about a week the scar may begin to feel a little itchy, but simple unscented emollient or calendula cream (see below) may help.

In general, it will take about six weeks for your superficial tissues to heal completely, but longer for the layers of muscle to knit together properly and for your scar to smooth out. In the meantime, you may notice some numbness around the wound, but full sensation should return as the nerve endings repair.

Regaining strength/caring for the scar
Nutrition

You need to rebuild your strength and eat plenty of foods that are rich in vitamin C, zinc and iron to help your body heal and fight infection and to prevent anaemia. You should also take a multivitamin supplement. These foods are rich in vitamin C, zinc and iron:

• Vitamin C is good for tissue repair, fighting infection and iron absorption. Good sources include citrus fruits, kiwi fruit, strawberries, blackcurrants, tomatoes and broccoli (see page 84).
• Zinc aids healing. Good sources include wholegrain foods, fish, poultry, beef, nuts, sweetcorn and bananas (see page 85).
• Iron prevents anaemia. Good sources include eggs, tinned bony fish, apricots, fortified cereals, raisins, prunes and red meat.

Complementary therapies/post-Caesarean care

Consult your midwife or doctor before you try any complementary therapies and make sure that your practitioners are fully qualified and accredited.

Aromatherapy

• For headache rub a few drops of essential oil (not diluted) of lavender on to your temples.
• For nausea sprinkle a few drops of essential oil of peppermint on to a clean handkerchief or tissue and inhale the scent.

Homeopathy Take care to follow the manufacturer's dosage instructions, but remedies are best prescribed by a professional homeopath to match your precise symptoms. Contact a registered homeopath.

You could try these remedies in the following dose: after delivery take one tablet every two to three hours for the first day and then a dose two or three times a day for the next two or three days, as needed.

• **Arnica 30c** For bruising and tearfulness. Ideally, start taking this before delivery (see page 211).
• **Aconite 30c** For shock and tearfulness.
• **Opium 30c** To help you to cope with feeling 'spaced out' after the anaesthetic.
• **Calendula** Can be taken orally in the 6c or 30c strength, but it can also be directly applied to the scar in the form of a cream, gel or tincture once the scar has begun to heal and if it feels itchy.

Western herbalism For an insufficient milk supply try drinking fennel tea.

Flower remedies Try Rescue Remedy if you feel a little tearful or olive if you feel exhausted.

TENS machine Try putting the pads above and below your scar to provide some natural pain relief.

Warning: If you have chills or fever, extreme fatigue or your wound is oozing or inflamed consult your doctor at once. You may have an infection.

SELF-HELP TIPS AFTER A CAESAREAN

Eat healthily and include plenty of fresh fruit and vegetables and foods rich in zinc – to assist healing

Keep your wound clean, but avoid using perfumed soaps, oils and shower or bath foams. Pat the area dry carefully with a clean, soft towel

Get plenty of rest and sleep. Be sure not to try to do too much too soon

Accept as much extra help as you can when you go home and concentrate only on essential chores

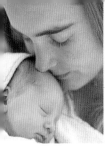

introducing the new arrival

THE FIRST FEW DAYS

Now it's time for the 'babymoon', so abandon the household chores, switch on the answerphone and give yourself time to recover. Enjoy being a new family together.

A s you return home you will feel pride in achievement and elation that you and your baby came through labour and birth. The true climax of your pregnancy was the arrival of your baby, but this is just the start of the real journey you are embarking on as a family. You are likely to be on an emotional rollercoaster as your body readjusts to your non-pregnant state and your new role as a mother prompts a new cocktail of hormones to be released into your system.

SOME ESSENTIAL TIPS

The responsibility of taking your new baby home can feel overwhelming – be prepared for this

Accept that your baby is likely to be unsettled on your first night or two at home and that you may not get much sleep

If your partner sleeps in another room, he or she may feel better able to deal with the baby next morning, while you catch up on lost sleep

Try to sleep whenever your baby does

Keep visitors and the time they stay to a minimum for a while and don't travel long distances just to show off the baby

Accept any help that is offered (especially cooked meals)

Only do essential housework

Don't try to lose weight or get back into shape just yet

Spend time as a family, so that everyone gets a chance to get to know the new baby

Dealing with 'baby blues'

The 'baby blues' (see pages 356–9) are very common among new mothers and tend to kick in when your breast milk arrives – around day three or four. You may feel weepy and overwhelmed at the reality of your responsibilities, but remember, becoming a parent means a lifetime of love, too, and there will be lots of people on hand to support you as your baby grows. Caring for a new baby can seem daunting, so don't be surprised if hormonal shifts and fatigue lower your spirits. You will soon pick up energy, but you need to help yourself. Eat well (see page 358), drink plenty of water, milk and diluted fruit juice and get as much rest as you can. When your baby sleeps don't try to catch up on chores – sleep, too.

Older children

If you have older children, you will want to give them attention, too, and in the first few days welcome them into bed with you to have a cuddle, but don't attempt to take them on outings at this stage. Your partner may be able to spend extra time with them while you and the baby sleep, but if not, enlist a friend or relative to take them out for a treat.

Friends & relatives

You are likely to have lots of friends and relatives keen to see the baby, but try to agree a policy of 'visiting times' with your partner so that you can have time to rest and be alone with your newborn.

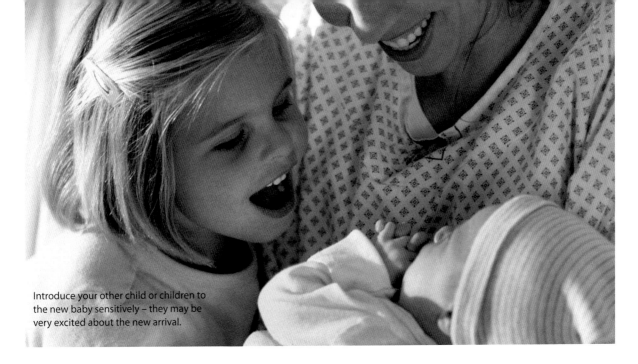

Introduce your other child or children to the new baby sensitively – they may be very excited about the new arrival.

HOW TO INCLUDE SIBLINGS

Make sure that your older child knows who will look after her when you go into labour (see page 217)

Before the baby arrives, include your child in your preparations and make her feel important

Be honest and try to explain that a lot of your time will be taken up with looking after the new baby and that you will be very tired at first. But explain that there will still be plenty of fun things that you and she can do together. If she knows what to expect she may be less upset at not having you all to herself any more

Let your older child choose a present that she would like to give to the new baby (encourage her to choose something lasting, such as a special blanket or soft toy)

Try to buy a present (in advance) that you can give to your older child 'from' the baby

When you return home with your baby (or your child visits you in hospital) make a big fuss of her and give her plenty of attention before you introduce her to her new sibling

Let your child gently stroke the new baby's feet or hands, but try to avoid criticising her if she is a bit clumsy at first

Once you are home, try to involve your child in caring for the baby (fastening nappies or helping to bathe her, for example)

When you are feeding the baby and things are calm, try to sit close to your older child and talk to her or read her a story

If your older child regresses and wants to be 'babied', try to be patient and indulge her with extra kisses and cuddles

Make sure that your older child still has her usual bathtime and bedtime routine – it will help make her feel secure

Jealousy is very common and natural. It is most likely to be strongest in children with an age gap of two years. A gap of just 18 months, or less, seems to be easier for the older child because she is likely to be more accepting of the new order of things. A gap of three years, or more, is also likely to be much more straightforward and you may be surprised by the maturity of your older child's attitude

If your older child does express anger or tells you that she wants the new baby to 'go away', try to keep calm. Encourage her to talk about her feelings and reassure her that you still love her and that things will get easier

Try to spend at least an hour a day alone with your older child and give her your undivided attention. This could be reading stories and playing games while you rest in bed

Never leave a young child alone with your baby unattended and do not let your child hold the baby unsupervised

If you planned your 'babymoon' (see page 221) before the birth you may have a cupboard, fridge and freezer full of food – and the understanding of others that you need time to yourselves.

Your midwife & health visitor

Your community midwife will visit you on the first day and again on the fifth and tenth. More frequent visits will only be made if necessary, though you may be able to attend a drop-in clinic if you have concerns. The midwife normally discharges you from her care on the tenth day, but visits may continue up to day 28. Your baby will be weighed and measured and if you have concerns don't hesitate to ask. The midwife will also want to know how you are feeling and will look out for signs of postnatal depression (see pages 356–9). Once the midwife feels you are coping well, she will hand over to a health visitor, who will visit and give you appointments to attend your local health clinic – so that your baby's growth and development can be checked.

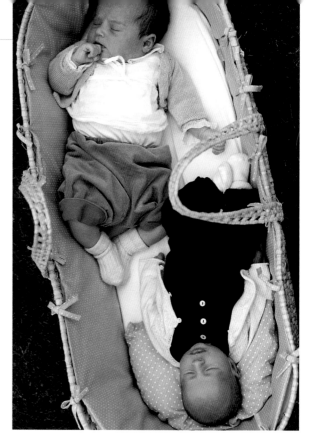

A moses basket is handy for daytime naps when you take twins on outings. Lay them on their backs with their heads at either end.

COPING WITH TWINS

Ask for, and accept, any extra help you can get. Bathtime and bedtime will be especially busy, so if nothing else, try to get some help for the evening period

Try not to panic. It can seem very daunting if you have two babies who are crying or needing to be fed at the same time, but you will soon learn to deal with them with confidence

Make yourself a 'nest' of cushions or buy a special nursing cushion (a V-shaped one to wrap around yourself). Then you can arrange a baby on each side while you feed them together. If one is not ready or finishes before the other, you can still hold her close while you feed the other

When one baby wakes in the night to be fed, consider waking the sleeping twin and feeding both of them together. Or feed one and put her back to bed and then wake the other to feed, too. If you don't feed them more or less together, the chances are, 20 minutes after you get back to bed, the second baby will wake and need feeding, too

If both babies are fretful and you cannot hold them at once, try putting one in a baby chair on the floor (secured with the safety harness), while you hold the other. You may be able to gently rock the baby chair with your foot as you soothe the baby in your arms. Have the other twin's chair at the ready, so that you can put the one you've been holding/feeding in it while attending to the other

Put your babies in a cot together to sleep. They will be comforted by each other's familiar presence. When they are very small, lay them next to each other at one end of it to sleep. Once they are a bit bigger, put one at each end (in the 'feet-to-foot position' – see page 340) so that their heads are together

Bathe your babies separately if you feel you can't cope with two in the water at the same time

Forget about all but the essential chores for the time being

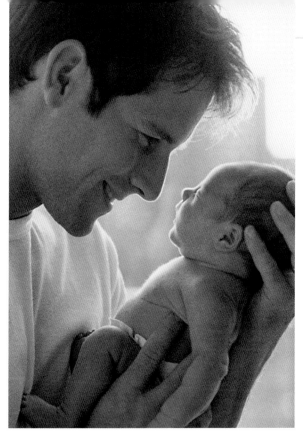

If you are the dad, take the time to bond with your new baby early on – you'll be creating the foundations of a strong relationship.

Caring for your baby together

Babies can seem very fragile and delicate and while it is important that you look after your newborn yourself, don't forget to let others take responsibility, too – especially the baby's father. It is common for new mothers to become fiercely protective of their babies, but try to remember that your baby belongs to both of you, so caring for your newborn should be a joint project. However, apart from handling your baby safely (see right) you and your partner will do some things differently. Try not to be critical of one another and involve your partner as much as you can (see pages 350–1).

Expressing feelings

Your baby needs plenty of affection from both of you and her father needs to express his feelings for his child, too. Research shows that if men are prevented from helping in the early days, they are unlikely to help later on and women end up doing the majority of the work. So let your partner soothe the baby if she has just had a feed and allow him to find his own way of doing things. If you have an older child who wants to hold the baby, make sure that she sits in a secure, supported place while she does so and that you are on hand to provide help.

Picking up your baby

You need to hold your baby carefully (especially her neck, which is not strong enough to support the weight of her head properly yet).

- Slide one hand under her head and neck and the other under her bottom and lower back.
- Draw her close to your chest, keeping her head slightly higher than her body.
- Slide the hand that is under her bottom further up her back, to her neck and head, while you bend your other arm so that she can nestle in both your arms. Her head then rests securely on the inner joint of your elbow.

Holding your baby

Your baby will feel safe if you hold her firmly, close to your body.

- Put her against your shoulder (this is especially good for gentle winding – see page 338) by holding her upright and supporting her bottom with one hand. You then put your other hand flat against her back, ready to support her head as she 'bobs' against you.
- She may also enjoy being held with her head over the crook of your elbow, but facing downwards. Your forearm can then support the length of her body and if you put your other hand between her legs you can support her tummy.

Your baby may like these positions at times, but at other times she may protest. You will only learn her preferences over time, so be patient and if one position is not working, try something different.

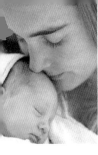

WHY BREAST IS BEST

You may have heard the saying 'breast is best'. This simple phrase is used to promote the benefits of breastfeeding, but it is no empty slogan. Breast milk and breastfeeding benefit your baby in so many ways and if you understand how and why, it may help you to get breastfeeding established.

Within each of your breasts there are around 15 to 20 chambers, known as 'lobes', and inside these there are smaller 'lobules' that have alveoli – smaller clustered cells that produce and store milk.

When you feed your baby the milk travels through your milk ducts and out through the 15 or 20 tiny openings in your nipple. When your baby sucks, the nerve endings in your nipple and areola send signals to your brain to release two vital hormones: oxytocin and prolactin. Oxytocin prompts the 'let-down reflex', which is the pins-and-needles-like sensation that you may feel as your milk begins to flow. Prolactin then stimulates further milk production, so the more your baby sucks, the more milk you produce – a perfect supply-and-demand system.

Triggering milk flow

When your milk starts to flow it may do so with force, so that it spurts, or it may simply drip. The signals that the nerves in your breasts send to, and receive from, your brain are so strong that you may be surprised to find that your milk flow can be triggered just by the sound of your baby crying. This can also happen when a feed is due, so if you don't want damp patches on your clothes use disposable cotton, or washable, breast pads inside your bra.

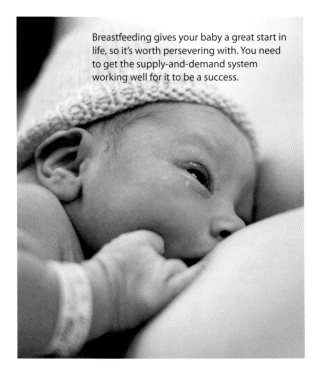

Breastfeeding gives your baby a great start in life, so it's worth persevering with. You need to get the supply-and-demand system working well for it to be a success.

Why breast milk is just right

When your baby feeds just after birth he receives colostrum, a rich, yellow liquid that not only contains all the protein, fats, vitamins and minerals that he needs for the first few days of life, but also the essential antibodies to help him fight off infections and kickstart his own immune system. Babies who receive colostrum also gain protection from allergies.

Many hospitals encourage mothers to give their babies their colostrum at the very least (even if they intend to bottlefeed), but if you can persevere with breastfeeding there is a range of important health benefits you can pass on to your baby. Research studies have shown that overall, breastfed babies seem to be less likely to have attention deficit hyperactivity disorder (ADHD), schizophrenia and asthma and they also seem to maintain greater intellectual capacity as they get older – possibly because breast milk contains the essential fatty acids so necessary for brain growth (see page 185).

Foremilk & hindmilk

Around three days after your baby's birth, your body will produce 'transitional milk', which is a mixture of colostrum and breast milk. Then within a few weeks this will change to mature breast milk, composed of two types of milk: the foremilk, which is thin, bluish and slightly watery and the richer, hindmilk, which is released as your baby continues to suck. To make sure that your baby gets enough hindmilk, try to make sure that he empties the first breast before he feeds at the other (see page 333).

Good-quality milk

Your breast milk is packed with proteins, vitamins, minerals, carbohydrates, essential fatty acids, salts and hormones and is perfectly suited to your baby's digestive system, but you need to be well nourished to create this extraordinary baby food. To produce plenty of good-quality milk and maintain your energy levels, drink lots of water and eat a varied but balanced diet (see pages 330–1) that will provide you with between 2,200 and 2,700 calories per day.

Supply-&-demand & quantity

Many women worry about how much milk their breastfed babies receive. It seems easier to be able to monitor how much milk a bottle-fed baby is taking because you measure it out in the bottle and you can

see how much your baby has consumed, but actually, with breastfeeding, the natural supply-and-demand system will ensure that your baby is getting enough. By feeding him whenever he seems hungry, you will stimulate your body to keep producing more. Don't be tempted to try to 'build up' your supply by delaying feeds. This may actually slow down and eventually lessen your supply, possibly even causing problems associated with engorgement (see page 335). If you are concerned that your baby still seems hungry at the end of a feed, try offering him your breast more often and make sure that he is latched on properly (see page 333).

Frequent feeds

Breast milk is digested quickly, so breastfed babies need to be fed often. At first, it can seem as if you are doing little else but breastfeeding, but be patient and remember that your baby is programmed to demand plenty of feeds in the first few days – as part of nature's way of getting the milk supply established.

You cannot 'spoil' a newborn baby by feeding on demand. Your own emotions can affect milk supply and even its flow, so you need plenty of support from your partner and family to get it going. The first few days may be hard work, but they will pay dividends. You will soon find that you are feeding your baby without even having to think about it and within a month or two your breasts may feel a lot less heavy, even though you are still providing sufficient milk.

Practicalities

By persevering in the early days you will find that you have great freedom when you go out with your baby because you don't have to prepare and keep milk at the right temperature. If you are worried about breastfeeding in public, invest in breastfeeding tops or drape a soft scarf over your shoulder so that you can feed your baby discreetly. Many shops have mother-and-baby rooms, where you can feed in private. Don't forget – you are doing what is natural and it is giving your baby a great start in life.

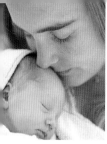

BREASTFEEDING NUTRITION

Maintaining a healthy diet now that you are feeding your baby with breast milk is just as important as it was when he was in your womb. Looking after a new baby is hard work, too, so you need to keep yourself well nourished and your energy levels topped up.

What to eat & drink

What you eat will determine the nutritional content of your baby's milk, so continuing to follow a healthy diet is essential.

You will also need to maintain your energy levels and keep your blood-sugar levels stable. It is vital, too, that you drink plenty of fluids – at least 1.5 litres (3 pt) of water per day, plus one or two cups of herbal tea and glasses of diluted fruit juices. Your diet should be based on:

- **Wholegrains** Choose brown rice, wholemeal bread, wholemeal pasta, quinoa (see pages 84–5).
- **Protein** You need to have an extra portion of protein each day. Try to get this essential building block from a variety of sources such as fish, poultry, meat, eggs, cheese, nuts, beans, lentils and seeds. Unless you are vegetarian/vegan, eat red meat at least weekly because the protein and iron is most readily absorbed from this source (see pages 84–5).
- **Fruit and vegetables** Aim for at least five, ideally seven or more, portions per day (see page 79).
- **Essential fats** In oily fish, avocados, nuts and seeds and oils including olive/rapeseed (see pages 80–1).
- **Calcium** You need about an extra 550 mg per day for your baby so that your total daily intake should be around 1,250 mg. This can be found in milk, yogurt and cheese as well as tinned bony fish such as sardines (you'll need to consume about six

SUPERFOODS FOR MILK PRODUCTION

Nuts Especially almonds, cashews and macadamias

Oats In savoury and fruit bakes and porridge

Barley Added to stews or served as an alternative to rice

Green, leafy vegetables such as kale, spinach and chard, as well as edible seaweed –try it sprinkled over salads or added to soups and stews

Herbs and (mild) spices Parsley, marjoram, basil, anise, dill, turmeric and fresh root ginger, as well as fennel (leaves, bulb and seed), caraway and fenugreek seeds

portions), but also in non-animal-derived foods such as leafy greens, beans, lentil, nuts and fruits such as apricots (see page 85).

Key nutrients

- **Vitamin A** To aid the development of your baby's hearing, vision and sense of taste and boost his immune system (for good sources see page 84).
- **B vitamins** These will help to prevent fluctuations in blood-sugar levels and improve your milk flow (for good sources see page 84).
- **Vitamin C** For the absorption of iron, making blood vessels, connective tissues, collagen and improving the immune system (for good sources see page 84).

- **Vitamin D** You will need to increase your intake of this vitamin to boost absorption of calcium and building and maintaining healthy bones. It is now recommended that all pregnant and breastfeeding women should take a supplement of 10 mcg per day (for good sources see page 84).
- **Vitamin E** Essential for brain and nerve development and tissue repair (for good sources see page 84).
- **Vitamin K** Needed by your baby for blood clotting (for good sources see page 186).
- **Calcium** You will need to replenish the calcium that your baby takes from your breast milk so that your bones are not at risk of developing osteoporosis (for good sources see page 85).
- **Iron** You and your baby need iron to manufacture haemoglobin and to help you fight infection (for good sources see page 85).
- **Zinc** Needed for the healing of tissue, production of hormones and to help prevent postnatal depression (for good sources see page 85).
- **Omega-3/docosahexaenoic acid (DHA)** This essential fatty acid is crucial to the development of your baby's brain (for good sources see page 185).

Your energy requirements

For the first six months after delivery you need around 450 to 500 calories per day more than your normal intake – for each baby you are breastfeeding. Even at this rate, you will probably lose weight at a rate of about 500 g–1 kg (1–2 lb) per month because breastfeeding and looking after a new baby burn up a lot of energy. If you feel you have gained excess weight during pregnancy, don't try to lose weight rapidly by eating less, because you and your baby could be deprived of vital nutrients. Aim to eat little and often, to help keep blood-sugar levels steady (see page 147). This helps maintain energy levels and keep stress hormones under control – it may therefore help to prevent postnatal depression (see pages 356–9). Breakfast is a particularly important meal, but make sure you have at least three

FOODS TO AVOID

Alcohol Don't drink alcohol while breastfeeding. It can impair your let-down reflex, but it is passed on in your milk and the baby's liver cannot process it. Alcohol levels peak in your system around an hour after consumption and it takes several hours to be eliminated from your body (therefore your breast milk, too) so you cannot avoid passing it on to your baby

Caffeine Avoid caffeine (found in coffee, colas, energy drinks, teas – including green tea – and chocolate). Fruit and herbal teas are better, but limit your intake to two cups a day. Over-the-counter cold remedies contain high levels of caffeine

Transfats and partially hydrogenated fats Found in highly processed foods, such as margarines and spreads, commercially made cakes, biscuits, pastries and crisps

Artificial sweeteners These are linked to a range of health problems – especially in babies (see page 88). Check labels if your baby has phenylketonuria (PKU). Babies in the UK are tested using a heel-prick test (see page 363)

COLIC

If your baby suffers from colic (abdominal pain that seems to be associated with wind after feeding – see page 343) you may want to try avoiding eating the following foods:

Common allergy-causing foods such as eggs, peanuts, soy, wheat and gluten, strawberries and chocolate

Cruciferous vegetables: cabbage, broccoli and cauliflower

Cow's milk (also avoid soya and goat's milk, although rice milk may be a possible alternative)

good meals a day, with healthy snacks, too. Aim to combine protein and complex (slow-release) carbohydrates (see page 79) as well as fruit or vegetables in each meal/snack. Avoid eating refined carbohydrates such as white rice, bread, pasta and sugary foods such as sweets, cakes, biscuits and fizzy drinks because your body converts these into glucose rapidly, which causes blood-sugar peaks and dips.

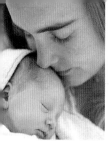

HOW TO BREASTFEED

Breastfeeding can feel blissful – when you get it right – but although it may look easy (and it is once it is established), it does take a little practice and knowledge of one or two key techniques. Here are a few tips for getting started.

Firstly, make sure you are comfortable. There are a variety of positions to use – try them out to see what works for you in particular situations. Most commonly you will probably want to feed your baby sitting up, but there will also be times when you may want to feed him while lying down (see opposite). Whichever position you adopt, you will need to bring your baby to your breast, not the other way around. If you are sitting, you could try using a V-shaped feeding cushion or a pillow to elevate your baby to the right height – so that his head is level with your nipple. You need to keep your back straight and avoid bending over your baby, so use pillows or cushions behind you, too.

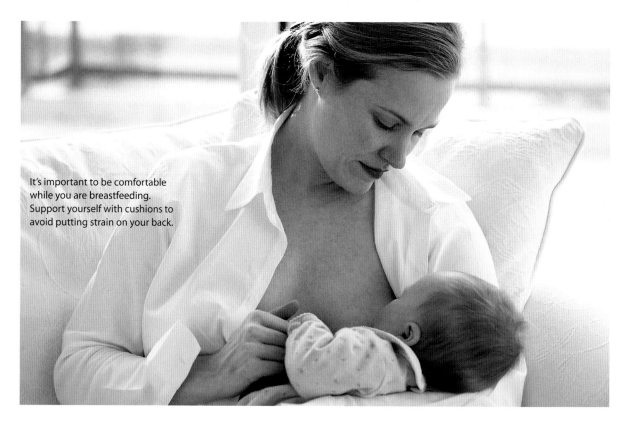

It's important to be comfortable while you are breastfeeding. Support yourself with cushions to avoid putting strain on your back.

Latching on

You need to get your baby to latch on to your nipple properly (babies must breastfeed not 'nipplefeed') and this is key to successful breastfeeding, which may take a little practice. Breastfeeding should not be painful, so if you notice sharp pain, or blistered or cracked nipples it is a sure sign that your baby is not correctly latched on. Once you and he have mastered the technique, it will feel just right and this 'perfect fit' will be easier to recognise. Try this technique:

- Once you are both comfortable, stroke your baby's cheek with your finger or nipple to stimulate his rooting reflex (see page 307), and encourage him to turn and open his mouth wide.
- As he opens his mouth, quickly bring him to your breast. Aim your nipple towards the roof of his mouth and try to ensure that he takes all of your nipple and most of your areola, too.
- You should feel his chin pressing into your breast

BREASTFEEDING POSITIONS

Lying on your side This can be especially useful for night feeds or when you are feeling very tired or sore after the birth. Use some soft pillows to support your head and neck, but keep your baby away from them. Lay him on his side, facing you, with his mouth in line with your nipple and your arm supporting his head. Draw him to your breast and make sure that his tummy is pressed against yours

Sitting upright If you have had a Caesarean section and are feeling tender, make sure that you use a soft pillow to support your baby's body and cushion your wound

Try the rugby hold You will need to put a pillow to one side of your body while you sit upright. Then lay your baby along the pillow, so that his head is level with your nipple and get him to latch on in the usual way (see above). If you are feeding twins, use a pillow on either side of you, or invest in a V-shaped feeding cushion and you will be able to feed both babies at the same time

and his tummy touching yours. His bottom lip should be curled back. Make sure that his nose is free of your breast so that he can breathe easily (he will not feed properly if his breathing is obstructed or uncomfortable).

- If your baby is properly latched on, you should see his cheek muscles working rhythmically and hear him swallowing. If his cheeks draw in when he is sucking, he is not latched on properly, so you need to break the suction by gently inserting your little finger into the corner of your baby's mouth and then starting again.

In the early days, your baby may be satisfied by feeding at just one breast, but as he grows, he may empty both. If he does only feed from one breast, start the next feed with the other. To help you to keep track of which breast to use, wear a loose elastic band on your left or right wrist when you feed your baby and swap it over each time you change breasts.

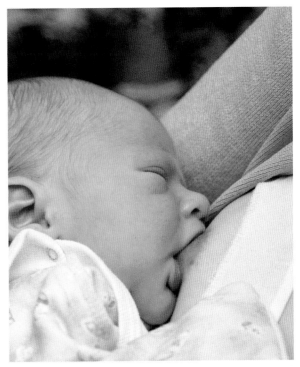

If your baby is properly latched on, his bottom lip should be curled back against his chin.

EXPERT BREASTFEEDING TIPS

1 Take time to get breastfeeding established. Don't have too many visitors in the early days – they are tiring – and make sure you are resting, eating and drinking plenty of fluids to help milk production. Watch how your baby feeds and learn the difference between effective sucking (slow, deep and rhythmic), which means he is getting milk and ineffective sucking (shallow and irregular), which means he is not

2 When your baby has had a full feed he should fall into a contented sleep and stay asleep when you put him into his cot. If he keeps on crying every time you put him down this is a sign that he is probably still hungry, so carry on feeding him

3 Breastfeeding should be pain-free, right from the outset. Sore nipples are nearly always caused by incorrect latching on. This will make your baby's sucking less effective, so he will find it harder to get enough milk, which may result in him being hungry and unsettled – even after long feeds. An experienced midwife or breastfeeding counsellor will instantly be able to show you how to correct your latching-on technique – so be sure to ask for help

4 If your baby can't latch on easily, give him a helping hand. If he is not opening his mouth wide and/or you have very large breasts, help him latch on by using the balls of your fingers to squeeze your breasts gently on either side of the areola. This should make your nipple protrude, making latching on easier

5 Identify problems and seek help. If your baby is crying a lot and/or not settling after feeds, don't assume this is part-and-parcel of breastfeeding, but seek medical advice. It might be that your baby is suffering from a problem such as reflux, which requires treatment

6 Enjoy breastfeeding! When it goes well it is a wonderful way to feed a baby, both emotionally and nutritionally. But if it is going badly and no one is able to give you the advice you need to improve the situation, you should not feel a failure if you have to give up. The most important thing is that you and your baby are happy and thriving, and that he gets enough milk

(Provided by Clare Byam-Cook)

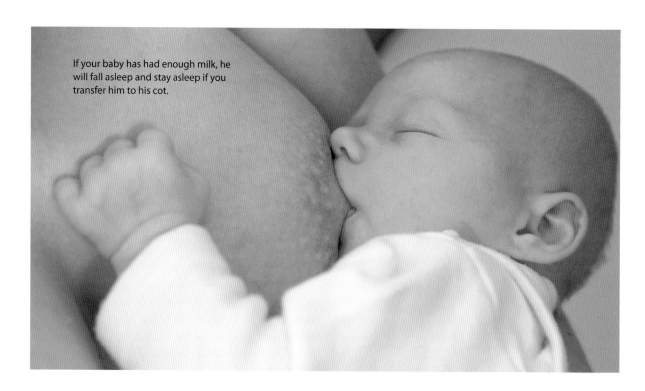

If your baby has had enough milk, he will fall asleep and stay asleep if you transfer him to his cot.

POSSIBLE BREASTFEEDING DIFFICULTIES

Engorgement

When your milk first comes in your breasts may become 'engorged', which means that they seem hard and are painfully swollen with the sudden influx of milk. Breastfeeding more may be the best way to prevent this happening again, but if your breasts are painful, this can be difficult. Try soaking yourself in a warm, relaxing bath for a few minutes. You may find that your breasts 'leak' some milk and so the pressure will be eased. You can also try covering your breasts with a warm flannel and massaging them to express a little of the milk to achieve the same effect (see below).

Blocked ducts and mastitis

Your milk ducts can sometimes become blocked if you have missed a feed for some reason. Perhaps your breast was not sufficiently emptied last time or your baby was not latched on properly (see page 333). If this happens, you may notice red or very 'hot' patches on your breast and/or lumpiness. Try feeding your baby as often and as regularly as you can, using a warm flannel to encourage the milk to flow, or expressing some milk at the end of a feed if your baby is not draining your breast sufficiently. If bacteria finds its way into the blocked duct it can become infected and inflamed. This condition is known as mastitis and the symptoms can appear very quickly. The breast will be red or inflamed, lumpy and painful, but you will also feel shivery, feverish and possibly nauseous. You are also likely to have quite severe aches and pains all over your body – as if you had flu.

You should contact your doctor immediately because you will need antibiotics to clear up the infection. You will be prescribed a type that is safe to take while you are breastfeeding, along with some analgesics such as paracetamol. Continue breastfeeding and the problem will clear quite quickly. If it does not improve after 24 hours speak to your doctor again to rule out the possibility of there being an abscess.

Expressing milk

It is best to avoid using bottles during the first month or so of breastfeeding or until it is well established. However there may be times when you want to store some of your milk so that your baby can be fed in your absence. The most effective way to express milk is to invest in an electric breast pump. However, if your breasts are engorged, you may also want to express a little milk to ease the pressure. You may be able to do this by massaging and stroking your breast from the top to the areola, then rhythmically squeezing your breast around the areola.

Getting enough rest

Fatigue is thought to be one of the most common causes of insufficient milk production, so it is important to get as much rest as you can. Try to sleep when your baby does and keep your body hydrated. Get plenty of fresh air by going for a walk for 20 or 30 minutes a day – it will benefit your baby, too (but make sure that he is well wrapped up. Exercise is good for circulation and digestion and it will lift your spirits. High-intensity exercise is not recommended and a strenuous workout can even change the flavour of your milk (some women find that their babies reject it).

Feeding your baby with love

Breastfeeding your baby gives you an ideal opportunity to rest, relax and concentrate just on him. You will be giving the warmth and nurturing comfort that will help him feel secure and loved and you will be able to deepen your relationship with him by picking up on those subtle cues that he gives as he gazes at you. Breastfeeding enables you to be confident that you are giving your baby the perfect food in the right conditions and you can feel proud that you are doing this.

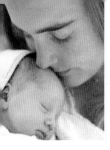

BOTTLEFEEDING

Whether you have chosen to bottlefeed from the outset or are doing so because you have moved on from breastfeeding (or have had to), you can make feeding an emotionally and physically rewarding time for both you and your baby.

Formula feeds have improved enormously over the past few decades, but you need to select one that is appropriate for your newborn, since there are different types for the various ages and stages. Organic formula will be best because it does not contain any traces of pesticides or chemicals, but you may need to try out one or two brands to see which suits your baby best. You will also need to experiment with different-shaped bottles and teats

and see which suit him best. Your newborn baby is likely to need a slow- or medium-flowing teat to begin with, but as he grows he will want to take more milk at a time and so you should gradually change to faster-flowing types. Silicone teats are more durable, but latex ones are probably more similar to a real nipple. Check that your baby does not have to work too hard to get his milk, because if he is sucking very hard he may be taking in excess air.

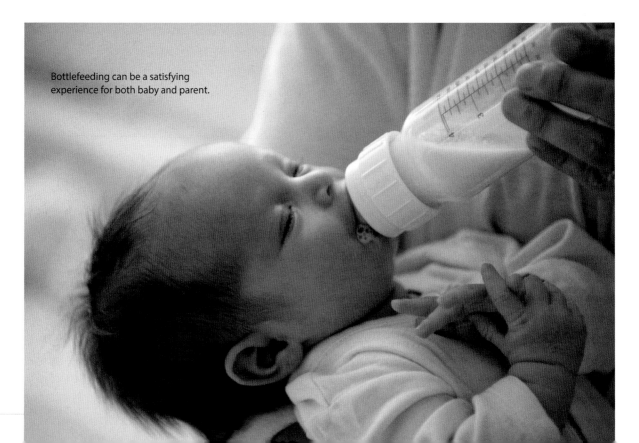

Bottlefeeding can be a satisfying experience for both baby and parent.

To make up a feed you should follow the manufacturer's instructions on the packaging precisely and never be tempted to add a little more formula or water for any reason – your baby could become either constipated and dehydrated or failing to get the correct balance of nutrients.

Make sure that you always use freshly boiled tap water (not mineral or bottled water – see below) and that it is cooled to a safe temperature before you give it to your baby. To test the temperature accurately, shake a little on to the inside of your wrist. It should feel warm, but not hot.

BOTTLEFEEDING HYGIENE

Babies have very sensitive digestive systems and are susceptible to bacterial infections, so for the first 12 months of his life, you must sterilise everything that your baby drinks or feeds from. Hygiene is of the utmost importance with bottlefeeding, so one of the most important pieces of equipment you need is a steriliser. Remember that everything you use to make up your baby's feed, from the bottle to the teats, caps and the milk-powder scoop itself will need to be washed properly in hot, soapy water using a bottle brush and then rinsed before being sterilised. To sterilise the feeding equipment you can either immerse everything in a pan of water and boil for 10 minutes or invest in an electrically operated steam steriliser or a chemical one. Microwave ovens and dishwashers are not suitable for sterilising baby bottles and equipment as they can contain 'cold spots', where bacteria are not destroyed.

Making up several bottles of formula at once and keeping them refrigerated until needed is practical, but it can cause stomach upsets and gastroenteritis if you do not follow the strictest hygiene standards. You must treat formula milk just the same as you would any perishable fresh food/drink. It's best to make up fresh formula for each feed, but if you do make batches in advance, remember that bacteria multiply in warm milk, so store bottles in the back of the fridge (not in the door) for no longer than 24 hours, at below 5°C (41°F). Follow a few simple rules:

How much/how often should you bottlefeed?

In general, newborn babies usually take around 60–120 ml (2–4 oz) of formula per feed in the first two or three weeks after delivery and are likely to be hungry every two to four hours. This means that you can expect to give your baby around six or seven feeds in a 24-hour period. This may seem a less-frequent 'schedule' than many breastfed babies, but that is partly because formula milk takes longer for babies to digest than breast milk. However, if your baby still seems to be hungry at the end of his feeds, offer another 60 ml (2 oz) at the next one.

Warm the bottles by placing them in a container of hot water or by using a bottle-warmer

Throw away unfinished milk If your baby does not take all his bottle, discard the contents – do not keep it for the next feed. Start the next feed with a clean, sterilised bottle and freshly made milk because bacteria grow rapidly in warm milk

Take care when you are out and about If you are away from home, use a sealed vacuum flask to store boiling water to make up a feed and ensure that the powder is kept in a sealed, sterile container. Alternatively, use cartons of ready-made formula, but make sure that your hands are clean when you open them and that the bottle teat and cap have been kept sterile

Set a use-by time If you make up a bottle of milk and transport it in a cool pack with an ice block, make sure that the milk is used within four hours – at the most

Use only freshly boiled water Do not use water that has been boiled repeatedly as it will contain raised levels of salt and minerals. Water from water-softening systems may also have high levels of sodium, so it should not be used either. Do not use purchased bottled water as it may contain bacteria and some mineral waters also have sodium levels that could be harmful to your baby

How to give your baby a bottle

Make sure that you are comfortably seated and that your back is well supported. You may want to use a feeding cushion or place a pillow underneath your baby's body (especially if you are sore after a having a Caesarean section).

Hold your baby by cradling him in your arms so that his body is in a semi-upright position and touching yours. His head should be slightly raised and he should be able to see your face. Tilt the bottle so that the formula fills up the top part of the bottle and the teat. You need to make sure that no air enters the teat because this could give your baby excess wind and cause him considerable discomfort. He may need a short break every so often to be winded (see below). Do not feed your baby formula when he is lying down as it could enter his sinuses or middle ear and cause an infection. Never leave your baby unattended with a bottle propped up, either, as there is a danger that he might choke and suffocate. He needs to be held while he is being fed, not only so that you can monitor how he is taking his feed but also because he needs to feel loved and secure.

There are different shapes and styles of bottle available on the market – some are made specially for newborns, but you will need to experiment.

HOW TO WIND YOUR BABY

Whether you breastfeed your baby or use a bottle, you need to 'wind' your baby at regular intervals to make sure that excess air does not get trapped in his digestive system. If this does happen it can make him extremely uncomfortable and may result in him bringing up part of his feed, should a large amount of air be finally released.

It is also thought that the abdominal pain of 'colic' is the main cause of the prolonged and distressing crying that some babies seem prone to in the early months of their life (see pages 342–3).

Bottlefed babies are naturally more prone to excess wind because the action of sucking the milk from a bottle rather than a breast means that they swallow more air. So you may need to interrupt some feeds to free the air in your baby's tummy.

Be prepared for 'possetting', which is when a small quantity of the swallowed milk comes back up with the burp. Before you wind your baby, drape a soft muslin cloth or towel over your shoulder to protect yourself.

Hold your baby upright and against your shoulder (see the picture, right). Support his head and gently rub and pat (do not bang) his back, working up from the base to the top repeatedly. You may even be able to feel the air bubble making its way up and out, but you should certainly be rewarded for your efforts with a burp. If your baby seems to be in distress and frequently brings up a large amount of milk forcefully, talk to your midwife or doctor because your baby may have a gastric infection or reflux that will need to investigated and treated.

You will soon get to know what your baby needs – he may not tolerate having his feeds interrupted for winding or he may prefer being held more horizontally across your forearm to expel the excess air (see page 327). As his neck and back muscles begin to strengthen, you could also try winding him in a sitting up position on your lap. You will need to support his head and neck by placing your hand under his chin and leaning him forwards slightly. With your other hand, you should then rub his back gently.

If your baby does not seem to be ready to burp and is not in distress, it may be that he simply does not suffer from much wind, so do not spend too long trying to get him to expel it and allow him to burp (or not) in his own time.

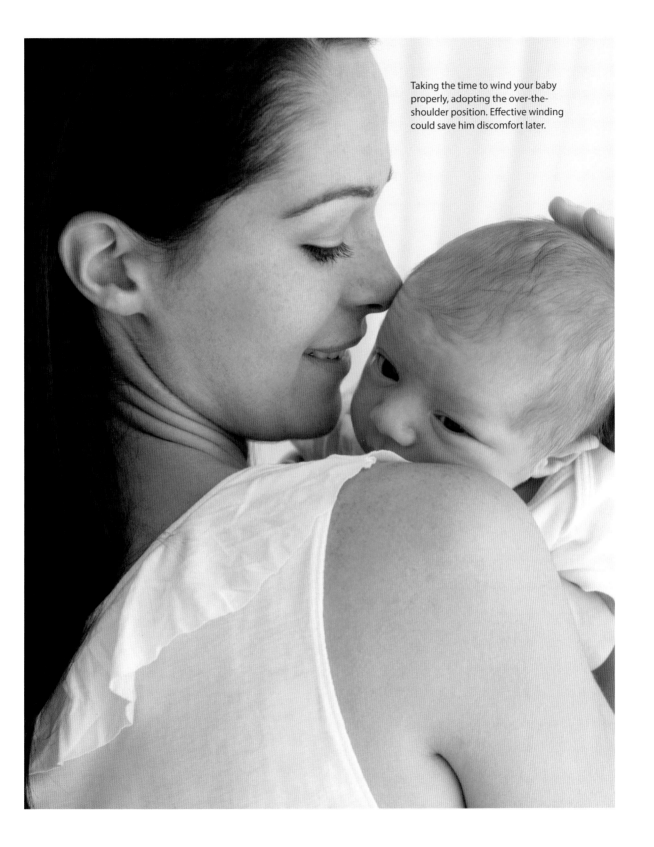

Taking the time to wind your baby properly, adopting the over-the-shoulder position. Effective winding could save him discomfort later.

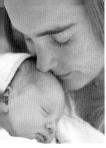

YOUR BABY'S SLEEP

Sleep can be elusive in the early days of life as a parent. Your baby needs plenty of sleep, but because he also needs food at regular intervals, he may only snooze for short periods at first. With a few gentle cues, however, you can soon help your baby to differentiate between day and night and encourage him to drift off happily.

Newborn babies take a while to settle into a sleeping pattern and often feel more secure in a smaller 'bed' such as a Moses basket. If your baby begins sleeping like this, as he grows you can try placing the basket inside his cot so that he becomes used to it before he outgrows the basket altogether. You might also consider using a 'bedside cot', which is attached to your bed on one side and allows you to attend to your baby without getting out of bed yourself. Resist the temptation to pick him up every time he makes a noise – on most occasions he will simply drift back to sleep by himself.

SUDDEN INFANT DEATH SYNDROME (SIDS)

SIDS – also known as 'cot death' – is when a baby dies suddenly without there being an obvious explanation. It is rare, but babies are at highest risk before they are four months old – although they may still be at risk until they are four years of age. The exact cause is unknown, but research has found that by taking certain steps it is possible to minimise the risk. You might want to use an under-mattress sensor, as these devices monitor your baby's movements and sound an alarm if his breathing dips to unacceptable level or stops completely.

Always put your baby to sleep on his back, with his feet at the foot of the cot (this is known as the 'feet-to-foot' position)

Put your baby to sleep in your bedroom for the first six months and make use of a baby monitor or mattress pad

Do not smoke, or allow anyone else to smoke in the house or anywhere near your baby. Avoid smokers when you are out

Use a baby sleeping bag to prevent your baby from being accidentally covered up by bedding. If you use blankets, choose cotton cellular ones, tuck them in at the bottom of the cot and make sure that they only reach up to his chest

Do not leave your baby to sleep on soft surfaces such as cushions, where he may become smothered or trapped

Do not use a cot quilt until he is at least 12 months old and do not leave sheepskins or large soft toys in his cot

Make sure that his room is not too hot – your baby should not overheat – so around 18°C (64°F) should be fine

Keep your baby's mattress clean, dry and well-aired. Do not use a plastic cover on it. Never use a second-hand mattress

If your baby is unwell or has a fever, keep him cool and seek medical advice

Do not share a bed with your baby if you have been drinking alcohol, taking medication or recreational drugs

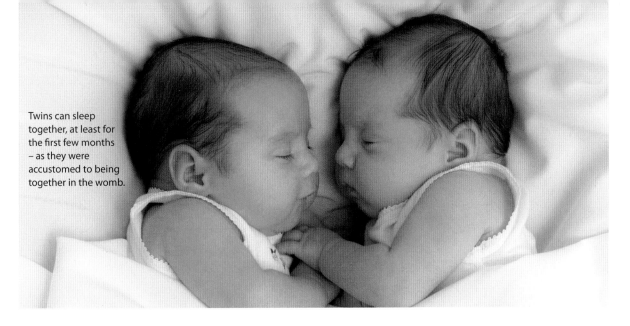

Twins can sleep together, at least for the first few months – as they were accustomed to being together in the womb.

TOP 10 TIPS FOR PROMOTING GOOD SLEEP

1 Babies learn and adopt the habits that we teach them, including the bad ones, so try not to set up confusions in your baby's mind about when he should sleep. It is important that he learns how to tell the difference between night and day, feeding and cuddling, and playing and sleeping

2 Remember – sleep breeds sleep! Many parents are surprised how much sleep their baby needs and may think that if their baby sleeps less in the day he will sleep better at night. However, the opposite is likely to happen, resulting in an overtired baby – unable to feed, settle or sleep properly

3 By establishing a sleep pattern in the first few weeks of his life, your baby will quickly begin to understand and accept a daily routine. For example, following the same routine of a bath, a feed and lullaby or story in the evening becomes a clear signal that sleepy-time is approaching

4 How much sleep each baby needs varies, but in general, in each 24-hour period a newborn needs 16–18 hours

5 Differentiating between day and night early is vital in establishing good sleep patterns. Wake your baby to stay on track with the feeding schedule during the day, but leave him to sleep through the night, only feeding when he wakes hungry. Never wake him at night, unless for a medical reason

6 Getting your baby used to sleeping independently from the start will help him make positive associations with sleep. He needs to learn to self-settle and soothe and be able to fall asleep in his own cot without 'sleep crutches' such as a dummy. Putting him down when still awake and allowing him to fall asleep unaided teaches him the art of independent sleep

7 Ensure that his bedroom is reasonably dark all night. It is not necessary to use 'blackout blinds', though – most ordinary curtains/blinds will do. If babies are used to complete darkness, a change to a lighter environment, say on holiday, may cause settling and sleep problems

8 Don't put toys into your baby's cot – his bed should be a peaceful rather than a stimulating place, plus it is not safe to put toys there

9 In the early weeks, when night feeds are still necessary, keep room lights low, don't over-stimulate your baby and try to carry out the whole process with minimum fuss. You could try not talking or looking at him, though your baby will feel reassured by loving words spoken quietly and a quick cuddle

10 If your baby is unable to self-settle or never seems able to sleep comfortably consider other symptoms (feeding and/or behaviours), as he may be suffering from gastro-oesophageal reflux. Acid reflux is one of the most common reasons why a baby may be unable to sleep comfortably – it can cause pain and this condition needs to be managed before you can expect him to sleep peacefully

(Provided by Alison Scott-Wright / www.alisonscott-wright.com)

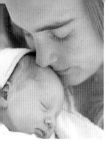

WHEN YOUR BABY CRIES

Your baby's cries are his key to survival and are natural. So try not to be upset when he cries, but respond promptly and calmly – you will soon learn to understand what his various kinds of crying mean.

Crying is the only way that your new baby can communicate his needs to you, so although the noise can be hard to cope with sometimes, try to look upon crying as a 'request' for help rather than a 'demand'. Babies can make a surprisingly loud noise in relation to their size and you may feel embarrassed and upset if he cries in public. Try not to take your baby's crying personally, but respond confidently. If he seems to be working himself into a red-faced fury when you are out, try to stop what you are doing and attend to him. Ask someone for help, if necessary, and get them to assist while you find out what the problem is and what you can do to calm him down. Most people will understand and be willing and able to help.

Timing is vital

Try to remember that the longer you leave your baby to cry, the longer he will take to calm down. Also the stress hormones (see pages 146–7) that his body will release while he is left uncomforted are not good for his short- or long-term physical or mental health.

If a baby is repeatedly left to cry, he may be unable to regulate his response to stress properly and react to even minor problems with fear and aggression, so it is really important that he is comforted when he is upset. You cannot 'spoil' a young baby by soothing his distress – he is unaware that he may be inconveniencing you; he only knows that he is uncomfortable or unhappy. You may not hit upon the correct solution straight away, either, so be prepared

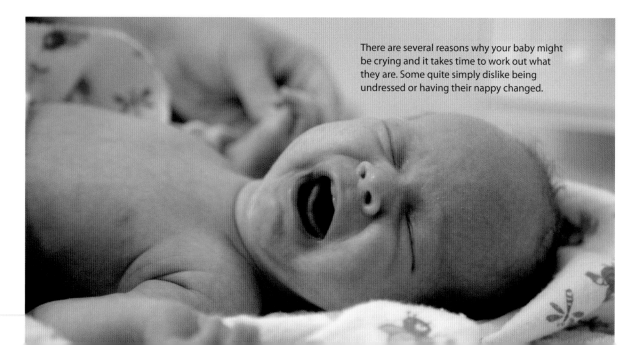

There are several reasons why your baby might be crying and it takes time to work out what they are. Some quite simply dislike being undressed or having their nappy changed.

WHY IS YOUR BABY CRYING?

The most common cause of crying is hunger. So first of all, try feeding your baby

Perhaps your baby has wind and is uncomfortable. Try putting him against your shoulder and rubbing his back (see page 338)

He may be uncomfortable or surprised when he has a bowel movement. Perhaps his nappy is wet or soiled – you may have only just changed him, but he may have just soiled it again – so it's worth checking

He may want to be held or rocked because that is what he was used to in the womb. Try carrying him in your arms or putting him in a baby sling or carrier that you can strap to your body. That way, he may be soothed while you get on with a few other things. Alternatively, put him in his pram and go for a walk

If he seems to wake suddenly and cries immediately, he may be jerking himself awake. Babies' immature nervous systems can cause them to twitch and jerk so much that they wake themselves too soon. Your baby may feel more secure if you gently wrap him in a soft blanket so that his hands are free, but he feels safely enclosed

Check that he is not too hot or too cold by feeling his face and the back of his neck

Perhaps he just wants some attention. Hold him close to you and talk to him softly. Play a gentle game with his fingers or toes and make plenty of eye contact

He may be over-stimulated by visitors or too much going on around him. Take him to a quieter place, such as your bedroom, and try lying quietly with him

Sometimes he may be 'overtired' and so needs some quiet or some 'white noise' to soothe him to sleep. Try putting on soft music or even the washing machine – sometimes simple, rhythmic noise can help overwrought babies to 'switch off'

If your baby's crying seems to happen around the same time each day and is accompanied by him drawing up his knees to his abdomen, as if he is in pain, he may have 'colic'. Talk to your doctor or midwife – they may recommend anti-spasmodic drops. Try winding your baby more often, too, changing his formula if he is bottle-fed or avoiding foods in your diet that may induce wind (see page 331) if you are breastfeeding. You could also give him a gentle massage before a feed

If he often cries or seems to want to feed almost incessantly between 5 and 10 pm, perhaps you need to do a little less during the day. It may be that you feel tired by early evening and so your milk is less satisfying by that time, or he may be picking up on your fatigue and stress as you anticipate his periods of prolonged crying – a vicious cycle. Try to eat a really nutritious lunch and have an afternoon nap or at least a rest. Eat an energy-boosting snack mid-afternoon and have some quiet time with your baby before the evening arrives

to try several things to see what the trouble is (see above). It can be frustrating to find, too, that what works wonderfully one day is of no use the next – one solution will not fit all circumstances every time. Try to remain flexible and talk to your baby softly – he may stop crying in order to hear your voice!

Taking a break

Occasionally, you may even find that your baby simply needs to cry for a while to express frustration and that trying to make him stop makes things worse. If you find his crying is hard to cope with,

try handing him over to your partner or a relative for a while so that you can have a little respite. If you are on your own, take your baby for a brisk walk. The movement and fresh air may be just what he needs to distract him and help him to calm down. You are bound to feel better for it, too.

If your baby has frequent, prolonged bouts of crying, don't suffer in silence – it can make you feel isolated and even depressed, so enlist the help of friends and family and talk to your health visitor or doctor so that any physical cause can be ruled out and you can get some extra support.

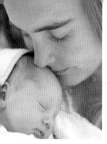

CLEAN & COMFORTABLE

A bath can be relaxing for your baby, but at first you do not need to bathe him every day. The main thing is to keep him clean and comfortable and you can do this by bathing, or topping and tailing.

Bath time

Giving your baby a bath can be relaxing for him, and a useful way to signal the end of the day, but it is not always necessary. Some babies protest at bath time and do not like being undressed or immersed in water, so if you feel that baths are distressing, top and tail your baby instead (see opposite). Take care, too, that frequent baths do not dry your baby's delicate skin. Plain, warm water is fine, but if you want to add anything to it, opt for natural (organic) products for babies that are suitable for sensitive skins.

How to bathe your baby

Make sure that the room is comfortably warm and have soft, clean towels and a flannel ready, along with a clean nappy and fresh clothes. You will also need cotton wool and a bowl of boiled, cooled water for washing his face. It is best to use this rather than bath water, to avoid any risk of infection.

Wash his face Before you put your baby in the bath, wash his face. You could undress him, but leave his nappy on and wrap him in a towel. Then wet a pad of cotton wool and gently wipe his eye from the nose outwards towards his ear. Wash the other eye using a fresh piece of cotton wool. Then use more fresh cotton wool to wipe around his mouth, nose, ears and neck. Pay attention to the folds of his neck.

Wash his hair Keep your baby firmly wrapped in the towel and tuck his legs under your armpit while you support his body with your other forearm. Then lean his head over the bath or washbasin and use a clean flannel to gently wet his hair. Use a few drops of gentle baby shampoo and rinse it off using the flannel or cup some water in your hand. Pat the hair dry with a soft towel.

In the bath

- When the water is the correct temperature, remove your baby's towel and nappy and by sliding your hand and arm across his back, hold the arm furthest away from you. Use your other hand to support his bottom and thighs as you gently lift and lower him into the bath. Make sure his head and neck are supported and keep his face free of the water.

BATH-TIME SAFETY

Never leave your baby unattended in the bath – even for a second – because babies can drown in tiny amounts of water very quickly. If you have to leave the room, pick your baby up, wrap him in a towel and take him with you

Run the cold water into the bath first. Once you have added the hot water, check the temperature carefully by dipping your elbow into it (it should be warm, but not too hot) or use a baby-bath thermometer

If you use a plastic baby bath make sure that it is sitting on a firm, non-slip surface. It may be easier for you if it is set at your waist height, but make sure that you hold your baby securely as you lift him in and out of the bath

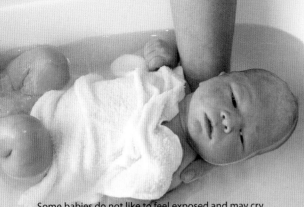

Some babies do not like to feel exposed and may cry when they are uncovered. If this is the case, use a flannel to cover his body in the bath – particularly his chest.

CORD STUMP CARE

It will take between five and 15 days for your baby's umbilical cord stump to dry and drop off. When it does so, there will be a small wound underneath that will take a few more days to heal.

After he is born, your baby's cord stump will be clamped with a plastic clip. Your midwife and health visitor should check how it is healing up when they come to visit you at home, but you will also need to know how to treat it. The most important thing is to keep the area around the stump clean and dry and to fold down the front of your baby's nappy at the very top so that it does not 'catch' the stump and cause irritation.

It is quite normal for the stump to blacken and for it to look a little yellowish, or even green, while it is healing, but if it becomes smelly or there is redness or discharge, ask your midwife or doctor's advice. Clean around the area with plain, cooled, boiled water and a clean flannel or cotton wool pad (avoid using cotton-wool balls as fibres can get wrapped around the cord and cause infection). Do not use lotions, powders or other products on it and try to expose the stump to the air to help it to dry out.

- Keep your baby supported with one hand while you use the other to gently wash his body with a flannel, starting at his shoulders and working your way down. Pay special attention to folds or creases, where perspiration, urine or faeces may collect.
- Lift him out, using both hands in the same way as you lowered him in and put him straight on to a clean, dry towel. Cover him with both sides of it and gently pat him dry, making sure that the creases at the tops of his legs are dried, too.
- Put a clean nappy on, but keep his chest covered with a towel if he seems distressed while you are fastening his clothes.

HOW TO TOP & TAIL YOUR BABY

Make sure that you always wash your baby's face first and his bottom last and that you use fresh cotton-wool pads, or separate, easily identified flannels for each task. They must be boil-washed after every use

You can either use two separate bowls of water (but always use the same one for washing your baby's face), or one bowl of water. Keep your baby away from any draughts and lay him on a dry, flat surface where he cannot roll off (such as a changing mat covered with a soft towel on the floor)

Wet his face flannel or cotton-wool pad and wash his face gently (as left)

Use another part of the flannel or fresh cotton-wool pads to

clean his neck and between his fingers and across his chest and upper tummy, but take special care to avoid his cord stump (see above)

To wash the lower part of his body, use the other flannel or a fresh pad of cotton wool to clean his legs and feet and then the creases at the top of his legs and around his genitals. Make sure that you always clean your baby's bottom from front to back and not the other way around. This is especially important for baby girls, to avoid introducing bacteria from around the anus to the vulva, where it could cause an infection. Lift your baby's legs up and clean his bottom (by wiping away from his anus towards his back)

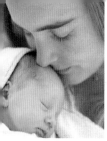

CHANGING & DRESSING

You may be surprised by how often you will need to change and dress and undress your new baby, but with a little advance preparation, you can help these times run smoothly.

You will need to change your baby's clothes and nappies frequently, so it is worthwhile making such mundane tasks as fun for you and your baby as possible. Try to use these times as an opportunity to talk, sing and play games with your baby. He will tolerate being wiped and cleaned and dressed more readily if the process is accompanied by engaging eye contact, smiles and chat. Changing time can also give him the chance to watch your face and mouth as you speak, so he can observe how you form sounds with your lips and tongue. Eventually he will begin to try to copy you.

Safety & convenience

Always dress or change your baby on a secure surface where he cannot roll off. Never leave your baby unattended on a changing table or another surface that is raised off the ground. A plastic changing mat placed on the floor is ideal, but its surface may feel cold, so it may be a good idea to put a soft towel over the upper half where his head and back rests, but keep the lower half uncovered, so that you can clean it up easily.

When dressing your baby try to have everything ready. Babies can find it distressing to have their chests uncovered, so it is a good idea to have a small towel to drape over his torso as you change the rest of his clothes. Try to find garments that open all the way down the front or cross over his chest and buy vests with envelope necks that are relatively easy to

put on over his head. When easing clothes over his head, stretch the garments to avoid dragging them over his nose or ears. To put his arms through sleeves, hold your baby's wrists gently and guide them through one at a time. Cut off labels that may irritate and ties that may pose a choking or strangling risk.

Choosing & changing nappies

It is up to you whether you use disposable nappies or washable, re-useable ones or perhaps a combination of the two. However if you opt for disposables, try to select those that are environmentally friendly. Many are now made using biodegradable materials and manufactured without bleaching agents.

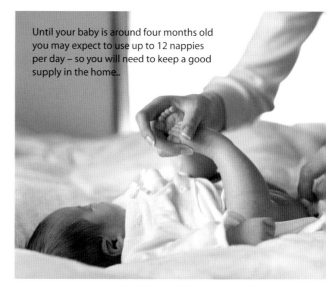

Until your baby is around four months old you may expect to use up to 12 nappies per day – so you will need to keep a good supply in the home..

How to change a disposable nappy

Clean your baby's bottom from front to back using gentle baby wipes or clean water.

Lift your baby's legs together and as you raise his bottom off the changing mat, slide the clean nappy underneath. The tabs at each side should be just level with his waist. If your baby is a boy, try to make sure that his penis is pointing downwards, to avoid the urine being deposited at the top of his nappy. Bring the front of his nappy up between his legs.

Make sure that the nappy fits snugly, then smooth out the front and fold it over, if necessary, to avoid it touching the cord stump (see page 345). Draw the tabs across the front of the nappy and fasten them, making sure that the nappy is snug, but not too tight.

Changing a reusable nappy

There is a variety of fastenings available to choose from. Some nappies are held in place by plastic pants, while others have clips or clamps, while some are pre-shaped and feature Velcro strips or poppers. It is much easier to deal with messy bowel movements if you use nappy liners. Some reusable versions have a waterproof backing, but if they do not, you will need to use waterproof pants over the cloth nappies.

If you are not using a pre-shaped nappy you will need to fold the cloth. Form a rectangle by folding the nappy in half, then fold one of the shorter sides around one-third of the way down. This will create a thicker part, which is more absorbent, to place at the front of the nappy for a boy and at the back for a girl. Keep the top edge level with your baby's waist. Now bring the cloth between your baby's legs and secure the sides before putting on the waterproof pants.

To wash the nappies you will need two buckets (one for urine-soaked nappies, the other for faeces-soiled ones). Fill both buckets with sterilising fluid and soak for a minimum of six hours. Remove the nappies with tongs and place them in the washing machine. Wash at 60°C (140°F). Dry them outside, if possible, and then put them in a tumble dryer with a fabric softening sheet to re-fluff and keep them soft.

YOUR BABY'S NAPPY

In the first few days your baby will pass meconium, the dark greenish-black substance made up of waste matter accumulated in his bowels before birth (see page 178). If your baby is breastfed his stools will be soft and almost liquid, yellow or possibly slightly yellow-green in colour and containing white lumps resembling cottage cheese.

Once breastfeeding is established your baby's nappies will be bright yellow, which will turn green if the baby is hungry (nature's way of telling us to give more feeds). If your baby is taking formula milk he will probably have slightly fewer bowel movements (formula takes longer to digest) and his stools are likely to be darker and firmer. They may also smell more strongly. If your baby's stools are hard or dry, or he seems to have difficulty passing them he may be constipated or dehydrated. Consult your midwife or doctor and increase your own fluids and frequency of feeds if you are breastfeeding. If you are using formula, speak to your doctor or midwife, but check that the proportions are correct or consider using a different brand and encourage your baby to drink more. If there is mucus or blood in your baby's stools, contact your doctor now.

NAPPY RASH

Nappy rash can be extremely uncomfortable for babies and is caused by their skin coming into contact with urine or faeces. The best way to prevent it is to make sure that you change your baby's nappy frequently. Try to let him have some time without his nappy on, too, so that the air can freely circulate over his skin.

Opt for fragrance-free wipes or plain water when you clean his bottom and if you are using reusable cloth nappies, make sure that they are properly rinsed to eradicate any traces of detergent.

You could also use a barrier cream on his bottom occasionally, but it should not be essential at every change.

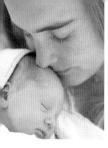

looking after yourself

SELF-CARE

Try not to put too much pressure on yourself. You have just been through a life-changing experience, so you may need a little time to settle down. If you are ready to go out with your new baby, then do so, but listen to your body and do whatever feels right for you.

A s you begin to recover after the birth of the baby, you may notice further changes in your body and your feelings. Try to give yourself time to adjust. Rest as much as you can and continue to eat a healthy, balanced diet, especially if you are breastfeeding (see pages 330–1). Once paternity leave is over for your partner and you are alone with your baby, things can sometimes seem a little overwhelming. Try to talk to friends and family and accept any offers of help – or simply ask for it if it is not volunteered.

Support systems

Use the support of your health visitor, too, she will be keeping an eye on your progress (see pages 360–1), but if you are concerned about something, ask for advice. It will take a while for you and your partner to really get to grips with your new roles as parents (see pages 350–1), but in the meantime one of the best ways to deal with new parenthood is to keep the channels of communication open and keep talking. Going for regular short walks together with your baby can be a great way to talk over issues and get away from nagging chores. Fresh air and exercise can do wonders for your spirits, but don't overdo it.

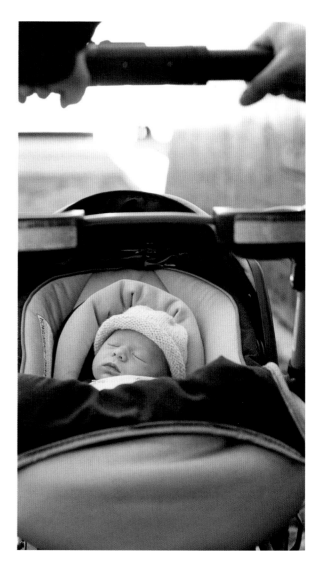

Wrap your baby up snugly and go out for a gentle walk together. It will do you both the world of good.

SELF-CARE Q&AS

"I seem to be sweating almost all the time – especially when I breastfeed my baby. Is there something wrong with me?"

This is perfectly normal and is a result of your body getting rid of all the excess fluid that it has been carrying around during pregnancy. Your metabolic rate speeds up with breastfeeding, so you will perspire more then, too.

Expect to perspire like this for up to six weeks, but do not try to limit your fluid intake. In fact, you can help the process along if you drink plenty of water and diluted fruit juice. Take regular showers or baths to keep feeling fresh and wear cotton fabrics next to your skin (try to wear cotton nursing bras, in particular). If you feel shivery or have a fever, though, contact your doctor to rule out any illness or infection.

"Every time I brush or wash my hair it seems to come out in handfuls. Should I see my doctor about it?"

You could have your iron levels checked, but usually hair loss is nothing to worry about and is perfectly normal after giving birth. You may remember that your hair seemed unusually thick and strong during pregnancy, when you probably shed less of it than usual. This is just what you would have lost over those nine months and is due to dramatic changes in your hormone levels. Try to treat your hair gently until it recovers, so use mild shampoos and do not brush it too vigorously.

"It is two weeks since my baby arrived, but now that she has, my lovely round bump has turned into a sagging, flabby lump. When will my body get back to normal?"

Try to be patient with your body – it has been through a lot! On average, most women lose around 5 kg (12 lb) when they give birth, but it takes a while for the skin that has been stretched so far to tighten up again. Your uterus will be gradually contracting to its normal size and position (if you are breastfeeding this process will be speeded up), but you will still have some fluid retention, which may take up to six weeks to eliminate and your muscles are not yet ready to be toned back into shape. Do not be tempted to go on a weight-loss diet – your body needs to recover and you should try to eat a really nutritious menu of food to regain your strength. Looking after your new baby will burn up plenty of calories and when you are stronger you can start some gentle exercise. However, for now try to relax and concentrate on getting to know your newborn.

"My friend, who had a baby last year, says that my baby should already be following a set routine so that I can get chores done while she sleeps. But I feel too exhausted to know where to start – should I be making more of an effort?"

If you are looking after your baby and taking time to rest and recuperate from labour and birth, you are doing exactly the right thing. In many cultures (especially in the Far East), it is common to believe that a new mother should do nothing around the house except just be with their baby for the first six weeks! It is really important that you spend this precious time with your baby and that you do not wear yourself out, because exhaustion will make you much more susceptible to postnatal depression (PND – see pages 356–9).

Sadly, I know from personal experience that it is easy to get hung up on trying to do everything and being 'superwoman'. With my second child, I was up and about too soon to take care of myself properly and I ended up with PND.

Talk to your partner and if he is unable to take on more of the domestic tasks, see if you can get some help with the chores – if the state of your home is bothering you.

Eat well and get plenty of rest and ask your doctor to test you for anaemia, just in case. Draw the curtains and sleep whenever you baby does. Try not to worry about what other people do or think, but instead concentrate on your baby.

By being attuned to his needs in the vital early days you will be laying solid foundations for a good relationship with him in the future and that is far more important than a clean kitchen floor.

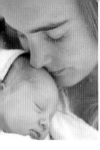

the transition to parenthood

FINDING A NEW BALANCE

After the euphoria of birth and the arrival of your baby, the early days of being new parents can present you with a steep learning curve. Being responsible for your baby 24 hours a day can feel challenging – a new experience that can affect you in different ways.

In the early days of parenthood it is common for men to feel very protective towards their partners and babies, while women often feel emotional and weepy. Some men then feel that they should be able to 'fix' things and become frustrated when there is no simple solution. In return, women are perplexed by what they see as the inability of their partners to respond to emotions.

In many spheres of life it is common for men and women to react to things differently, but when this is combined with the exhaustion of early parenthood, it can make relations between couples tense. Try to recognise that lack of sleep causes frayed tempers.

IF YOU ARE ON YOUR OWN

There is no doubt that having a baby on your own can be tough, but that doesn't mean yours won't have the best of upbringings. Whether you are a single parent by choice or not, you still need support. Make use of networks such as mother-and-baby groups and ask friends and family to help out so that you have time to yourself sometimes. Making decisions can seem daunting if all responsibility falls on you. However your health visitor may be able to connect you with other single parents or organisations (see Resources) who can offer advice. Ensure you are getting any available financial help and if you are in contact with your baby's father, try to involve him in your baby's life – you may be able to work together as parents.

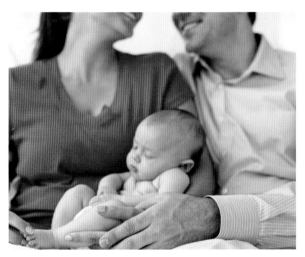

Take time to nurture your relationship as a couple while you are getting used to being a family.

If you become irritable, remember that this is a passing stage. Your relationship as a couple may change and while things shift it may feel strange, but you will find a new balance to accommodate you all.

The division of labour

It will help if you talk about what expectations you have of each other regarding chores and baby care and it may be useful to list jobs that need doing. Find out what jobs you both like and split those you don't, prioritising what has to be done and what is less important. Care for your baby together, remembering that he belongs to both of you. Even if

MAKING LIFE EASIER

Clear your diaries and restrict visitors

Try to sleep whenever your baby sleeps

Ask grandparents or friends to take your baby out between feeds so that you can rest properly

Sleep in separate rooms for a while so that one of you gets some uninterrupted sleep and can relieve the other for a while in the daytime. Make sure, though, that you talk about this first and agree on it as a temporary measure

Fill the freezer with lots of easy-to-cook food

If family or friends offer to help, ask them to make a meal or shop for food. If they don't offer, ask them to help anyway

Investigate online shopping deliveries and set up shopping lists that you can simply update when you need to

Order baby necessities, equipment and clothes online

Lower your standards; don't fret if your home is not as clean as you would like. Consider employing someone to help

you breastfeed, your partner can help settle the baby afterwards. Accept caring as a joint project and try not to be critical of each other – you cannot expect perfection – from yourselves or each other – and you need to accept that you will do things differently.

Your finances

Babies change the financial balance in the family and this can lead to issues surfacing regarding money and work. Women can find it hard to accept financial dependence and men may be resentful of the new demands and financial pressures that are placed on them. It's good to talk about money issues before the baby is born. Remember that you are a partnership.

You as a couple

The well-being of your relationship is very important and it is not selfish to take time to talk and listen to each other. Try to stop resentments building up by expressing positive feelings to each other whenever issues arise. Make time to have fun and be friends and lovers as well as parents.

It may be months before your sex life resumes and there may be physical discomfort at first, so be prepared to be patient. Also coping with tiredness and the demands of your baby may lead to a loss of libido –it's worth noting that many women experience a certain satisfaction if they are breastfeeding and so may feel less desire for sex.

THINKING ABOUT FINANCES

Draw up a budget, including income and expenditure, before and after the baby is born

Be honest about any debts and build them into your post-baby budget

Talk to each other about how you view financial dependence and responsibility

Work out how your personal expenses will be managed and how money should be organised between you

DON'T FORGET GRANDPARENTS

When you start to think about returning to work or resuming a social life, you may want to ask grandparents to help. Most will be pleased to be involved, but do respect the fact that they have their own lives, too. Try to involve them in positive ways:

Make grandparents feel wanted and welcome. Some are reluctant to offer help in case they seem interfering

Don't assume that grandparents can drop their own plans at a moment's notice and make sure that you thank them

If grandparents take on regular caring duties, make sure you discuss your expectations of feeding, sleeping and 'discipline' so that there is less room for misunderstanding

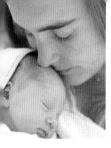

INTERACTION

Although the first weeks of parenthood can seem a bit of a blur and you may begin to wonder how you will ever get back to some sort of routine, this time – slowly but surely getting to know your baby – is time well spent.

Just as you stimulated your baby when he was in your womb (see pages 188–9), so he needs interaction now, too. Babies are born with a surprising array of reflexes (see page 307) and are ready-programmed to learn – your baby will learn more in his first year of life than at any other time. Play is the essential tool for learning and if you can help him with age- and stage-appropriate activities you will be setting up a life-long love of learning.

Encouraging development

Although his vision is not yet fully developed he can focus on objects 20 to 25 cm (8 to 12 in) away and even in the early days, he will love to do this, though he will prefer his parents' faces above all else. By talking to him as you carry out everyday tasks, such as changing his nappy, you will give him the chance to watch you as you form words. By the time he is six or eight weeks old you may notice that he responds to what you say and is increasing the range of sounds he can make. Keep talking to him – give him a commentary on what you are doing or tell him a funny story and build in some pauses so that you enable him to respond. Although he cannot yet form words, he is trying to communicate with you and if you allow him to contribute, you will be having your first 'conversations'. Very soon, too, perhaps as early as four or five weeks after his birth, you may be rewarded with his first smile.

Ways to have fun with your baby

- Your baby needs 'tummy time' to help his neck and back muscles develop, so put him on a soft mat or baby gym for a few minutes each day.
- Choose a baby gym with contrasting colours and shapes, with 'noisy', textured fabrics and hanging toys. At first, your baby may just look and listen, but once he is two or three months old he will realise he can bat at the toys.
- Play music, but keep the volume low. Try tunes you played while when you were pregnant. See how he reacts. Hold him close and gently dance to the rhythm. If he is fractious, choose soothing tunes.
- Repeat rhymes and tap out the rhythm of the words on his feet and hands so that he 'feels' the language.
- Show him patterns on a soft cloth book. A black and white one is easiest for him to see. In time, he will hold it and run his eyes over each page.
- Give him a soft rattle. By three months he may hold it for himself if you put it in his hand – though he will not yet know how to let it go (see page 365).
- Exaggerate your facial expressions, gently tickle him and bicycle his legs. Sing songs to him about his body and touch each part as you say it.

Note: Some babies are easily over-stimulated and become distressed when they feel bombarded with too many sensations. If your baby cries when you play with him, choose a quieter activity.

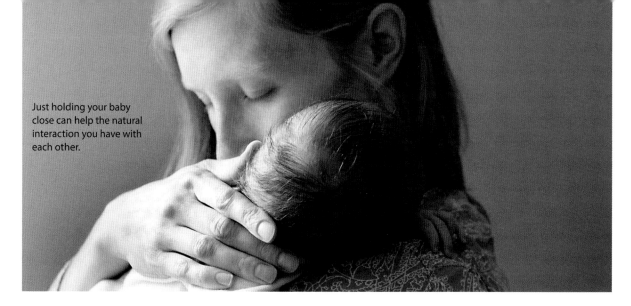

Just holding your baby close can help the natural interaction you have with each other.

BABY MASSAGE

Touch is vitally important for your baby and massage is an excellent way to build a better relationship with your baby. Studies have shown that it benefits babies in a number of ways and that premature babies who are regularly massaged are stronger than those who are not.

Massage also seems to help to prevent postnatal depression (see pages 356–9) by strengthening the bond between mother and baby. Not only does gentle massage help you to establish a close physical relationship, but it also improves your baby's circulation, flexibility and coordination. It may help him to sleep more peacefully and expel excess wind (making it especially useful for babies who suffer from colic – see page 343).

You and your partner do not need to learn special massage techniques, although a baby massage class can be a good way to get to know other babies and parents and pick up valuable skills. The main thing is to use soft, gentle, rhythmic strokes and to take your cues from your baby.

You could use a simple oil such as sweet almond oil, grapeseed or olive oil to make your strokes more even and smooth, but avoid essential oils (unless they are recommended by a qualified aromatherapist experienced in treating babies). Make sure that no oil is used near your baby's eyes, mouth or genitals.

Ensure that the room is really warm and that your baby is not placed near a draught. When he is very tiny you can massage him on your lap, but it is easiest if you spread a soft towel on his changing mat. If he seems unhappy at the start, then cover him again and wait for a better moment. Let his reactions guide you.

If you are using massage oils, make sure that you warm them on your hands first

Place your baby on his back and use long, gentle rhythmic strokes from head to neck, then down his arms and all over his hands (paying attention to fingers and thumbs). Stroke his chest and tummy and then move your hands in a clockwise and anti-clockwise direction over his tummy (and back again when you turn him over). Stroke his legs, feet and toes

Gently turn him on to his tummy, so that his head is facing to one side and repeat the process down his back. If your baby suffers from colic, you can try paying special attention to the muscles in his lower back. Taking care not to press too hard, use the flats of your hands to make circular movements over the area

When you have finished, cover your baby with a towel (and make sure that he does not get cold while you are massaging him). If you have used some oil, make sure that you wipe off the excess so that he is not too slippery to handle when you pick him up

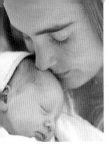

when to call a doctor

COMMON CONCERNS

All babies get ill from time to time, but it can be worrying when yours is unwell for the first time. Keep calm and monitor your baby carefully. Contact your doctor if you continue to be concerned.

As you get to know your baby better you will notice if anything seems unusual. Perhaps your baby is crying more than you are used to or seems reluctant to feed. If you suspect that your baby may be ill, keep a close eye on his symptoms. All babies have to go through some illness in order to strengthen the immune system, but if you are worried, call your doctor. Trust your instincts and remember that you know your baby better than anyone else.

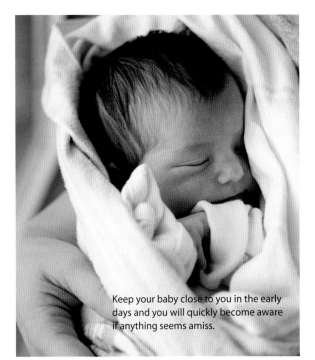

Keep your baby close to you in the early days and you will quickly become aware if anything seems amiss.

WHEN TO CALL A DOCTOR

As a new parent it is often hard to know whether your baby is ill or not – you are unsure about symptoms and you feel very anxious and your gut feelings come into play. Newborn babies can become ill very quickly and so it is important to keep a close eye on your baby if he seems ill. If you are in any doubt, call the doctor and particularly if your baby has any of the following symptoms:

A fever of 100.4°F (38°C) or higher

Unusually pale skin or bluish colouring around the mouth

A floppy or stiff body

Projectile vomiting

Vomiting that lasts for more than five hours or is accompanied by diarrhoea or fever

Diarrhoea that is producing more than six watery soilings per day

Blood in the stools

Redness or tenderness around the tummy

Refusal to feed over a period of several hours

Pink or bloodshot eyes, sticky white discharge from the eye or eyes that seem stuck together

White patches in the mouth

A severely blocked nose that makes it difficult to feed

Crying for an unusually long period or in an unusual manner

COMMON ILLNESS Q&AS

"My newborn baby is only four days old and seemed fine in the hospital, but now that we have taken him outside in daylight I think he looks yellow. Could he have jaundice?"

It is very common for babies to develop neonatal jaundice shortly after birth (as many as 50 per cent of babies born in the UK may be affected). It is caused by a build-up of bilirubin, which is a natural waste product of the blood. If your baby was bruised during birth he may be more susceptible to jaundice, because the extra blood under the skin has to be broken down. Talk to your midwife about it. Most commonly, neonatal jaundice clears up by itself after a few days or so, as the baby's liver begins to work more efficiently. If your baby does require treatment he may be given controlled amounts of safe ultraviolet (UV) light, which breaks down the excess bilirubin. Treatment is usually given in hospital by using a 'biliblanket', which swaddles the baby while he is receiving treatment in the cot on the ward.

"We took our newborn out for a short walk a few days after he was born and he was well wrapped up, but now I feel terrible because he has developed a nasty cold. His nose seems to be blocked and it's difficult for him to feed. Does he need antibiotics or something?"

Colds are all too common in new babies. Most babies can expect to catch at least eight to 10 in their first year of life, so try not to worry and don't feel guilty about taking him out. Make sure that your baby's head is covered outside at all times and that the rest of him is warm. You cannot completely protect him from every bug. Try to sit him a little more upright when he is feeding and if he is very snuffly, sit in the bathroom with him and run a warm bath. The steam from the tap may help to unblock his nose and enable him to breathe more easily. Antibiotics will not do anything to get rid of a cold, but keep an eye on him and call your doctor for advice if he seems to have a fever or a cough.

"My baby had perfect-looking skin, but he has now got a red rash on his face. Could he be allergic to something?"

It is extremely common for new babies to develop spots and rashes. Their delicate skin has been protected from the air until birth, so like the rest of their body, it now has to cope with the unfamiliar elements of the outside world. Many babies have milia, which are white spots caused by blocked sebaceous glands, sometimes called 'milk spots', or they may have a rash that sounds similar to your baby's. Both problems are partly due to some of your hormones remaining in your baby's body after birth and should disappear of their own accord after a few days. It is very unlikely that your baby's rash is an allergic reaction or an infection, but if it persists or you are concerned, ask your health visitor or doctor to examine it.

"My baby's eyes seem to have a yellow discharge and one is red and swollen in one corner. What should I do?"

Conjunctivitis is sometimes known as 'sticky eye' and is usually caused by a viral infection, such as a cold, but it is sometimes caused by a bacterial infection developed in a blocked tear duct. Keep your baby's eyes clean by using a separate pad of new, clean cotton wool for each eye. Moisten the pad with cooled, boiled water and wipe from the inner corner to the outer part once and then throw the pad away. If the eye is still not clear of discharge, repeat, but use a fresh pad each time. If his eyes do not clear in a day or so, see your doctor. You may need some antibiotic drops to clear up an infection.

"My baby has been reluctant to feed for a couple of days and has white patches on his tongue. He also has a nasty nappy rash. Might he be allergic to my breast milk?"

It is mostly likely to be oral thrush. You may have had a vaginal infection that was passed on during birth. See your doctor – you will need oral medication and antifungal cream for your nipples. The infection should clear up quickly but you should try to get more rest and eat less sugar and refined carbohydrates (see page 79). It is also a good idea to drink plenty of water, eat live probiotic yogurt and avoid coffee and alcohol. Bathe your baby's sore bottom with plain water and ask your doctor for some cream to soothe it.

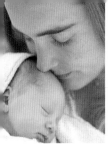

'BABY BLUES' & PND

Early parenthood can be a bumpy ride. One minute you might feel euphoric, the next hopeless and overwhelmed. Most mothers experience a short period of feeling low, but bounce right back, but some find things more difficult. However, prompt help can make a huge difference and life can become much happier again.

If you did not fall in love with your baby the instant that you saw him, don't blame yourself. The bonding process doesn't happen instantly for every mother, and if you had a difficult labour and birth it may be that you need time to recover before you are able to connect properly with your baby. But don't worry – it will happen. Bonding with your baby is a process and for some mothers it starts more slowly – but just because it takes longer, it does not mean that it is not happening and it doesn't mean that you are a 'bad' mother. You will bond with your baby over time and it will happen because of the difficult periods as well as the happy ones, so try not to expend precious energy fretting about it.

What are 'baby blues'?

The 'baby blues' are extremely common and affect around 85 per cent of all mothers shortly after birth. In fact this phenomenon is so common that midwives and health visitors almost expect to see some signs of low spirits on day three or four after the delivery of the baby.

Baby blues are not the same as postnatal depression (PND), though. The blues are short-lived and are primarily caused by fluctuating hormones, so they usually start just as your milk comes in. You are probably at your most tired and uncomfortable at this point and it may seem odd that just when you expected to feel euphoric you suddenly feel tearful and overwhelmed. Baby blues usually resolve themselves within a few weeks, when your hormones start to settle down and life begins to seem a little less chaotic. For some women, though (around 10 to 15 per cent), the blues do not go away, but deepen into a depression that typically reaches its peak at about ten weeks after delivery.

The bonding process may not happen instantly. Give yourself time to recover from the birth first.

POSTNATAL DEPRESSION (PND)

Signs and symptoms may include:

Anxiety

Guilt

Tearfulness

Lack of enthusiasm or enjoyment of motherhood

Indifference towards people you usually love (also feelings of hostility towards them)

Irritability

Disturbed sleep and early-morning waking

Listlessness and exhaustion

Difficulty in making decisions and feelings of confusion

Loss of appetite and a dry mouth

Low self-esteem, feelings of self-disgust and a lack of confidence in being a mother

Complete loss of libido

Shame at the lack of feelings for your baby

Fear of harming yourself or your baby

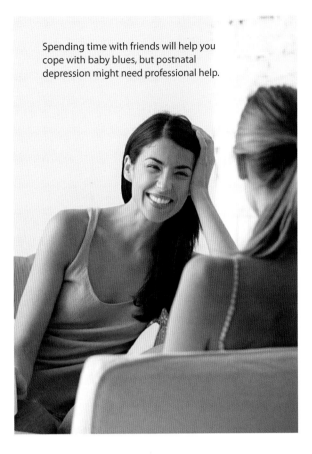

Spending time with friends will help you cope with baby blues, but postnatal depression might need professional help.

What is postnatal depression (PND)?

Many women who are affected by PND feel ashamed that they cannot enjoy their babies as they expected to and so find it hard to admit that they have a problem. However, midwives and health visitors are trained to spot signs of PND and when they come to visit you at home they will take care to find out about all aspects of your recovery after your baby's birth. You will probably be asked how you are finding life as a new mum and you may be given a questionnaire to fill in. If you suspect that you are finding it difficult to bounce back, talk to your midwife, health visitor or doctor, because prompt treatment can make a huge difference.

If your PND is fairly mild, it may be that you simply need more practical and emotional support from those around you and that once some of your difficulties have been addressed your depression will be short-lived. If your PND is more serious, it may require treatment with antidepressant medication that is safe to take while breastfeeding (if you are doing so) as well as counselling or psychotherapy. If you had a complicated delivery or have suffered from depression in the past you are more likely to develop

SELF-HELP TIPS FOR PND

Eat healthily and include plenty of fresh fruit and vegetables, and foods containing B vitamins (see page 84)

Be kind to yourself. If you cannot manage to do everything yourself, set realistic, achievable targets and stick to them

Get help – don't suffer in silence

Get some gentle exercise out of the house

Talk to a health professional

PND, but there may be other triggers such as a longer-lasting hormonal imbalance, genetic factors or personal circumstances such as financial worries, relationship difficulties or bereavement. The symptoms may not become apparent until after your postnatal check and can develop during the first year after the birth. It can be debilitating and while you have the illness it may be difficult for you to be objective and recognise how much it is affecting you.

High expectations

Quite often, women who have had high-flying careers and are used to being in control can be surprised to find they are feeling low and vulnerable. It may be that they are expecting too much of themselves and because they are high achievers they aim for perfection in motherhood. If this sounds like you, try to remember that there is no such thing as the 'perfect' mother. The important thing is to be an attentive, responsive parent, but even with the best will in the world, this can be difficult and extremely tough when suffering from depression.

Effects on the baby

While you are affected by the condition it may be hard to feel you are worthy of help, but it is important that you do get some for your baby's sake as well as your own. Studies have shown that when mothers are suffering from PND some babies become withdrawn and stop seeking attention – they are beginning to learn that it will not be given. Other babies are far more demanding, crying more loudly and more often and even showing signs of rage. This can make things even harder for a mother who is already struggling. The aim of your healthcare team is to get mothers and babies back on track and to help them to enjoy their relationship, so do not to hide your difficulties. Some women also experience changes in their thyroid function after they have given birth and the lethargy and other symptoms associated with such a problem can be mistaken for depression, or may even contribute to its

development. PND is an illness, so it is not your fault if you get it and it does not betray weakness in your character. The important thing is to be honest with your healthcare provider because the more information they have about the nature of the problem, the better they can treat your illness and help you to overcome it quickly.

Nutrients

There are deficiencies in certain nutrients that have been associated with depression: specifically essential fatty acids and especially omega-3 (DHA). Building up stores of these during your pregnancy will help. In addition, lack of vitamin D, iron and zinc can leave you feeling low.

Complementary therapies

Consult your midwife or doctor before you try any complementary therapies and make sure that your practitioners are fully qualified and accredited.

Acupuncture An acupuncturist may aim to improve your flow of qi (see pages 38–9). Consult a practitioner experienced in treating PND.

Aromatherapy A few drops of essential oil of jasmine, mandarin, grapefruit or bergamot, diluted first in some carrier oil (such as sweet almond, or grapeseed oil) can be added to your bath water or used as a massage oil.

Homeopathy Take care to follow the manufacturer's dosage instructions, but remedies are best prescribed by a professional homeopath to match your precise symptoms. Contact a registered homeopath.

- For tearfulness (that does not give you relief), feelings of hopelessness and sleeplessness: sepia 30c.
- For low self-esteem and fear of failure: lycopodium 30c.
- To help with mood swings and difficulties adjusting to the reality of motherhood rather than its idealised version: ignatia 30c.
- For deep disappointment and tearfulness, dismay at being unable to enjoy motherhood: pulsatilla 30c.

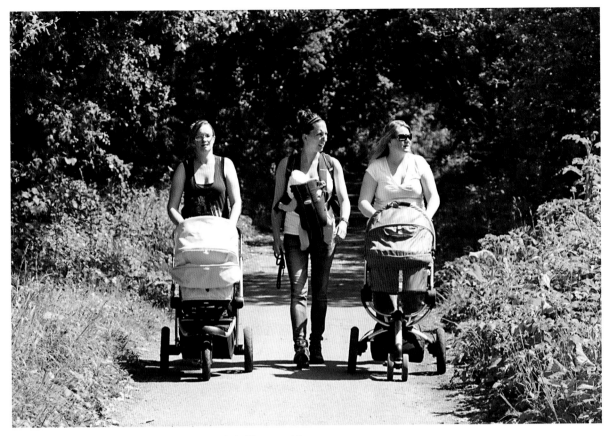

Getting out of doors with other new parents can help lift your spirits.

WAYS TO COPE WITH PND

Try to get out of the house at least once a day – to avoid becoming isolated. Even a quick trip to the shops will help. At the very least, make sure that you get dressed every morning

Get help in the home so that chores don't overwhelm you

Meet up with other new mothers as often as you can – you will probably find that they are facing many of the same difficulties as you and you may be able to help each other

Don't keep your problems to yourself – talk to your partner, friends, family and accept any offers of practical help that others give you. Seek help and support from friends

Talk to your midwife, health visitor or doctor – they are experienced in dealing with such problems and are there to help you. No one will judge you. Consider counselling

and therapies such as cognitive behavioural therapy (CBT), hypnotherapy and acupuncture. A psychologist will help with your mindset, if necessary

Take regular, gentle exercise. Arrange to exercise with others

Eat regularly and have nutritious snacks throughout the day to keep your blood-sugar levels stable. If you go without food you will feel low and lethargic

Ask your partner for a massage (perhaps with some uplifting essential oils such as mandarin, rose or jasmine). Gentle touch can be very therapeutic and will help you to reconnect with your partner and your happier self

Arrange a few treats for yourself and get a friend or relative to babysit for a little while

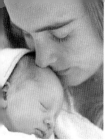

YOUR POSTNATAL CHECK

Between six and eight weeks after delivery, you and your baby will see your doctor for a full check-up. Your postnatal check is designed to ensure that you and your baby are both physically and emotionally well and it offers you an important opportunity to ask about any concerns that you may have.

At this postnatal appointment you can expect to have the following important physical and emotional checks:

- Your blood pressure will be taken.
- You will be asked to provide a urine sample to test for the presence of protein or blood.
- You may have a blood test to check for anaemia and thyroid function.
- You will be weighed and given dietary advice.
- Your breasts and nipples may be checked.
- Your abdomen will be examined and your uterus palpated to make sure that it has fully contracted. If you had a Caesarean, your scar will be examined.
- Your perineum will be examined if you had tears or an episiotomy.
- Your vagina will also be examined to make sure that it has healed and that you have no pain or discomfort. If you had a complicated or difficult delivery, you may also have an internal examination.
- A smear test – if you are due one.

Expect to be asked:
- What was your labour and delivery like and how do you feel about the experience?
- Are you breastfeeding? Do you have any concerns?
- Is your perineum healing well?

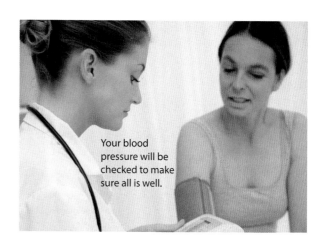

Your blood pressure will be checked to make sure all is well.

- Do you have any discharge, discomfort or pain?
- Are your bladder and bowels functioning normally?
- Have you had sex? You may be worried about resuming sex, especially if you have had an episiotomy. If you have pain or discomfort speak to your midwife or doctor. What form of contraceptive are you using or planning to use?
- Are you getting practical and emotional support?
- How are your moods and how are you sleeping?
- What is your diet like and are you taking exercise?
- Are you doing pelvic floor exercises and have you had any stress incontinence?
- Do you have any concerns about your baby?
- Does your baby seem to be content and responsive?

Exercise in company. Seek out mum-and-baby exercise groups in your area and start to make new friends for yourself and your baby.

GETTING SOME EXERCISE

You can get back to doing pelvic floor exercises (see page 141) almost immediately after the birth of your baby (or as soon as is comfortable for you) and more general exercise is a good idea once you have recovered from labour and birth. If you have had a Caesarean you should take care not to do abdominal exercises too soon (ask your midwife or doctor about when this should be), but if the birth was quite straightforward you may want to think about getting back into shape from now on.

Take things gently

Begin with some very simple stretching exercises. You can try these when your baby is sleeping or while he is in his bouncy chair (see page 166). Don't forget, though, that the muscles and ligaments in your body will have softened in preparation for labour and birth, so you must take care not to overstretch them and put too much strain on them. Once you have stopped bleeding (see page 312) you can go swimming, which is an ideal way to get active again. The water will help to support your body and soothe any aching back or limbs. Swimming and exercise in general, provided it is not too strenuous, will relax you and encourage the release of endorphins, the 'happy hormones' that raise your spirits and lighten your mood.

Exercise for strength

Try to exercise for strength rather than for weight loss. If you are breastfeeding you will need to eat really well to ensure a good supply of milk for your baby as well as energy for your own body to function at its best. Breastfeeding burns up a lot of calories – in fact just looking after a new baby does that, so you need to eat a balanced nutritious diet.

A little regular exercise will boost your metabolism and actually give you more energy, but be careful not to overdo it. You could try joining a mother-and-baby exercise class, where you can do some simple stretching exercises and yoga or pilates alongside your baby. These have the added bonus of bringing you together with other new mums.

Try to concentrate on rebuilding your strength and stamina. If organised classes seem a step too far at this stage, then try getting together with a friend or two and take your babies out for walks. As time goes on (and if you have a robust enough buggy) you could jog while pushing your babies along. Choose the kind of exercise that you will enjoy and try to meet up with other people to do it – you are more likely to continue with it if you commit to meeting up with others – and you and your baby can make new friends at the same time.

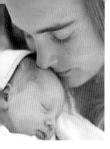

HEALTH & DEVELOPMENT

During the next few years of his life, if you live in the UK, your baby will be given a series of appointments with health professionals to test and assess his health and development. These are a good way to keep an eye on his progress and explore any concerns you may have.

Your baby's six-week check

At the same time that you have your six-week postnatal check, your baby will also be examined. He will be given a full physical check and an assessment of his developmental progress. Checks will include:

• Your baby's weight and length will be measured and recorded in the Personal Child Health Record (see opposite).

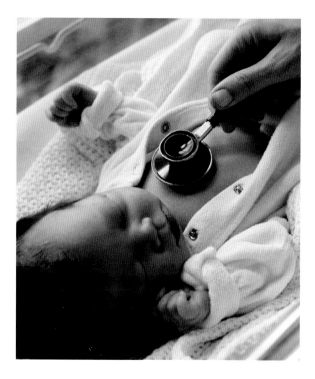

• Your baby's head circumference will be measured and the fontanelles (see page 302) will be checked.
• His eyes, ears and mouth will be checked (there will be hearing and vision tests carried out at separate appointments – see below).
• Your baby's breathing, lungs and heart will be listened to, using a stethoscope.
• His abdomen and the major organs, such as the liver and kidneys, will be gently felt.
• Your baby's genitals will be checked (if he is a boy, the doctor will check that his testes are properly descended).
• His hips will be checked for proper alignment and their stability will be tested.
• Your baby's reflexes (see page 307) will be carefully tested, including the grasp reflex, your baby's muscle tone and his head control.

You will also be asked about your baby's general well-being and details about how he is feeding and sleeping, and what the contents of his nappies are like. This is a good opportunity for you to discuss any concerns you may have and to gain more information about the schedule of health checks that will be offered to your baby, including vaccinations (see opposite).

A stethoscope will be used to check your baby's breathing, heart and lungs.

YOUR BABY'S HEALTH CHECKS

Besides being weighed and measured, your baby will be given a number of tests and reviews to make sure that all is well. Between his birth and his first day at school you can expect the following:

One to three days Newborn Checks – a general physical examination that includes checking your baby's head, mouth, heart, lungs, hands, feet, legs and arms, abdomen, hips and spine (see pages 306–7). It is usually carried out by a paediatrician in hospital, but may be done by a trained midwife in your own home

One day to one month Newborn Hearing Test – This is to check that your baby's hearing is normal. It may be carried out either before you leave hospital after the birth or by a health visitor in your home or at your local clinic

Five to eight days Newborn Heel-Prick Test – This is a blood test for phenylketonuria, congenital hypothyroidism, cystic fibrosis and sickle cell disorders and is done by taking a tiny sample of blood from your baby's heel

Six to eight weeks The Six-Week Postnatal Check – This is a full physical examination and assessment of your baby's health and progress (see opposite)

Eight weeks onwards Routine Vaccinations – In his first two years, your baby will be offered a number of routine vaccinations and will then receive 'booster' vaccinations before he starts school

Six to eight months Hearing Assessment – This is a second hearing test, but if your baby did not have a newborn hearing test, he may also be offered a distraction test at this assessment

Between eight and 36 months General Health Review – You may be offered a general review of your baby's health and progress sometime between eight and 12 months after birth, and again when he is two years of age

Between four and five years School Entry Screening – This will include vision and hearing tests and a height and weight check as well as a review of your baby's vaccinations and general health

The Personal Child Health Record

Your midwife or health visitor will give you a Personal Child Health Record (PCHR), which you should take to all appointments.

Your baby will usually be weighed about once a month until he is six months old, and then once every two months until he reaches his first birthday. He may also be weighed whenever he has his routine vaccinations (see page 364) and more often if there is concern. Regular weighing is important because steady gain is a sign that your baby is feeding well and is generally healthy. In the first week or so after birth, it is common for babies to lose weight, so he will be weighed to make sure he regains his birth weight. Two weeks after birth, four out of five healthy babies will have regained birth weight or exceeded it, but if your baby is not gaining weight as steadily, your health visitor will discuss how feeding is going, and look at his health in general.

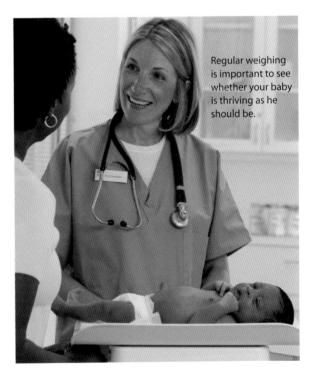

Regular weighing is important to see whether your baby is thriving as he should be.

The centile charts

Your baby's weight, length and head circumference will be recorded on centile charts in your PCHR. These printed graphs show the pattern of growth that healthy children should follow and are based on breastfed babies from a range of countries. They show a series of curves (centile lines) that represent the range of weights and lengths of most children. If your baby's weight is on the 50th centile, for example, this means that if you took the measurements of 100 babies of the same age in order, from the lightest to the heaviest, your child would be number 50 and right in the middle of the group. There is no 'normal' line on the chart, and every baby is different, so do not worry if your baby begins on the 10th centile, or even the 5th. The chart allows you and your healthcare professional to monitor

your baby's progress, so that any sudden change can be spotted. It is common for babies to gain weight quickly in the first six or nine months and to slow down after that. If your baby is ill for a while, too, he may lose some weight, but as long as he begins to add more by the time he is weighed again, there should be no cause for concern. If he continues to lose weight, the problem can be swiftly addressed.

Your baby will also be regularly measured and these figures, along with his vaccinations or other important health information, will be recorded in his PCHR. Take it with you to any appointments with your doctor, health visitor or other health professional. Add any relevant information, such as illnesses, accidents and medication. This can be useful if your child ever has to go to an A&E department of a hospital and his health records need to be accessed.

YOUR BABY'S ROUTINE VACCINATIONS

The childhood vaccination programme in the UK has been designed to protect babies from the most serious childhood diseases.

It can be upsetting to see your baby being given injections, but since many diseases can be fatal or produce life-long health complications, there are very good reasons for vaccinations to be given. However, the issue is still a concern for many parents and has been the centre of much debate. But parents need to be aware that it is vital to protect children – so it is an issue for serious consideration.

If your child has been ill or has a fever and is due a vaccination speak to your doctor first. Afterwards, if there are any medical issues or unusual reactions, speak to your doctor. You will probably be asked to wait in the doctor's surgery or clinic for ten minutes, or so, to make sure that your baby is fine, but it is common for babies to have a raised temperature after vaccinations and for them to cry a little more than usual. An appropriate dose of baby paracetamol usually helps, but if your baby has a high fever, vomiting or a rash, call your doctor.

VACCINATION TIMETABLE

Two months The five-in-one vaccination for DTaP/IPV/Hib. One injection is given to protect against five separate diseases – diphtheria, tetanus, pertussis (whooping cough), polio and haemophilus influenzae type B (also known as Hib), a bacterial infection that can cause pneumonia or meningitis in babies and young children, plus pneumococcal infection

Three months The five-in-one, second dose of DTaP/IPV/Hib (see above) and meningitis C

Four months The five-in-one, third dose of DTaP/IPV/Hib plus the second dose to protect against pneumococcal infection and meningitis C

Between 12 and 13 months Hib and meningitis C booster. Administered as a single jab containing the third dose to protect against meningitis C, and the fourth dose to protect against Hib. There is also a third dose to protect against pneumococcal infection. The MMR vaccine (measles, mumps and rubella) is also given as a single injection

Around three years and four months The second MMR is given (single injection). Your child will be offered a four-in-one pre-school booster (DtaP/IPV) containing vaccines to protect against diphtheria, tetanus, pertussis and polio

YOUR CHILD'S MILESTONES

In the first year of your baby's life, although the exact timing may differ, you can expect him to reach the following milestones:

At six to eight weeks:

If you place him on his tummy for short periods of time (which is important for the development of his neck and back muscles) he will bring his arms forwards in front of his head and should lift his chin

He may show alarm and be startled by a sudden or loud noise

He may follow a moving object with his eyes up to 50 cm (19 in) away

He should respond to your voice when he hears you. He may also increase the range of sounds that he makes

He may give you his first smile

At three months:

If he is placed on his tummy he may try to lift both head and shoulders, using his arms for support

He will grasp any object that is put into his hand, but will not yet know how to let go of it

He will obviously enjoy making different sounds and may coo when you speak to him

He may look in the direction of sounds and turn his head towards them

He may use different cries for when he is hungry, tired, frustrated or in pain

At six to seven months:

He may push up on his elbows or hands when he is placed on his tummy. He may be flexing his legs, in readiness for crawling and he may roll over

If he lies on his back, your baby may reach for his legs and feet

He may be able to sit if you support him and even 'stand' on your lap for a few minutes if you hold his hands

He may be able to reach out for objects with either hand and pass them from one hand to the other

He will put objects to his mouth where his sensitive nerve endings will give him more information about them

He will coo and gurgle with pleasure and can deliberately 'play' with objects

At nine months:

Your baby may sit unsupported and start to crawl

He may also pull himself up to a standing position and use pieces of furniture to 'cruise' around the room

Your baby may now be able to drop an object as well as grasp it

He may be able to hold smaller objects and may develop a pincer grip so that he can hold things between his thumb and forefinger

He may recognise his own name and he may understand simple words and concepts such as 'no'

He may be able to play 'peek-a-boo' and clap his hands together. He can feed himself with simple finger foods

He may now become anxious when separated from you and be more wary of people he is unfamiliar with

At one year:

Your baby may be able to stand and even walk a short distance (although he will be unsteady for some time)

He may be able to give objects back when you ask for them and may be able to roll a ball towards you. He will love repetitive games and rhymes

He may be able to use a spoon and drink from a beaker

Your baby may be able to say 'Mama' or 'Dada'

He may be able to wave and have his own names for people he knows well

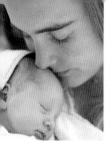

LOOKING AHEAD

Your baby will grow and develop at an astonishing rate and there is so much to look forward to. Ensure that you take the time to appreciate your baby and enjoy life together as a family.

There's no doubt that the first few weeks of parenthood can be pretty exhausting, but just as you may begin to feel that looking after your baby is almost all hard work, you will be rewarded with your baby's first smile. When this happens, you will probably be able to forget all the broken nights and dirty nappies – very soon you will realise that this is just the start of your baby's responses to you, which will become increasingly sophisticated as time goes by.

Encouraging your baby

While your baby was inside your womb, you were doing your best to nurture and stimulate him. Now that he is in the outside world, his brain is receiving all kinds of stimuli that it is trying to process, sort and assimilate. The way that you interact with him is vital to his ability to manage all these signals and key to his further development. So that by smiling, cuddling and talking to him, you help your baby to associate human contact (both physical and verbal) with comfort and pleasure. By doing this, not only are you encouraging more connections (synapses) to be made within his brain (see pages 182–3), but you are also laying solid foundations for his emotional security and well-being. If he feels emotionally secure he will have the best environment in which to make further progress and learn. Try to find ways to stimulate all his senses – the more you do so, the more he will want to learn. Studies show that babies

who are rarely spoken to (or listened to), and infrequently touched and played with develop fewer parts of the brain – perhaps as much as 30 per cent of it is left unstimulated. This does not mean that you should start playing foreign-language tutorials to your tiny baby. The stimulation that you give must be age- and stage-appropriate always, but just as there were critical opportunities to boost your baby's health and growth in the womb, so in this first year, when his brain is developing at a phenomenal pace, there is a wonderful chance for you to help him reach his full potential.

'Tuning in'

The most important thing that you can do to help your baby in this period is to 'tune in' to him. Observe what makes him happy, sad, anxious or excited and respond sensitively to the cues that he gives you. Cuddle him and talk to him as much as you can (babies who have had this kind of parenting have been found to have significantly higher IQ scores than children who have been rarely spoken to). You may have to make a more conscious effort to talk to begin with, and you might even feel a little as if you are talking to yourself, but look carefully: although your baby may not have the spoken vocabulary to respond yet, his little kicks, eye movements and arm-waving will tell you that he is desperate to have a 'conversation' with you – and before you know it he will.

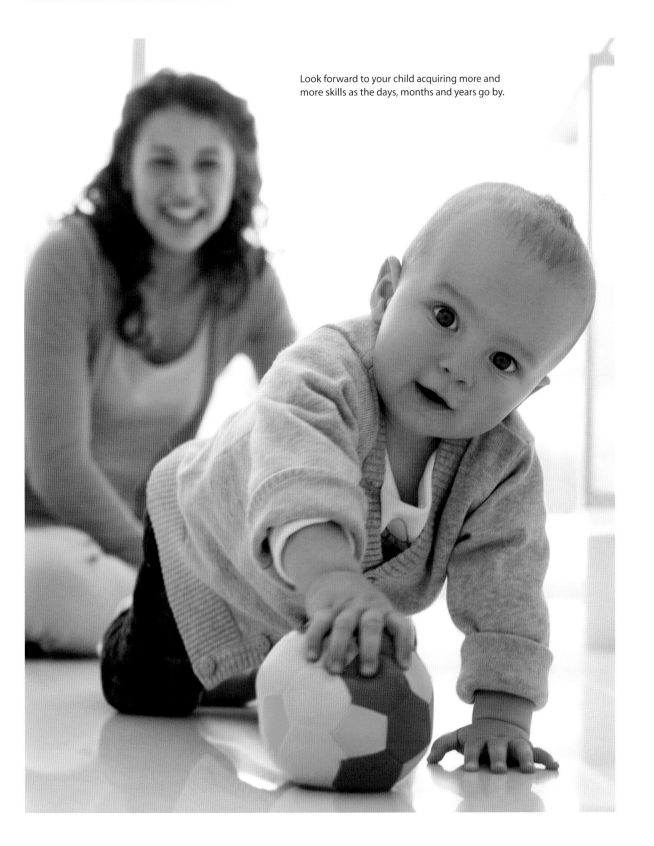

Look forward to your child acquiring more and more skills as the days, months and years go by.

RESOURCES

Preconception help
The Zita West Clinic
020 7224 0017; www.zitawest.com

Human Fertilisation and Embryology
Authority
www.hfea.gov.uk

Pregnancy
National Childbirth Trust
0870 444 8709; www.nct.org.uk

TAMBA (Twins and Multiple Birth
Association)
Twinline 0800 138 0509;
www.tamba.org.uk

Royal College of Obstetricians and
Gynaecologists
020 7772 6200; www.rcog.org.uk

Royal College of Midwives
www.rcm.org.uk

NHSdirect
www.nhsdirect.nhs.uk

Antenatal results and choices
(Information and support for parents
during the antenatal testing process)
020 7631 0285; www.arc.uk.org

Independent Midwives UK
0845 4600 105;
www.independentmidwives.org.uk

Nutritional advice
www.eatwell.gov.uk

The British Dietetic Association
www.bda.uk.com

British Nutrition Foundation
020 7404 6504; www.nutrition.org.uk

The Eating for Pregnancy Service
www.eatingforpregnancy.co.uk

Information on vegetarian diets during
pregnancy and for babies and children
www.vegsoc.org

Smoking and Health
QUIT Quitline 0800 002 200;
www.quit.org.uk

NHS advice on stopping smoking
www.smokefree.nhs.uk

Drinkline: The National Alcohol
Helpline
020 7307 7450; www.drinkaware.co.uk

FRANK (Information and support for
drugs and alcohol problems)
0800 776 600; www.talktofrank.com

Institute of Complementary Medicine
0845 345 5977; www.bcma.co.uk

British Acupuncture Council
020 8735 0400;
www.acupuncture.org.uk

British Homeopathic Association
01582 408 678;
www.britishhomeopathic.org

British Hypnotherapy Association
020 8942 3988;
www.hypnotherapy-association.org

British Chiropractic Association
0118 950 5950;
www.chiropractic-uk.co.uk

General Osteopathic Council
020 7357 6655; www.osteopathy.org

The Sutherland Society (The UK
Organisation for Cranial Osteopathy)
www.cranial.org.uk

British Reflexology Association
www.britfrelex.co.uk

British Wheel of Yoga
www.bwi.org.uk

National Institute of Medical Herbalists
www.nimh.org.uk

The Shiatsu Society
www.shiatsusociety.org

Society of Teachers of the Alexander
Technique
www.stat.org.uk

Pilates Foundation
www.pilatesfoundation.com

British Foreign and Commonwealth
Office (Information and advice for
travel during pregnancy)
www.fco.gov.uk

Royal Society for the Prevention of
Accidents (Information on safety
standards and legal requirements for
child car seats etc.) www.rospa.com

The Hospital for Tropical Diseases
www.thehtd.org

Labour & Birth

BirthChoiceUK
www.birthchoiceuk.com

Doula UK (Support for women during labour and birth) 0871 433 3103; www.doula.org.uk

Home Birth
www.homebirth.org.uk

Caesarean Support Network
www.caesarean.org.uk

The Birth Trauma Association
www.birthtraumaassociation.org.uk

Association of Breastfeeding Mothers
08444 122 949; www.abm.me.uk

Breastfeeding Network
0844 412 4664;
www.breastfeedingnetwork.org.uk

La Leche League
0845 120 2918; www.laleche.org.uk

International Association of Infant Massage (UK)
www.iaim.org.uk

Association for Postnatal Illness
www.apni.org

PNI (postnatal depression)
www.pni.org.uk

Support Groups

Fatherhood Institute
0845 634 1238;
www.fatherhoodinstitute.org

Gingerbread (Single parents, equal families) 0808 802 0925; www.gingerbread.org.uk

Relate (Relationship counselling) 03000 100 1234; www.relate.org.uk

Home Start (Support and friendship for families) 0800 068 6368; www.home-start.org.uk

Family Lives (Support for families) 0808 800 2222; www.familylives.org.uk

Twinsclub (Support for parents of twins and multiples) www.twinsclub.co.uk

Tommy's (Pregnancy research and information) 0800 0147 800; www.tommys.org

Bliss (Premature and special care babies) 0500 618 140; www.bliss.org.uk

Diabetes UK
www.diabetes.org.uk

SCOPE (Information and advice on cerebral palsy) 0808 800 333; www.scope.org.uk

St. Thomas' Lupus Trust
www.lupus.org.uk

Mencap (Understanding Learning Disability) 0808 808 1111; www.mencap.org.uk

Mind (National Association for Mental Health) 0300 123 3393; www.mind.org.uk

Sense (National Deafblind and Rubella Association) www.sense.org.uk

Contact a Family (Support for families with disabled children)
www.cafamily.org.uk

Down's Syndrome Association
www.downs-syndrome.org.uk

Association of Spina Bifida and Hydrocephalus Helpline
0845 450 7755; www.asbah.org

The Miscarriage Association
www.miscarriageassociation.org.uk

The Ectopic Pregnancy Trust
www.ectopic.org.uk

SANDS (Stillbirth & Neonatal Death Society) 020 7436 5881; www.uk-sands.org

Cruse Bereavement Care
0844 477 9400
www.crusebereavementcare.org.uk

Rights & Benefits

Department for Work and Pensions
www.dwp.gov.uk

ACAS (Advisory, Conciliation and Arbitration Service) www.acas.org.uk

Citizens' Advice
www.citizensadvice.org.uk

Equality and Human Rights Commission
www.equalityhumanrights.com

Maternity Action
0845 600 8533;
www.maternityaction.org.uk

GLOSSARY

A

Acupuncture A form of Traditional Chinese Medicine (TCM) in which fine needles are inserted into the skin to redirect the qi or energy flow.

Active birth Labouring and giving birth using upright positions or movement.

Amniocentesis A semi-surgical procedure whereby a sample of amniotic fluid is taken from the uterus by passing a needle through the abdomen. The fluid is then tested to diagnose foetal abnormalities.

Amniotic sac also known as the amnion, the membrane that surrounds the foetus and the amniotic fluid.

Amniotic sac/fluid The fluid that surrounds and cushions the foetus in the uterus.

Anterior position The back of the baby's head (occiput) is against the mother's abdomen.

Anti-D injection Antibodies administered to women who have a Rhesus Negative blood group but have been exposed to rhesus positive blood cells.

Apgar score Test carried out within one, five and 10 minutes of a baby's birth that assesses skin colour, breathing, pulse/heart rate, movements/muscle tone and reflexes.

Areola The circle of dark pink-brown skin that surrounds the nipple.

Aromatherapy The practice of using natural plant 'essential' oils to enhance psychological and physical well-being.

B

Bilirubin Red-blood cells (haemo-globin) broken down by the liver.

Blastocyst The fertilised egg when it has divided into around 100 cells.

Body mass index (BMI) A way of measuring body fat based on height and weight.

Braxton Hicks' contractions 'Practice' contractions that are noticeable towards the end of pregnancy.

Breech presentation The position of a baby in the uterus where the bottom is presenting first (rather than the head).

C

Cardiotocograph (CTG) An electronic monitor that tracks the mother's contractions and the baby's heartbeat during labour.

Catheter A thin, flexible plastic tube that may be used to give fluids such as saline in an IV drip, to administer anaesthetic into the epidural space, or to drain urine from the bladder.

Cephalic presentation Also known as 'vertex', when the baby is head down in the uterus so that it is presenting first.

Chloasma Uneven, darker patches on the skin.

Chorion The membrane that surrounds the foetus and the placenta.

Colostrum Protein and antibody-rich fluid that is secreted by the breasts after birth.

Complementary medicine A range of therapies that fall beyond the scope of conventional scientific medicine, but may be used alongside it.

Corpus luteum Formed in the ovary after fertilisation, it produces progesterone, which prompts the development of the placenta.

Crowning The appearance of the baby's head at the entrance to the vagina.

Cystic fibrosis An inherited disease that affects the internal organs, especially the lungs and digestive system.

D

Dilatation The progressive stretching or opening of the cervix during labour.

Doppler A hand-held device that is used to listen to the foetal heartbeat.

Doula A non-medically trained female helper during labour.

Down's syndrome Also known as trisomy 21. A condition caused by the presence of all or part of an extra 21st chromosome.

E

EDD The baby's expected delivery date.

Edward's syndrome Also known as Trisomy 18. A genetic disorder caused by the presence of all or part of an extra 18th chromosome.

Electroencephalogram (EEG) A method of monitoring the electrical impulses of the brain by attaching an electrode to the scalp.

Embryo The developing organism after fertilisation is known as the embryo from 10th day to around the 10th week.

Endometrium The lining of the uterus.

Engorgement Breasts that are over-full with milk.

Epigenetics A modification of a gene that is independent of the DNA sequence of a gene.

Episiotomy A surgical cut in the perineum.

Essential fatty acids (EFAs) 'Good' fats required by the body that must be eaten as they cannot be synthesised.

F

Foetal distress Lack of oxygen being received by the baby.

Foetus The developing baby when it has moved on from the embryonic stage at 10 weeks until birth.

Folic acid A vitamin of the B complex that is needed in pregnancy for the foetal neural tube to form properly.

Follicle-stimulating hormone (FSH) Hormone released by the pituitary gland that prompts the egg follicle to form each month and is often used in fertility treatments such as IVF.

G, H

Genes A unit of heredity that is passed on from parent to child.

Homeopathy A system of medicine involving treating with highly diluted substances with the aim of triggering the body's natural system of healing.

Hormone A chemical messenger in the blood.

Human chorionic gonadotrophin (hCG) The hormone released into the woman's bloodstream by the growing placenta. It is detectable in the urine from the early days of pregnancy.

Huntingdon's Disease An inherited disease of the brain.

Hyperemesis gravidarum A severe form of morning sickness.

Hypertension High blood pressure.

Hypnobirthing Self-hypnosis techniques used for labour and birth.

Hypotension Low blood pressure.

I

Implantation When the fertilised egg embeds itself in the wall of the uterus.

Induction Artificial triggering and maintenance of labour.

Intravenous drip Fluids introduced through a vein.

In vitro fertilisation (IVF) A form of assisted conception where fertilisation occurs outside the uterus before the embryos are transferred back into it.

L

Lanugo Fine hair that covers the baby in the uterus.

Linea nigra A line of dark, pigmented skin that runs down the centre of the abdomen in pregnancy.

M

Meridians The pathways through which the life force or 'qi' flows through the body according to traditional Chinese Medicine (TCM).

N

Nuchal fold translucency scan (NTS) A screening test that uses ultrasound to measure the amount of fluid under the skin at the back of the baby's neck. An increased amount may indicate a higher risk of Down's syndrome.

O

Occipito anterior The position of the baby in the uterus where the back of its head (occiput) is against the mother's abdomen (anterior).

Occipito posterior The position of the baby in the uterus where the back of its head (occiput) is against the mother's back (posterior).

Oedema Swelling as a result of fluid retention.

Oestrogen A hormone produced by the ovaries and the placenta.

Opioids Also known as narcotics. Painkilling drugs that are opium-based or synthesised versions.

P

Palpation Feeling the uterus or unborn baby through the mother's abdomen.

Pelvic floor The sling of muscles that support the bladder and uterus.

Perinatal The period from the 24th week of pregnancy to the first week after delivery.

Perineum The tissue around the vagina and between the vagina and rectum.

Placenta An organ attached to the lining of the uterus during pregnancy that keeps the unborn baby's blood supply separate from its mother's.

Postnatal After the baby's birth.

Postpartum After delivery of the baby.

Pre-eclampsia A medical condition that causes high blood pressure and other symptoms in pregnancy.

Premature A baby delivered before the 37th week of pregnancy.

Presentation The part of the baby that is pressing against the cervix and so will be delivered first.

Primigravida First pregnancy

Progesterone A hormone produced first by the corpus luteum, but then also by the placenta.

Prostaglandins Substances that trigger labour contractions.

Q, R

Qi The energy or life force that flows through the body according to Chinese Traditional Medicine (TCM).

Recessive gene A physical trait carried by one or other parent of a baby that is not immediately obvious such as blue eyes in a baby born of two brown-eyed parents.

Reflexology Also known as 'zone therapy', it is an alternative therapy based on the idea that areas of the feet that correspond with organs in the 'zones' of the body.

Rhesus negative/positive factor All humans have either rhesus negative or rhesus positive blood. A rhesus-negative mother's body may send antibodies to the baby if it is rhesus positive, but this can be prevented by anti-D gamma globulin.

Rooting A baby's instinct to feed at the breast.

S

Show Bloodstained mucus that has come away from the cervix before labour.

Spina bifida A birth defect in which the backbone and spinal canal do not close before birth, affecting the brain, spine and central nervous system.

Spotting Light bleeding in pregnancy.

Still birth The delivery of a dead baby at 24 weeks or later.

Surfactant A detergent-like substance that coats the alveoli of the lungs and prevents the walls sticking together, so allowing them to expand.

T

Tay-Sachs Disease A rare and usually fatal genetic disorder that progressively causes damage to the nervous system.

TENS machine Transcutaneous Electrical Nerve Stimulation delivers small electrical impulses that are thought to interrupt the pain signals to the brain and encourage the production of natural painkilling chemicals – endorphins.

Teratogens Harmful substances that cross the placenta and therefore can affect the baby.

Traditional Chinese Medicine (TCM) An ancient medical system that looks at the mind, body, spirit and emotions when treating illness and that tries to restore the harmony of all the elements

Transducer An instrument that is used to build up an ultrasound image.

Transition A phase of labour that occurs between the first and second stages or labour.

Trial of labour A period of time allowed to a woman whose circumstances indicate that she may need a Caesarean section labours – to see whether vaginal delivery is possible.

Trimester Name for the thirds that pregnancy is divided into.

U

Ultrasound scan High-frequency sound waves are sent through the abdomen to the uterus, where they bounce off the foetus. The echoes are then turned into an image on a screen.

V

Varicella syndrome Congenital abnormalities caused by the same virus (varicella) as chicken pox, a common childhood disease.

Vernix White, waxy substance that coats a baby's skin to protect it in the uterus.

Z

Zygote An egg that has just been fertilised.

INDEX

Author's acknowledgements

I have had the most amazing team of editors, who have made this book not only possible but were a real pleasure to work with. Susanna Abbott, Julia Twaites and Sarah Bennie at Vermilion; Claire Tennant-Scull has been absolutely amazing to work with and put her heart and soul into the project; Jo Godfrey Wood for editing and Peggy Sadler for designing this book – making it a pleasure to read.

Oriane Abbonizio, Leonora Bamford (for useful advice on baby sleepwear), Sarah Bearman, Clare Byam-Cook, Claire Caisson, Dr Harry Chummun, Zoe Garrod, Oliver Gillie, Ann Joseph, Brigitte Lacombe (for the photograph of Kate Winslet, page 8), Isobelle Obert, Alison Scott-Wright (www.alisonscott-wright.com, for information from her book *The Sensational Baby Sleep Plan*), Denise Tiran, MSc RM RGN ADM PGCEA, Jack West for great diagrams and illustrations, Robert West.

Publisher's acknowledgements

The publisher would like to thank Sarah Bearman (consultant midwife) for reading proofs and answering queries and for supplying the partogram diagram (page 274), Justine Taylor for proofreading and Charmian Parkin for indexing, Lucy Howells (a mother – caesareans and twins), Deborah Lloyd (BSc Homeopathy, LCHE, MARH) and Pippa Jones (NHS midwife).

Picture credits

Key: t-top, r-right, l-left, b-bottom, c-centre

Getty Images: 238; George Doyle 7t; Brandy Anderson 7bc; Focus_on_Nature 7b Ghislain & Marie David de Lossy 11; Image Source 19b, 305, 357; B2M Productions 19t; Datacraft Co Ltd 28–9; Dorling Kindersley 33, 208; Lisa Romerein 39; Bloom image 40; Ruth Jenkinson 41, 87, 96, 99, 140, 142, 143, 276l, 302; JGI/Jamie Grill 43; Jerome Tisne 44; Tetra Images 47, 226, 267; JGI 48; Rhea Anna 49; Zephyr 51b; Mehau Kulyk 53tl; Dr Najeeb Layyous 53bl; Lost Horizon Images 58–9; Dorling Kindersley 61; Sam Edwards 73; Philippe Desenrck 79; Ian Hooton 80, 163l, 245, 254, 272; Martin Poole 82; Glow Images, Inc 89; Altrendo Images 92; John Carleton 93; Erik Isakson 95l; Stockbyte 97, 104, 107, 350; Cultura/Judith Haeusler 101; Sian Irvine 103; Fotosearch 110; Jose Luis Pelaez 115l; Assembly 115r; Chris Cole 116; William Reavell 117; G Williamson 125; Tetra Images 126; Paul Bradbury 127; Vincenzo Lombardo 133b; Mark Alberhasky 133t; MSW 137; Nancy Brown 141; Mimi Haddon 145, George Diebold 149; Vanessa Davies 151, 165, 166b, 182; Liam Norris 153; Rachel Weill 158; Britt Erlanson 161; Smith Collection 162; Michael Mahovlich 168; Marcy Maloy 169; Jonathan Knowles 170-1; Denny Cody 179b; Jamie Grill 181; Philippe Desenrck 184; Susanna Blavarg 186; K. Miller Photographs 187; Peter Cade 191; arabianEye 195; RubberBall Productions 207; Andersen Ross 220; LWA 225; Nancy Brown 227; Leanne Temme 228; John Lamb 229; Radek Detinsky 233; Monkey Business Images 237; Ian O'Leary 241l; Joy Skipper 241c; Harald Walker 241r; Roderick Chen 247l, 328; Karen Cochrane 247r; Imagemore Co., Ltd. 257; Jupiterimages 261; Science Photo Library 266, 280; Chris Ryan 268, 339; Hans Neleman 273, 275, 278; Cristian Baitg 276r;

Design Pics/LJM Photo 281r; Blend Images/Ariel Skelley 283, 293, 310, 363; Patricia McDonough 289; Virginia Star 291; G Williamson 295; Widmann Widmann 298; ERproductions Ltd 300; Photodisc 301, 325; Damir Cudic 304; Rosanne Olson 306; Mike Kemp 308-9; Alex Bramwell 312; Mike Kemp 313; Lilly Dong 315; Kerry M. Halasz 316; Westend61 319; Jerome Tisne 326; Fuse 332; KidStock 336; Leanne Temme 341, 345; D-Base 346; Kirk Mastin 348; Lisa Spindler Photography Inc. 353, 354; soulsurfing – Jason Swain 359; Zia Soleil 361; Mel Yates 362; Sam Edwards 367

Alamy images: Corbis Premium RF 6b, 67; Radius Images 13; Tetra Images 15; i love images 16-17; Imageshop 46; Corbis Cusp 98; Allan Mcintyre 121; PhotoAlto 157; Tetra Images 205, 221; Catchlight Visual Services 217; Science Photo Library 253, 269; Janine Wiedel Photolibrary 281l; Shout 287; Picture Partners 303; Pat Savage 321; Corbis Flirt 327

Corbis Images: Image Source 2, 21; Dave and Les Jacobs/Blend Images 6tc, 56; Rick Gomez 26; Imagemore Co., Ltd. 27; Larry Williams 32; Michael A. Keller 37; Tetra Images 66, 94; Eric Audras/Onoky 83; Jose Luis Pelaez Inc/Blend Images 88; Monalyn Gracia 95r; Tomas Rodriguez 112; Jon Feingersh/Blend Images 122; Nancy Yuenkel 118; Studio/photocuisine 119b; Lois Ellen Frank 119t; Brooke Fasani Auchincloss 152.

Dorling Kindersley: 203, 211, 212.

Lennart Nilsson Image Bank: 52, 53tr, 53br, 54tr, 55bl, 178, 132, 134, 135.

Mother & Baby Picture Library: Ian Hooton 128–9, 159, 163r, 172, 200, 218, 222–3, 230, 249, 251, 256l, 270, 271; Ruth Jenkinson 166t, 234, 256r, 260; Verity Wellstead 219; Angela Spain 243;

Science Photo Library: 7tc, 189; 74; Ian Hooton 1, 123, 130, 175, 185, 196bl, 196br, 198, 239, 279; 3D4medical.Com 22, 25; Medical Rf.Com 23tl; Pascal Goetgheluck 23tr; Steve Allen 50; Edelmann 51tl, 62r; Dopamine 51tr; Scott Camazine 54l; Bernard Benoit/Kretz Technik 54b; Aj Photo 55tl, 177b; Kevin Curtis 55r, 179t; Ralph Hutchings, Visuals Unlimited 62cr; Carolina Biological Supply Co/Visuals Unlimited, Inc. 62cl; Sciepro 62l; Steve Allen 65t; Dopamine 65br, 65bl; Simon Fraser 176, 197r; Bsip, Kretz Technik 177t; Dr Najeeb Layyous 197l.

Shutterstock: Schalke fotografie/Melissa Schalke 6tl, 264; hartphotography 6c; kesipun 12; Valua Vitaly 30; Reflekta 69; AdventureStock 70; OtnaYdur 124; Pedro Salaverría 173; Shanta Giddens 259; Yuri Arcurs 262; Reynardt 288; Martin Valigursky 299; Valentin Mosichev 333; PHB.cz (Richard Semik) 334; Anna Jurkovska 342; Elena Yakusheva 356; wavebreakmedia ltd 360.

All illustrations and photograph of Zita West (page 10) by Jack West

Photograph of Kate Winslet (page 8) by Brigitte Lacombe

The Zita West Clinic

Following a career as a midwife in the NHS and several years in private practice as a fertility and pregnancy consultant on Harley Street, Zita founded the Zita West Clinic in Marylebone, London, in 2002. It is now one of the largest integrated clinics in the UK specialising in reproductive health.

Each year, the clinic's multidisciplinary team of specialist doctors, midwives and complementary therapists helps hundreds of couples to get pregnant, both naturally and through assisted conception, with innovative programmes designed to help boost natural fertility and to improve the chances of IVF success.

The clinic started its own assisted fertility programme in September 2011. It is the UK's first integrated IVF service offering not only the very latest medical treatments, but a more complete, holistic approach to both preparation and support. Our results so far have been very encouraging and we look forward to many more years of success

Services the clinic offers include:
• Fertility health checks and MOTs
• Pre-conception planning and support
• Sexual health screening
• Natural fertility coaching and enhancement
• Unique male programme with comprehensive semen analysis
• IVF planning, treatment and support
• Recurrent miscarriage clinic
• Early pregnancy care and support scans
• Private midwife support
• Antenatal and early-parenting training
• Postnatal care and support

The clinic also offers a range of complementary treatments, such as nutritional guidance, acupuncture, counselling, hypnotherapy and massage, each of which can be taken individually or as part of a coordinated programme of care.

Further details of the clinic's services can be found at www.zitawest.com or call 020 7224 0017

Zita West multivitamins, books & CDs

Zita has developed a comprehensive range of vitamin, mineral and essential fatty acid supplements to help support fertility, conception and pregnancy. Two new formulations have recently been added, specifically to help couples preparing for IVF.

She has also recorded a number of CDs to help prospective parents cope with the stress that can sometimes make a pregnancy seem so elusive.

Full details of the product range, the CDs and Zita's other books can be found at www.zitawest.com

Zita West affiliated network

The Zita West Clinic has also put together a network of affiliated acupuncturists across the UK and the Republic of Ireland offering specialist acupuncture treatment to help improve the chances of natural and assisted conception. Further information on the network can be found at www.zitawest.com; 020 7224 0017